# Th
# of
## Tow
## resea

*Edited*

Harry
Arthur
John W
Linda



BMJ Books

BMJ Books is an imprint of the BMJ Publishing Group



First published in 2002
by BMJ Books, BMA House, Tavistock Square,
London WC1H 9JR

www.bmjbooks.com

**British Library Cataloguing in Publication Data**
A catalogue record for this book is available from the British Library

ISBN 0 7279 1594 0

Typeset by SIVA Math Setters, Chennai, India
Printed and bound in Spain by GraphyCems, Navarra

# Contents

Contributors v

Foreword ix

1 An overview 1
*Arthur Kleinman, Harry A Guess, Joan S Wilentz*

**Section 1: Historical and ethical perspectives 33**

2 "Seeing" the placebo effect: historical legacies and present opportunities 35
*Anne Harrington*

3 Ethical issues in use of placebo in medical practice and clinical trials 53
*Sissela Bok*

**Section 2: Elucidating placebo effects: explanatory mechanisms 75**

4 Explanatory mechanisms for placebo effects: cultural influences and the meaning response 77
*Daniel E Moerman*

5 Explanatory mechanisms for placebo effects: cognition, personality and social learning 108
*Richard R Bootzin, Opher Caspi*

6 Explanatory mechanisms for placebo effects: Pavlovian conditioning 133
*Shepard Siegel*

7 Regression to the mean or placebo effect? 158
*Clarence E Davis*

**Section 3: Elucidating placebo effects: intervening psychophysiology 167**

8 Neuroendocrine mediators of placebo effects on immunity 169
*Farideh Eskandari, Esther M Sternberg*

9 Endogenous opioid and non-opioid pathways as mediators of placebo analgesia 183
*Donald D Price, Lene Vase Soerensen*

**Section 4: Use of placebo groups in clinical trials – methodological and ethical issues 207**

10 Placebo controlled trials and active controlled trials: ethics and inference 209
*Robert J Temple*

11 When is it appropriate to use a placebo arm in a trial? 227
*Kenneth J Rothman, Karin B Michels*

12 The pros and cons of non-inferiority (equivalence) trials 236
*Stuart J Pocock*

13 Use of placebo in large-scale, pragmatic trials 249
*Robert M Califf, Sana M Al-Khatib*

14 Placebo controls in clinical trials of new therapies for conditions for which there are known effective treatments 264
*Robert J Levine*

**Section 5: Priorities for future research 281**

15 The research and ethical agenda 283
*Joan S Wilentz, Linda W Engel*

Part I: Recommendations for research to further elucidate the nature of the placebo effect 286
*Fabrizio Benedetti, Susan M Czajkowski, Cheryl A Kitt, Michael Stefanek, Esther M Sternberg*

Part II: Recommendations for research on applying placebo effects in clinical practice 293
*Ruth L Fischbach, David Spiegel*

Part III: Recommendations for research concerning the use of placebos in clinical trials to test pharmacological and procedural interventions 300
*David W Feigal, Jr, Kathleen J Propert, David S Wendler*

Part IV: Recommendations for research concerning the use of placebos in clinical trials to test behavioral interventions 306
*Thomas D Borkovec, Lisa S Onken*

**Section 6: Conclusions and future directions 311**

16 Conclusions and future directions 313
*Stephen E Straus, Josephine P Briggs*

Appendix 317

Index 323

# Contributors

**Sana M Al-Khatib**, Associate in Medicine, Department of Medicine, Duke University Medical Center, Durham, NC, USA

**Fabrizio Benedetti**, Professor of Physiology and Neuroscience, Department of Neuroscience, University of Turin Medical School, Turin, Italy

**Sissela Bok,** Senior Visiting Fellow, Harvard Center for Population and Development Studies, Harvard School of Public Health, Cambridge, MA, USA

**Richard R Bootzin**, Professor, Department of Psychology, University of Arizona, Tucson, AZ, USA

**Thomas D Borkovec**, Distinguished Professor of Psychology, Department of Psychology, Pennsylvania State University, University Park, PA, USA

**Josephine P Briggs,** Director, Division of Kidney, Urologic and Hematologic Diseases, National Institute of Diabetes and Digestive and Kidney Diseases, National Institutes of Health, Bethesda, MD, USA

**Robert M Califf,** Professor of Medicine, Associate Vice Chancellor for Clinical Research, Director, Duke Clinical Research Institute, Durham, NC, USA

**Opher Caspi**, Research Assistant Professor, Program in Integrative Medicine, University of Arizona College of Medicine, Tucson, AZ, USA

**Susan M Czajkowski**, Social Scientist Analyst, Division of Epidemiology and Clinical Applications, Behavioral Medicine Scientific Research Group, National Heart Lung and Blood Institute, National Institutes of Health, Bethesda, MD, USA

**Clarence E Davis**, Professor and Chair, Department of Biostatistics, University of North Carolina School of Public Health, Chapel Hill, NC, USA

**Linda W Engel**, Special Assistant to the Director for Program Development, National Center for Complementary and Alternative Medicine, National Institutes of Health, Bethesda, MD, USA

**Farideh Eskandari**, Research Fellow, Department of Intramural Research Programs, National Institute of Mental Health, National Institutes of Health, Bethesda, MD, USA

**David W Feigal, Jr**, Director, Center for Devices and Radiological Health, US Food and Drug Administration, Rockville, MD, USA

**Ruth L Fischbach**, Senior Advisor for Medical Ethics, National Institutes of Health, Bethesda, MD, USA (currently Professor of Bioethics, Columbia University, College of Physicians and Surgeons, New York, NY, USA)

**Harry A Guess**, Vice President, Epidemiology, Merck Research Laboratories, West Point, PA, USA; Adjunct Professor of Epidemiology and Biostatistics, University of North Carolina, Chapel Hill, NC, USA

**Anne Harrington**, Professor of the History of Science, Harvard University, Cambridge, MA, USA

**Cheryl A Kitt**, Program Director for Pain Research, National Institute of Neurological Disorders and Stroke, National Institutes of Health, Bethesda, MD, USA

**Arthur Kleinman**, Professor of Social Anthropology, Harvard University; Maude and Lillian Presley Professor of Medical Anthropology and Psychiatry, Harvard Medical School, Cambridge, MA, USA

**John W Kusek**, Clinical Trials Program Director, Division of Kidney, Urologic, and Hematologic Diseases, National Institute of Diabetes and Digestive and Kidney Diseases, National Institutes of Health, Bethesda, MD, USA

**Robert J Levine**, Professor, Department of Medicine; Lecturer, Department of Pharmacology; Co-Chairperson, Yale University Interdisciplinary Program for Bioethics; Yale University, New Haven, CT, USA

**Karin B Michels**, Assistant Professor of Epidemiology, Harvard School of Public Health; Assistant Professor of Obstetrics, Gynecology and Reproductive Biology, Harvard Medical School, Boston, MA, USA

**Daniel E Moerman**, William E Stirton Professor of Anthropology, Department of Behavioral Sciences, University of Michigan-Dearborn, Dearborn, MI, USA

**Lisa S Onken**, Associate Director for Behavioral Treatment Research; Chief, Behavioral Treatment Development Branch, Division of Treatment Research and Development, National Institute on Drug Abuse, National Institutes of Health, Bethesda, MD, USA

**Stuart J Pocock**, Professor of Medical Statistics, London School of Hygiene and Tropical Medicine, London, England

**Donald D Price**, Professor, Department of Oral and Maxillofacial Surgery, College of Dentistry; Department of Neuroscience, College of Medicine, University of Florida, Gainesville, FL, USA

**Kathleen J Propert**, Associate Professor of Biostatistics, Department of Biostatistics and Epidemiology, University of Pennsylvania School of Medicine, Philadelphia, PA, USA

**Kenneth J Rothman**, Professor, Department of Epidemiology and Biostatistics, Boston University School of Public Health, and Section of Preventive Medicine, Department of Medicine, Boston University School of Medicine, Boston, MA, USA

**Shepard Siegel**, University Professor, Department of Psychology, McMaster University, Hamilton, Ontario, Canada

**Lene Vase Soerensen**, Department of Psychology, University of Aarhus, Denmark

**David Spiegel**, Professor and Associate Chair of Psychiatry and Behavioral Sciences, Stanford University School of Medicine, Stanford, CA, USA

**Michael Stefanek**, Chief, Basic Biobehavioral Research Branch, Behavioral Research Program, Division of Cancer Control and Population Sciences, National Cancer Institute, National Institutes of Health, Bethesda, MD, USA

**Esther M Sternberg**, Chief, Section on Neuroendocrine Immunology and Behavior; Director, Integrative Neural Immune Program, National Institute of Mental Health, National Institutes of Health, Bethesda, MD, USA

**Stephen E Straus**, Director, National Center for Complementary and Alternative Medicine, National Institutes of Health, Bethesda, MD, USA

**Robert J Temple**, Associate Director for Medical Policy, Center for Drug Evaluation and Research, US Food and Drug Administration, Rockville, MD, USA

**David S Wendler**, Head, Unit on Vulnerable Populations, Section on Human Subjects Research, Department of Clinical Bioethics, Warren Grant Magnuson Clinical Center, National Institutes of Health, Bethesda, MD, USA

**Joan S Wilentz**, Senior Science Writer, Bethesda, MD, USA

# Foreword

These proceedings grew from parallel discussions among staff of the National Institute of Diabetes, Digestive and Kidney Diseases (NIDDK) and members of the National Center for Complementary and Alternative Medicine (NCCAM) that reflected the somewhat different perspectives of each organization. The first perspective is that of clinical scientists who design and oversee studies aimed at providing rigorous evaluations of unproven therapies – placebos are generally seen as indispensable in many such studies. The second perspective is that of biologists and behavioral scientists who are fascinated by what might be the basis of the placebo effect, what it tells us about how people experience illness and recover from it, and whether placebo mechanisms could be harnessed to facilitate healing. It was only after each group of discussants learned that others at the National Institutes of Health (NIH) shared their interests in the placebo, that a plan began to unfold to collaborate on a broad-based multidisciplinary meeting.

Part of our charge at the NIH is to oversee research that aims to build the evidence base for the treatment or prevention of disease. At NIDDK, for example, we are concerned with burdensome chronic illnesses such as diabetes, urologic disease, progressive kidney diseases, and inflammatory bowel disease. We mount major clinical trials aiming to advance the state-of-the-art approaches to these diseases. When we in NIDDK began to think about convening a meeting on the placebo and started to plan it, the dominant issues were whether placebos are truly needed, how large their effects can be, how long they last – practical issues of the sort that dog the design of randomized clinical trials.

The randomized placebo controlled clinical trial has emerged over the past half century as a critical tool for evidence-based medicine for many good reasons. Hunches about what is good for patients commonly prove wrong, preliminary studies are often misleading, and unexpected harmful effects can overwhelm benefits, problems that become apparent through rigorous and unbiased evaluation with a randomized and blinded design. This must be balanced, however, with the ethical imperative of equipoise, which demands assurance that treatments being offered to participants are equally valuable. Yet, a treatment that is plausible enough to justify a large-scale trial has, quite inevitably, both its advocates and its detractors. Often what we call equipoise reflects a kind of truce between the believers and the skeptics, the enthusiasts and the nihilists. Sometimes new therapies can be compared appropriately to standard, established therapies; however, when there is no proven therapy, or substantive risk of withholding one, we opt to include a placebo control. In this situation we do suspect that we are committing the research subject to *nothing at all*, to a treatment with no promise of benefit. And, evolving ethical arguments question the acceptability of displacing active treatments with placebos. Paradoxically, and as is shown in the chapters that follow, many believe the placebo is not in fact neutral. It can convey startling therapeutic power, making it difficult to accurately measure the inherent effects of the active treatment above this "background" level of response.

In NCCAM, our charge is to critically assess whether increasingly popular herbal therapies, acupuncture, and myriad other traditional practices – what collectively are termed complementary and alternative medicine – are truly beneficial and safe. In some instances, the practices simply have not been well studied and can no longer be ignored. For others, however, the particular modalities are totally alien to contemporary Western scientific thought, both in terms of their approaches and the hypotheses underlying them. The cumulative evidence favoring the vast proportion of these modalities is far from compelling, and it has been cynically suggested that any benefits they may convey result merely from their roles as placebos. How could one begin to accommodate the purported effects of homeopathic remedies that can contain nothing but diluent? Only deliberate and exacting study can yield the data upon which as thorny a question as this could be fairly resolved. Thus, like our colleagues in NIDDK, in NCCAM we find ourselves concerned with the implications of the placebo for rigorous study design and conduct.

Yet, we in NCCAM are also fascinated with the mechanisms by which placebos might manifest their clinical effects. We know, for example, that drugs like naloxone antagonize the analgesic effects of morphine. Yet, these same drugs prevent placebo analgesics from relieving pain. Thus, there is something inherent in how we perceive pain, how we anticipate its relief, how we invest a particular touch or medicament with the power to heal, that serves us as if we were being given authentic morphine. What explains this remarkable ability to achieve something practical and beneficial from "nothing"? And, what of the instances in which placebo recipients felt less depressed, more powerful, less subject to recurrent infections, and more? One would have to postulate that placebos may be literally totipotent, affecting whole networks of inflammatory mediators, hormones and neurotransmitters. Contemporary technologies can now begin to address in elegant ways how placebos might possess such protean effects.

As we assembled a cadre of willing colleagues among the other Institutes and Centers of the NIH and other federal health agencies to help us plan a meeting about placebos, we came to realize that the issues we were addressing are fundamental to so much of biomedical research. They go beyond the practical, nitty-gritty issues regarding trial design and statistical analysis, and beyond the heady theories about placebo mechanisms that illuminate formidable mind-body connections. We were delving into fundamental questions about the limits of evidence-based medicine. Physicians trained in scientific medicine have still to confront the reality that extrapolating from statistical data to the management of an ill or dying patient is a tough business, and that the truths that emerge from evidence-based medicine are complex – and often only guardedly applicable to individual patients. Every experienced physician has a variety of strategies to simultaneously communicate truth and hope. What does the placebo effect tell us about all this, and how can health care professionals harness it for the patient's benefit?

To help us organize the remarkable body of data regarding placebos and effectively charge the meeting participants to project for us the key directions that future placebo research should assume, we commissioned the scholarly papers that constitute this book. The leadership of the meeting and the task of editing this compendium were left to two energetic and able colleagues, Linda Engel of NCCAM and John Kusek of NIDDK, and two extraordinary and visionary scientists, Arthur Kleinman of Harvard, and Harry Guess of Merck Research Laboratories and the University of North Carolina. We owe them our gratitude for their creative labors in the pursuit of fuller health.

*Josephine P Briggs*
*Director, Division of Kidney, Urologic and Hematologic Diseases, National Institute of Diabetes and Digestive and Kidney Diseases, National Institutes of Health*

*Stephen E Straus*
*Director, National Center for Complementary and Alternative Medicine, National Institutes of Health*

# 1: An overview

ARTHUR KLEINMAN, HARRY A GUESS,
JOAN S WILENTZ

## Introduction

A decade ago the idea of convening a conference on the placebo at the National Institutes of Health, the pre-eminent US government biomedical research establishment, would have been all but unthinkable. That the NIH hosted such a meeting on November 19–21, 2000 and that it attracted over 500 medical scholars, researchers, and clinicians from diverse fields marks a sea change. Not only were the participants eager to explore the *science* of the placebo, they were also keen to revisit the *ethics* of placebo use in the clinic and in clinical trials. Thus has the placebo been transformed in a few short years from a sham in medical practice and a control agent in clinical trials to a therapeutic ally. Some skepticism remains, however, as witness the May 24, 2001 article by Hrobjartsson and Gotzsche in the *New England Journal of Medicine*.[1] In their review of over a hundred clinical trials that included both placebo and no-treatment groups, the authors concluded that they "found little evidence that placebos in general have powerful clinical effects." In contrast, conference participants found that placebo effects – defined as the beneficial physiological or psychological changes associated with the use of inert medications, sham procedures, or in response to therapeutic encounters and symbols, such as the white coat – often appear to be real and significant, not make-believe; an emperor *with* clothes. This new legitimacy is altering and expanding the concept of the placebo from its pejorative 19th century definition as "a medicine adapted more to please than benefit the patient," to one that encompasses many features occurring in the course of patient–provider interactions that can positively affect health and wellbeing.

This difference in attitude is in itself the product of progress in science. Old boundaries between scientific fields and medical specialties are breaking down as cell and molecular biology studies detail extensive and reciprocal connections linking the nervous, endocrine, and immune systems. The black box of the brain itself is yielding to functional magnetic resonance imaging (fMRI) and positron emission tomography (PET) scans that show activation of specific brain nuclei and pathways following stimulation by placebos. Ironically, these advances – evidence of the spectacular success of reductionist biology in the latter half of the 20th century – are providing insights into a central question in biology: how do mind and body interact in orchestrating human experience – in particular, how do they affect the healing process?

Indeed, that question was a major stimulus for the conference. Initially, participants explored the nature of placebos and placebo effects from a variety of psychosocial, cultural, behavioral, and biological perspectives, citing evidence from a wide range of experimental studies. These considerations gave rise to the model of placebo effects as a dynamic function of positive features of patient–provider interactions. Next, conferees explored the ethical and methodological implications of the use of placebos in clinical practice and research. Here, there were differences of opinion on a number of issues, including whether placebos should ever be used in a clinical trial in place of proven safe and effective therapies. Finally, participants developed a research agenda for the further elucidation of the science of placebos and the ethical applications of this knowledge in clinical practice and research.

## The nature of placebos and placebo effects

### The historical background

Day one of the workshop set the stage for the conference by providing historical background and opening discussion of a concept of the placebo as a "meaning" response. Harvard medical historian Anne Harrington[2] reminded attendees that up to the 19th century only a handful of effective drugs were available to treat disease, so that the practice of medicine was essentially placebo-driven. The conundrum, then as now, was that pills and potions, whether recognized as placebos or provided as orthodox therapy in accordance with one or another system of medicine, often worked. Nevertheless, the scientific transformation of medicine in Western society over the past 200 years, and the emergence of an ever-growing armamentarium of potent drugs and medical procedures, saw the reputation of placebos severely tarnished. They were regarded as part of the "art" of medicine, separate from the wonders of modern medical science. By the 1950s and 1960s the idea of giving patients sugar pills or saline injections was derided as a sham and a deception; morally repugnant. This view was reinforced by the 1962 passage of amendments to the US Food, Drug and Cosmetic Act of 1937 requiring rigorous evidence of the *efficacy* of new drugs in addition to their safety. The new Federal regulations stated clearly, "The purpose of conducting clinical investigations of a drug is to distinguish the effect of a drug from other influences, such as spontaneous change in the course of the disease, placebo effect, or biased observation" (21 CFR 314.126).

The need to establish the efficacy of new clinical treatments led to improvements in the design and analysis of clinical trials and the emergence of the randomized double blind placebo controlled clinical trial as the gold standard in clinical testing, the most highly ranked type of study in any hierarchy of clinical evidence, and all but essential in order for drugs, biologics, and medical devices to gain approval by the US Food and Drug Administration. In the course of this evolution, investigators were encouraged to see placebo effects as potential spoilers of the data – "noise" that needed to be filtered out in the data analysis.

Harrington remarked that the idea that placebo effects are a sham still haunts medicine, as does the idea that placebo effects in clinical trials are noise to be subtracted out. In that simplistic equation placebo responses are regarded as a kind of second-order physiology that "floats like oil on water" on top of the fundamental physiological changes associated with the active treatment. In reality, placebo effects modulate active treatments as well as pharmacologically inactive ones and thus play a role in both the active and control arms of a trial. Regulatory requirements encourage study designs which enhance specific effects of active treatments, not those which enhance placebo effects. Yet in clinical practice both effects work together to benefit patients.

Beyond the traditional concept of placebos as pills or injections, Harrington presented evidence for the effects of phenomena she called "sightings." As an example she reported a study which showed that hospital patients whose post-surgical recovery took place in a room with a view had reduced pain and were released 7 to 9 days earlier than patients whose post-operative recovery took place in a room overlooking the hospital parking lot. Another sighting she described was associated with a negative placebo effect, or "nocebo" which is associated with a worsening of health and wellbeing. The example concerned Cambodian women refugees who had been forced to witness atrocities. These women, now living in California, are all blind and near-blind – not because doctors can find anything wrong with their eyes, but because they "cried until they could not see." She concluded with the hope that the new look at placebos would find investigators turning not to past *maps* that attempted to explain away placebo phenomena, but would lead them to explore the *territory* of the placebo – how it looks, when it happens, and under what conditions – not just in a clinical trial, but as a recurring touchstone for exploration. She quoted a Chinese proverb that speaks of a finger pointing to the moon, and exhorts the listener not to look at the finger but at the moon itself.

## Enlarging the framework: the meaning response

Harrington's admonition to enlarge perspectives on the notion of "placebo" and "placebo response" was amplified by medical anthropologist Daniel Moerman (University of Michigan, Dearborn)[3] who addressed social and cultural aspects of placebo effects. He introduced the term "meaning response," which he defined as "the physiological or psychological effects of meaning in the treatment of illness." Essentially, he described a process in which patients and providers ascribe meaning to a broad range of occurrences in the course of their encounters which affect the outcomes of treatment. These occurrences can be regarded as stimuli, and include:

- language – what is said and how it is said
- procedures – what is done and what explanations are offered
- settings – whether office, clinic, or hospital
- how the information and perceptions are processed and integrated into the personal history and social and cultural beliefs of the participants.

This emerging concept of placebo responses sees them as part of the much larger field of mind–brain–society interactions. Harrington used the metaphor of the theater to capture the dynamic qualities of the interaction: the patient-practitioner encounter she observed is like an ongoing drama, complete with sets, costumes, props and roles, in which the players write the script, spin the plot, and transform symbolic meanings into biological responses.

Moerman elaborated on the meaning response with examples from the medical and anthropological literature. That we implicitly attach meaning to color and quantity was seen in a study of medical students who were each given packets containing one or two pink or blue capsules. The pills were inert but the students were told that one capsule was a stimulant, the other a sedative. Student responses to a follow-up questionnaire indicated that the pink capsules acted like stimulants (pink = "up", "hot", "danger") while the blue capsules acted like sedatives (blue = "down", "quiet", "cool") and two capsules had more effect than one (two is greater than one).[4]

A British study that would seem to confirm the power of advertising involved 835 women who took over-the-counter analgesics for headache.[5] The women were randomly assigned to one of four groups. Group A was given unmarked placebo; B, placebo marked with a widely advertised brand name aspirin; C, the same aspirin in a plain package; and D, aspirin of a widely advertised brand. The women reported their pain relief on a six point scale (from –1, worse, to +4, completely better), one hour after taking the pills for successive headaches. All groups reported feeling better, averaging 1.78 for A; 2.18 for B; 2.48 for C; and 2.7 for D. The active drugs did better than placebos and the branded drugs did better than unbranded drugs – with branded placebo doing better than unbranded placebo. Moerman concluded that aspirin does indeed relieve headaches, but so does knowledge that the pills taken are good ones – which is learned from advertising.

No tangible placebo was operative in another study in which two groups were instructed on the benefits of aerobic exercise.[6] One group was told that their aerobic capacity would increase after 10 weeks while the other group was told that not only would their aerobic capacity increase, but their psychological wellbeing would be enhanced. Both groups improved in aerobic capacity, but only the second group reported improved self-esteem. "Words are not inert," Moerman observed.

Nor are traditional beliefs inert. Moerman cited a large study in California which found that Chinese-Americans, but not matched white controls, died younger if they had a combination of birth year and disease which Chinese astrology and medicine considers ill-fated than if the birth year and disease coded as cause of death were not so linked. The effect was stronger in Chinese-Americans with characteristics indicative of closer adherence to Chinese traditions. Thus, the California Chinese born in Chinese "Earth" years, associated with susceptibility to diseases involving lumps or tumors, were found to die of lymphatic cancer at an average age of 60 – four years younger than Chinese born in other years or Americans with comparable cancers. Similar differences were found for most other categories of disease matched with vulnerable birth-years.[7]

Moerman cited other examples of the ways in which providers and patients interact to affect disease outcomes, noting that beneficial placebo effects are more likely to be operative when the provider is enthusiastic and positive in contrast to more matter-of-fact and non-committal behavior. A particularly subtle example of provider effects was a double blind dental pain study that involved two sets of patients. All patients were told they may receive either a narcotic analgesic, a narcotic antagonist, or a placebo and that the treatments might decrease their pain, increase it, or have no effect. Clinicians who administered the drug and the pain questionnaires knew that one set of patients would be subdivided into three groups each of which would receive one of the above three treatments, while the other set would be subdivided into two groups who would receive either placebo or a narcotic antagonist. The patients were not aware of this. Only patients in the first set showed positive pain relief to the placebo. This study suggests that clinicians' knowledge of possible treatment effects may influence placebo responses even in a double blind study.[8]

Moerman's data included numerous studies of placebo effects that debunk popular myths and indicate how complex placebo phenomena are. For example:

- The oft-quoted figure from Beecher[9] that about one third of patients in any given study exhibit placebo effects is misleading at best. There is wide variability in placebo responses within individuals, within groups, across clinical trials, and by the disease condition and by the nature of the drug or procedure under study.
- Placebo effects – or meaning responses – occur in the course of active treatments as well as with placebos.
- Some investigators have reported a strong correlation between placebo effects and active treatment effects, i.e. the more potent the active pharmaceutical is, the more marked are the placebo effects of a

look-alike pill. The contribution to this correlation of measurement artifacts such as regression to the mean has not been established.

- Placebo effects vary by country and within countries by disease. How much of the variation may be explainable by other factors remains to be determined.[10]
- Good adherers to a regimen, whether that regimen be a placebo or active drug, do better than poor adherers to the same regimen.
- The meaning response may be higher in clinical than in experimental settings.

Moerman's interpretation and review of the literature enlarged the frame of reference for discussion of the placebo, emphasizing a process rather than a pill or other measure. He argued for research to understand the mechanisms that lie behind observations and capitalize on them for the benefit of patients. "The evidence suggests that treatments don't need very powerful specific effects to energize highly effective therapeutic systems. The application of a focused, meaningful theory to injury or disease … can make a huge difference … for patients in the objective and subjective dimension of their illness, regardless of the specifics of the treatment," he observed.

In his discussion of Moerman's paper, anthropologist Thomas Csordas (Case Western Reserve University) agreed with Moerman's main points, making reference to his own studies of Navajo healing ceremonies and Catholic Charismatic rituals to emphasize that these rituals are richly endowed with meaning and incorporate very specific themes and formal elements. Indeed, he showed how meanings organize the process of healing. A second discussant, Robert Hahn, an epidemiologist and anthropologist with the US Centers for Disease Control and Prevention, was also sympathetic to the meaning approach, but raised a concern about how meaning can be quantified and connected to specific health outcomes, citing, for example, the multiplicity of meanings attached to specific colors. He also criticized the implicit Cartesian dualism that affects the study of placebos. Western scientists are heirs to a mind-body dualism in which mental or psychological phenomena are judged to be subjective and less real than "objective" body effects and hence in need of explanations in terms of fundamental physiological (body) mechanisms.

## Explanatory psychosocial mechanisms

Attempts to explain why placebos work – when they work – have engaged biomedical and behavioral scientists for the past half century. Psychosocial and physiological explanations include theories of personality, cognition, social learning, and conditioning.

### *Personality, cognition, and social learning*

In parallel with Harrington, Moerman, and others, psychologist Richard Bootzin, University of Arizona,[11] welcomed enlarging the framework for conceptualizing the placebo. Initially, however, he pointed to several paradoxes that affect the use of placebos. On the one hand, clinicians see the value of maximizing placebo responses to enhance active treatments for disease. On the other hand, researchers aim to control for placebo effects in clinical trials. A second paradox consists in the need in the clinic to individualize treatments to maximize placebo effects in a particular patient. In contrast, subjects in a clinical trial are generally treated according to a standardized protocol to ensure that all patients are treated alike. "A better understanding of the psychological explanatory mechanisms that underlie placebo effects requires a systematic approach that examines both domains, the clinic and research settings," he said.

Toward that end, Bootzin noted problems with research methodologies in which trials testing for efficacy may be confused with trials to determine mechanisms of action. He also objected to the frequent characterization of the effects of active medication or of the particular school of psychosocial therapy employed as specific and theory-driven, while the effects of placebo controls (which in the case of psychotherapies are called "attention placebo controls") are non-specific, and characterized as psychological rather than physiological. This leads to the kind of oil-on-water thinking in which placebo effects are considered add-ons to some fundamental physiological effect.

Bootzin approached the role of cognition and behavioral mechanisms in placebo effects from a social learning perspective in which learning is seen not as a passive reaction to stimuli, but involves active selection, organization, and transformation of the input. In order, he discussed:

*Personality factors* Much of the 1960's and 1970's research on placebo mechanisms was based on studies that tried, unsuccessfully, to identify what kind of individuals were placebo responders. It is of some interest that many of these early studies depicted placebo responders in a negative light. As summarized by Shapiro and Shapiro,[12]

... personality traits found in one study differ from those reported in others. ... Some of the studies report, however, and it is commonly assumed, that (when compared with placebo nonreactors) placebo reactors are less intelligent; less educated; more frequently neurotic or psychotic; more frequently female; from lower social classes, more dependent, inadequate, immature, impulsive, atypical, depressed, religious, and stereotypic; and more likely to have symptoms of hypochondriasis, obsessive-compulsiveness, anger-hostility, bewilderment-confusion, and performance difficulties. In our studies and others there appear to be no consistent data relating either these variables or demographic variables such as age, sex, intelligence, race, social class, ethnicity, religiosity, or religious background in placebo reactions.

Bootzin observed that the current consensus is that the capacity to elicit a placebo response is probably inherent in everyone and may be a function of a "contextual situational phenomenon more than an enduring personality trait."

*The therapeutic relationship* Bootzin emphasized that it is not the provider per se, nor the patient, nor the treatment process, but the interplay of all these elements that can influence placebo responses. He cited numerous studies indicating that the placebo response is more likely to occur in the clinic when the patient regards the clinician as experienced, competent, and optimistic,[13,14] when the clinician expects the treatment to help,[8,15] and when both patients and physicians are of like mind.[16] He noted that a physician's positive attitude was more effective in eliciting a placebo response than writing a medication prescription,[17] and that the more frequently the provider and patient meet, in a supportive setting, the more likely is it that the patient will respond – possibly because the provider is seen to be more attentive to the patient's needs.[18]

Some studies have indicated that various schools of psychotherapy are about equally effective in achieving beneficial results. There are demurrers, however. Andrews and Harvey[19] found that behavioral therapies had a significantly higher effect size than verbal dynamic psychotherapies. Miller and colleagues[20,21] also found distinct differences between therapies that worked best and those which were least effective in treating alcoholism. Superior treatments were characterized by brief intervention, motivational enhancement, social skills training, and community reinforcement. Least effective were educational lectures/films, general alcoholism counseling, psychotherapy, and confrontational counseling.

*Hope* Some theories propose that a common element in healing is an action performed by healer that imbues the patient with hope. According to a leading proponent, Jerome Frank, interventions are important only because they provide a shared belief system between clinician and patient and give form to prescribed rituals.[22]

*Outcome and efficacy expectations* Outcome expectations refer to the consequences that follow actions, while self-efficacy expectations are beliefs that one can successfully perform the actions needed to achieve desired outcomes. To a large extent these contributions to treatment effects focus on the belief systems of the patient. Whatever occurs in the course of treatment to alter negative belief systems and empower the patient with coping skills can contribute to positive treatment effects. In the case of some chronic illnesses, for example, Bootzin notes that training to increase self-efficacy led to improved mood, less anxiety, reduced pain, and improved health status (for example, lower blood pressure; better metabolic control). A clinician's enthusiasm and prediction of a positive outcome has also been linked to improved functioning, although Bootzin cautions that unless the clinician's predictions are confirmed, the patient's expectancies will be subject to revision.

*Response expectancies* Some investigators believe that response expectancies, defined as expectations about one's emotional state and physiological responses, including idiosyncratic reactions to pain or anxiety, are the major determinants of placebo. In turn, they see response expectancies as dependent on the condition being treated and a number of situational variables. These include the plausibility of the treatment regimen and dosages as well as the likelihood that the treatment will produce the response expected. As evidence Bootzin cites an experiment of Kirsch and Weixel[23] using regular and decaffeinated coffee. One group of subjects was treated in a double blind fashion so that neither they nor the experimenters knew which type of coffee they would be served in the trial. However, a second group was told that they would be given regular coffee, when in fact they were served a decaffeinated brew. Results showed that subjects in the second group – with response expectancies associated with drinking real coffee – had higher pulse rates than those in the double blind condition who presumably had more equivocal expectancies. The groups also differed in ratings of alertness, tension, and systolic blood pressure.

Kirsch and Sapirstein[24] have proposed that response expectancies may be the key factor in the effects of drugs used to treat psychiatric disorders such as depression. Results of placebo controlled clinical trials of antidepressants generally show small or no differences between active drug and placebo. As a result of a meta-analysis of studies of antidepressant medications, these investigators suggest that antidepressant drugs may be little more than active placebos that reinforce patients' response expectancies insofar as they produce side effects.

*An interactive multi-dimensional model* Bootzin's own model for the placebo effect combines many elements of the patient–practitioner encounter with multiple explanatory mechanisms. In his view, the placebo effect is not static, but a dynamic, constantly changing variable co-varying with other variables, both psychological and physiological, that operate within the therapeutic process. The interactions are not predictable but operate synergistically with the active treatment (rather than simply adding to active treatment effects). He emphasizes that the meaning ascribed by the patient to the health problem and the treatment proposed provides a context in which a number of mechanisms may operate – conditioning, expectancies, information from the clinician, internal feedback – with reciprocal and recursive interactions. Thus, he postulates that the placebo effect operates:

- directly – by activating the body's innate healing mechanisms (acting through homeostatic processes)
- indirectly – mediated by the patient's behavior (such as adhering to a treatment regimen, possibly complemented by implementing other health-promoting behaviors)

- interactively – in the sense that active treatment and indirect effects operate recursively and synergistically in the course of care.

"In summary," Bootzin says, "the model supports the view that the placebo effect is a therapeutic ally that helps to improve outcome through various causal pathways."

*Classical (Pavlovian) conditioning*

Shepard Siegel (McMaster University)[25] reviewed an extensive literature demonstrating that some placebo effects can be attributed to classical (respondent, Type I, or Pavlovian) conditioning. In Pavlovian conditioning a neutral conditional stimulus (CS) is paired with a biologically significant unconditional stimulus (UCS). The UCS normally elicits an unconditional, often reflex response (UR). Following pairings, the CS becomes associated with the UCS and when presented independently, elicits the reflex response, now called the conditional response (CR). Siegel noted that environmental cues often serve as conditioned stimuli in drug administration, citing early studies by American and Russian investigators. In a 1925 study of chronic morphine administration in dogs, the investigators observed that in the course of the study the entry into the room of the experimenter was sufficient to cause copious salivation in the animals.[26] Pavlov reported similar observations by Russian scientists in 1927.[27] Later studies showed that following assorted drug treatments, animals could be conditioned to exhibit catalepsy, insulin-shock-like behaviors, and modification of circulating immunodefense mechanisms.

Conditioning has been studied as a factor in syndromes such as multiple chemical sensitivity (in which lower levels of irritants or other cues previously associated with irritants that caused allergy-like symptoms also trigger symptoms).[28,29] Conditioning has also been noted in subjects habitually using caffeine, nicotine, alcohol, and both illicit drugs and medically useful drugs. For example, the inveterate coffee drinker may respond with heightened alertness to decaffeinated coffee.[30] Siegel cited as an example of conditioning to a prescription drug a study of the immunosuppressant drug cyclophosphamide. The drug was given by injection to multiple sclerosis patients who first ingested an anise-flavored syrup. In a double blind test study the patients ingested the syrup but were infused with an amount of cyclophosphamide that was less than one per cent of the effective dose. Nevertheless, 8 out of 10 patients showed decreased peripheral leukocyte counts.[31] Results like this suggest that conditioning could be used to reduce the dosages of potent drugs, prolonging their useful life by lowering toxicity and side effects. This point of view has been championed by Robert Ader, a pioneer in the field of placebo conditioning. In an experiment in the early '80s Ader and Cohen[32] showed that rats susceptible to an autoimmune systemic lupus erythematosis-like disease also demonstrated immunological conditioning. The mice received CS paired with cyclophosphamide presentations interspersed with the CS alone. The conditioned mice experienced delays in the onset of disease comparable to mice which had received twice as much cyclophosphamide and no CS.

Siegel noted that conditioning as an explanatory mechanism for some placebo effects is plausible insofar as it satisfies a number of established principles of conditioning. These include the sequence effect: the need to present the UCS (the effective drug) first, stimulus generalizability (the CS such as environmental cues need not be identical in repeated trials), and extinction (repeated presentations of the placebo should show decreased effectiveness over time). He noted that conditioning is also possible on a single trial and also when there is a delay between presentation of the UCS and the CS. But there are also complicating factors in which placebos are seen to modulate the effects of the active drug. In early morphine studies in dogs for example, it was observed that repeated conditioned responses enhanced the effects of morphine when it was administered, a phenomenon described as reverse tolerance or sensitization. Perhaps even more surprising is that placebo conditioned responses can sometimes produce effects opposite to the effects of the active drug. This has been interpreted as an adaptive preparation for the impending pharmacological perturbation. Siegel cited several examples of such compensatory CRs, including an *increase* in activity following training with the potent tranquilizer chlorpromazine[33] and hyperglycemia after inert injections following training with insulin.[34,35,36] Similarly, some studies have shown that CRs to morphine result in hyperalgesia.[37,38,39,40] More complicated yet are mixed responses. Amphetamine results in increased activity and increased temperature, but reported effects of CRs to amphetamine indicate increased activity but lower body temperature.[41]

Siegel concluded that the major advantage of conditioning as an explanation of placebo effects is that drug responses are readily conditionable and can be studied in non-human animals for clues to the physiological mechanisms involved. But they cannot be the whole explanation – not only because of the problem of compensatory CRs, but also because of the many instances in which people experience placebo effects in the absence of previous drug experiences. Thus there are probably a variety of placebo effects with conditioning accounting for a subset.

In commenting on Siegel's paper, Robert Ader, University of Rochester, distinguished between placebo conditioned pharmacologic and placebo conditioned pharmacotherapeutic effects, stating that the psychophysiologic state of the individual was a critical factor in conditioned placebo responses. If the subject is a healthy volunteer in a study, the CR to a pharmacological intervention could go in the same direction as the UCR.

With certain drugs on certain occasions, however, the response might be compensatory – in anticipation that the UCR might upset the body's normal homeostatic balance and thus compensate for it. If the subject is a patient whose homeostatic balance is already upset by the pathologic process, the pharmacotherapeutic CR should favor a restoration of balance and thus go in the same direction as the UCR. To do otherwise, would "violate the wisdom of the body."

## Intervening psychophysiology

Psychosocial factors such as personality, cognition (including, expectancy), social learning, and conditioning are presumed to activate psychophysiological events that involve not only the nervous, endocrine, and immune systems, but also the cardiovascular, gastrointestinal, and other systems. The mechanisms by which placebo interventions are able to convert meaning into the modification of physiologic responses is not known. Indeed, no studies have fully traced the pathways by which cognition/expectancy, personality, social learning, and psychosocial interactions may affect psychophysiological responses. The two mediating physiological processes that have been studied extensively in relation to placebo effects are the immune system and the opioid and non-opioid nervous system mechanisms of pain control.

### *Psychoneuroendocrine immunology*

Work in the field of psychoneuroimmunology, which studies interactions between psychological/mental states and the endocrine, immune, and other effector systems, has been instructive in delineating pathways and molecules leading to conditioned placebo effects as a result of learning and emotional input. For example, in a paper which appears in this volume (but was not presented at the conference)[42] Farideh Eskandari and Esther M Sternberg from the National Institute of Mental Health (NIMH) review research on the hypothalamic-pituitary-adrenal (HPA) axis and autonomic processes in response to stress. The HPA axis dampens immune inflammatory responses via the secretion of potent anti-inflammatory glucocorticoids from the adrenal glands, while branches of the autonomic nervous system regulate immune organs regionally through their innervation of immune organs such as the spleen and thymus. Peripheral nerves also influence immune responses at sites of inflammation by the release of neuropeptides that stimulate immune cells. The cross-talk among neurons, endocrine and immune cells made possible by reciprocal connections and an extensive population of neurotransmitters, neuropeptides, neurohormones and immunocytokines enables a fine tuning of immune responses. While the pathways remain to be specified, it is reasonable to assume that signals from cognitive and emotional centers in the cortex tapping into these systems are the means by which learning and emotion affect immunity and the body's response to illness.

*Pain as paradigm*

In the search for explanatory mechanisms, pain research occupies a special place in placebo studies. Because pain is a subjective experience, investigators have long recognized the problems inherent in developing standard measures of both its sensory and emotional qualities and applying these measures in clinical trials of analgesics. Indeed, pain research has been a source of the well-reported phenomenon that the potency of placebo effects often varies directly with the perceived potency of the placebo vehicle; a placebo injection generally elicits a more powerful placebo effect than a pill that is swallowed, while the effects of sham surgery can exceed both. Now, thanks to several major advances in pain research over the past 35 years, there is a growing body of evidence that brain activity can change under various placebo manipulations.

The first major advance was the discovery of descending pain-modulatory pathways in the central nervous system. One pathway uses endorphins, a family of endogenous opioid neurotransmitters, which operate at cortical and subcortical levels to inhibit the transmission of nociceptive (pain) information relayed from the dorsal horn of the spinal cord. The endorphin receptors on neurons involved in these pathways also respond to various forms of exogenous morphine. These pathways can be inhibited by administration of the morphine antagonist naloxone. There are also non-opiate, pain-modulatory pathways that use other neurotransmitters, such as serotonin, which are not inhibited by naloxone. A second major advance was the development of neuroimaging technology using PET or fMRI scans that enable visualizing which parts of the brain are activated under various experimental and pathological conditions. These brain maps have been used to show that hypnotic suggestion can alter brain activity in experimental pain studies. For example, brain scans of subjects responding to the suggestion that the pain they are experiencing will be reduced either in intensity in one manipulation or unpleasantness in another, show corresponding reductions in brain activity in somatosensory cortex or limbic areas.

In his presentation, Don Price,[43] a pain researcher at the University of Florida, noted that pain modulatory pathways in the hypothalamus, the amygdala, and the midbrain periaqueductal grey are involved not only in pain, but also in learning and memory, and in threat-induced defensive behavior ("stress analgesia"), suggesting that these systems might be activated not only by tissue damage, but as a result of cognitive and emotional input. As an example, he described the analgesia in rats that follows their exposure to inescapable noxious footshock when placed in an experimental apparatus. The analgesia subsides, but when rats are re-introduced to the test apparatus the environmental cues alone serve as a conditioning stimulus to induce stress analgesia. Interestingly, this type of analgesia can be blocked by naloxone.[44]

Price reviewed a number of animal and human experiments in which placebo analgesia was achieved, enumerating a range of possible cognitive, psychological, and biological mediating mechanisms, including classical conditioning, expectancy, desire for pain relief, and anxiety. In one experiment Voudouris[45,46] exposed volunteers to electric shock in successive test sessions. In the first session subjects experienced painful shock. They were then told that test two would follow the application of a pain-reducing cream. Instead, the intensity of the shock was lowered and a placebo cream was applied. In the third test the placebo cream was again applied but the intensity of shock was raised to match the level of test one. Subjects reported pain relief. However, it was not clear whether the placebo analgesia occurred because of classical conditioning, or as a result of information given to human subjects eliciting a "response expectancy," or some combination of both. With regard to the pain experiment the information given would elicit the response expectancy that their pain would be reduced. In attempts to distinguish conditioning from expectancy, subjects in a later experiment of Kirsch and Montgomery[47] were divided into two groups. Both groups were told that the placebo cream would reduce their pain and both were subjected to shock on test one and to application of the cream under reduced shock intensities on test two. However, one group was told that the shock level would be lowered prior to test two, in effect, controlling for response expectancy. Results of the third test, showed that only the uninformed group showed placebo analgesia. The experimenters concluded that conditioning may cause a placebo effect as long as the subject does not know about the manipulation, but they maintain that when conditioning does result in placebo analgesia, it is still mediated by expectancy.

Price reported on research to study the pain-modulating pathways involved in placebo analgesia. In a conditioning study using an arm tourniquet as the painful procedure and pain tolerance as the outcome measure, Amanzio and Benedetti[48] used repeated injections of either morphine or a non-opioid analgesic, ketorolac, followed by placebo injections, to elicit placebo analgesia. Interestingly, the placebo analgesia conditioned by morphine was reversed by naloxone, while the analgesia conditioned by ketorolac was not naloxone-reversible. In an experiment testing expectancy, subjects injected with saline solution were told they were being given a potent analgesic. The placebo analgesia obtained was reversed completely by naloxone. Price also noted that placebo analgesia is highly specific and quantifiable. He and co-workers,[49] in a variation on the Montgomery and Kirsch model, selected three adjacent sites on the forearm of subjects. They applied either a "strong" placebo cream to site A, a "weak" placebo cream to site B, or a control agent to site C, all sites being initially subjected to painful skin temperature stimuli. On test two they varied the reduction in thermal intensity so that the temperature at site A was reduced the most; site B, less, and site C not at all. In test three all three sites were subject to the equally high temperatures used initially. The placebo effects were graded in proportion to the extent of stimulus lowering in the second test. Moreover, since the skin sites were adjacent, it would appear that placebo analgesia is somatotopically organized. This experiment was also revelatory in terms of memory distortion. When placebo effects were measured concurrently with the placebo trials, the effects were modest. When participants were questioned only a few minutes after the trials were over, placebo effects were magnified three to four times over what had been reported during the tests.

## Placebo effects and measurement artifacts: a composite

Conference participants were mindful that some or all of the improvements in a patient's health and wellbeing, whether the individual was a subject in a controlled clinical trial or a patient being treated by a clinician, may not be the effect of an active treatment nor a placebo, but due to other factors. Indeed, some of the difficulty – and skepticism – that attends placebo research derives from critics who say that what is deemed a placebo effect is really the result of such other factors. It follows that the studies of placebo effects must be designed to avoid these pitfalls and tease out actual biological effects of placebo from various artifacts.

### *Natural history*

Chronic diseases such as multiple sclerosis and some cancers, and many conditions where pain is a prominent feature, exhibit a relapsing, remitting course. In such circumstances, the patient who shows improvement may reflect the natural history of the disease and not the effects of any treatment (or placebo) given prior to the amelioration. The inclusion of "no-treatment" groups in randomized, placebo controlled clinical trials provides one way to evaluate natural history as a cause of improvements. However, the issue is complex because few, if any, patients experience "no treatment" in the strict sense of the term. Individuals may diet, exercise, or take home remedies or over-the-counter medications. They may try various herbals or dietary supplements and even prescription medications left over from other episodes or obtained from others.[50] In addition, most experiences of illness take a social course in the sense that social factors such as economic costs, access to care, quality and type of treatment, and ongoing stress and social support influence the everyday experience of an illness.[51]

### *Patient bias*

Some patients may exhibit a response bias, especially in the case of subjective reports of symptoms – a reduction in pain and suffering, enhanced wellbeing. They either consciously or unconsciously want to show that they are good patients and appreciate the care they are given and so may report positively to questions about symptom improvement. Some investigators refer to this as the patient's placebo – the patient's desire to please the care provider. Patient bias may also affect participation in the trial. In order to satisfy inclusion criteria, the patient may exaggerate symptoms. Another factor that can contaminate results may be the concomitant use of other medications that may affect the condition under study.

*Investigator bias*

If an investigator knows which subject has been given the active drug and which a placebo in a study, he or she may be disposed, and possibly have a vested interest, in seeing that the active treatment works better than placebo. Such expectancies can lead to measurement errors, faulty judgments of symptom relief, and so on. The problem can affect double blind studies since in the course of the trial investigators and patients may both become unblinded as they perceive notable differences in reactions and the presence of side effects.

*Regression to the mean*

CE Davis, a biostatistician at the University of North Carolina, provided a detailed analysis of the regression to the mean,[52] a statistical phenomenon that refers to the tendency that a variable found to be extreme on one measurement will be closer to the mean on a subsequent measurement. The degree to which regression to the mean occurs in a study depends on the reliability of the measurements and the extent to which patients are selected into the study on the basis of extreme measurements.[11] In a study of cholesterol levels, for example, an individual selected for inclusion in a trial because of high blood cholesterol will tend to have a slightly lower cholesterol reading at a second later measurement, mimicking a placebo effect. In fact, regression to the mean often appears together with the placebo effect in clinical trials, since the criteria for inclusion of a participant often require selection for being extreme. Some statisticians have argued that much of what are regarded as placebo effects in clinical studies actually result from regression to the mean.[53] This is an important distinction, since regression to the mean is a statistical artifact of measurements subject to random error and does not reflect any biological effect.

## Ethical and methodological implications of placebo use in clinical practice and research

While the nature and underlying operative mechanisms of placebo effects – the what, when, where, how, and why of the processes involved – dominated discussion during the first part of the conference, ethical and methodological issues related to the use of placebos in the clinic and in clinical trials dominated the second part. Participants agreed that the introduction of randomized double blind placebo controlled clinical trials a generation ago established the gold standard for testing clinical efficacy. But, as several speakers argued, that was *then*. In the interim a burgeoning pharmaceutical industry has produced prodigious numbers of safe and effective disease-specific drugs. Why, they asked, should placebo controls ever be used in trials of new drugs where an effective intervention already exists? Why deny patients the benefits of treatment?

## The ethical issues

Moreover, Harvard bioethicist Sissela Bok,[54] among others, raised concerns about the increasingly global scale of placebo clinical trials, the adequacy of informed consent and reviews by Institutional Review Boards (IRBs), differing standards for trials conducted in developing countries, and other ethical issues. Prior to the present pharmaceutical era, she noted that it was not uncommon for practitioners to give patients placebos. The practice was condoned along with an authoritarian attitude that it was all right to lie to patients or to withhold information if it was perceived to be in the patient's own good. Only in 1980 did the American Medical Association add to its Principles of Medical Ethics the instruction to physicians to "deal honestly with patients and colleagues".[55]

No doubt the new emphasis on truth-telling reflected the changing climate of medicine. Today there are over 5000 prescription drugs and countless over-the-counter preparations that can treat disease or allay symptoms. Physicians can do more for patients; they have reason for greater optimism and less need for deception. At the same time, patients' expectations are higher; they are better informed and less passive in dealing with health problems. This combination of events can work to the patient's advantage when it leads to a constructive dialogue and cooperation between patient and provider, for example, in working out a treatment plan. Observations that such positive features of provider-patient interactions are among those associated with placebo responses – yielding positive effects on the patient's health and wellbeing – are among the reasons for a revived interest in the nature of placebos and the placebo *process*. In turn, the growth of research studies elucidating a physiological basis for mind–body effects is providing a rationale for learning how best to elicit placebo effects in patient care. This renewed interest has also been fueled by changes in health care in the United States, characterized by a dissatisfaction with managed care systems and an increased popularity of complementary and alternative medicine (CAM) approaches. CAM practitioners are widely perceived as espousing a philosophy that health can be promoted and disease prevented and treated by marshaling the body's natural healing systems, in this way encouraging placebo responses.[56]

While the potential for exploiting placebos and placebo responses in clinical practice is promising, it is not without ethical dilemmas. The deceptive use of pharmacologically inert placebo medications may be much less common in American medical practice today than in the past, but the use of active medications prescribed for their supposed placebo value appears to be widespread. A familiar example is the indiscriminate use of antibiotics. Ironically, this practice may be driven more by patient demand than physician desire. The global increase in bacterial antibiotic-resistance may be in part attributable to inappropriate use of antibiotics for their placebo effects. Indeed, the word placebo is a misnomer in this instance since antibiotic drugs are far from inert. The same can be said for the use of invasive diagnostic procedures for a supposed "placebo" effect. Moreover, placebos, whether inert or active, can harm patients. Risks include delaying diagnosis and treatment of an unrecognized condition and, in some cases, addiction to the placebo.

Clearly the use of placebos in practice, inert or otherwise, has not disappeared, nor have occasions for deception. What are practitioners to do, for example, asked conference participant Howard Spiro of Yale University if, upon entering a hospital, they are confronted by the sight of one of their patients being rushed into surgery with what appear to be mortal wounds and the patient asks, "Hey doc, am I going to make it?" Such situations serve as a reminder that the standard of truth-telling cannot be absolute. There are grey areas and there are increasingly complex ethical issues arising out of today's sophisticated medical technology.

Bok observed that we know very little about how practitioners behave today. How common is the provision of placebos? She proposed that when placebos are given they be fully documented in the patient's file, suggesting that such record-keeping would discourage placebo use. How well and truly do providers inform patients of their diagnosis, the benefits and risks of proposed therapies, and possible prognoses with or without treatment? Should a patient seeking treatment for disease be recruited to a clinical trial where randomization might mean assignment to a placebo control? All that can be done should be done to improve communications, clarify consent forms, and prevent coercion, she said. What are health professional students taught about placebos and placebo use? A useful first step would be to examine medical texts and training manuals.

In raising these ethical questions Bok and others underscored the changing climate of health care, the growing emphasis on patients' rights, and the need for safeguards against medical error, the misuse of placebos, and reported examples of less-than-forthcoming communications by providers or research investigators. These issues were aired throughout the conference and came to the fore in discussions about the use of placebos in clinical trials.

A focal point for discussion was the *Declaration of Helsinki* resolution, issued by the World Medical Association* as a guideline for clinical research. Article II.3 of the fifth revision of the Declaration, issued in 1996, states:

> The potential benefits, hazards and discomfort of a new method should be weighed against the advantages of the best current diagnostic and therapeutic method.
>
> In any medical study, every patient (including those of a control group, if any) should be assured of the best proven diagnostic and therapeutic method. This does not exclude the use of inert placebo in studies where no proven diagnostic or therapeutic method exists.

A sixth revision of the declaration, published in October 2000, states as Article 29:

> The benefits, risks, burdens and effectiveness of a new method should be tested against those of the best current prophylactic, diagnostic, and therapeutic methods. This does not exclude the use of placebo, or no treatment, in studies where no proven prophylactic, diagnostic or therapeutic method exists.

It should be noted that all conferees agree that placebo controls should not be used in trials of agents for serious or life-threatening conditions, such as acute infectious diseases or cancer, under circumstances where proven safe and effective therapy would otherwise be available. Also, all agree that placebos can appropriately be used in trials in the absence of any effective treatment. Where the main disagreement lies is in the use of placebos and not known effective agents as controls in trials in which temporary deferral of treatment would pose no long-term threat to health or wellbeing. While some investigators interpret both the 1996 and the 2000 revisions of the *Declaration of Helsinki* as prohibiting the use of placebo in any clinical trial where there is an existing therapy of proven safety and effectiveness, others see the 2000 revision as more definitively prohibiting use of placebo instead of an active control of proven safety and effectiveness in any clinical trial. It did not escape notice among participants that the Declaration's strong proscriptive statement was occurring,

---

* In light of the notorious World War II Nazi medical experiments on concentration camp prisoners, the 1947 Nuremberg Code set forth initial standards for protection of human participants in biomedical research, emphasizing the requirement for voluntary consent and respect for human rights. The *Declaration of Helsinki*, first issued by the World Medical Association in 1964, deals comprehensively with ethics in all aspects of human biomedical research, providing guidelines for investigators to follow in research involving human subjects. The Declaration has been revised five times, the most recent being the October 2000 revision. World Medical Association leaders have indicated they may consider further refinement of the provisions of the Declaration concerning use of placebo.

ironically, at a time when the power of placebo effects and the recent studies to elucidate underlying psychophysiological mechanisms had been one of the factors in deciding to hold the placebo conference in the first place.

In support of the use of placebos, clinical researchers note that many conditions for which drugs are developed involve symptoms which vary considerably within patients over time and which often appear to be responsive to placebo therapy in carefully designed experiments. The problem of distinguishing between placebo effects and active therapy is especially critical in the early stages of drug development when there are no reliable objective markers of efficacy. (An exception is the development of new antibiotics where *in vitro* markers of antibiotic sensitivity can provide guidance). Early in drug development experimenters are not sure that the new drug has *any* more clinical efficacy than placebo, nor do they know what the minimal effective dose should be.

## Clinical trial design and analysis

Experts on both sides of the placebo issue are aware of the levels of complexity and uncertainty that challenge the design, conduct, and analysis of all clinical trials – whether the trials use placebos, historical controls, no treatment, or active controls. To use a randomized clinical trial to show that a new treatment is effective, investigators may either show that it is superior to a placebo or active treatment, or that it is no less effective (within a pre-defined margin) than a treatment previously proven to be effective. The former type of trial, known as a *superiority trial*, is by far the most common way to establish effectiveness of a new therapy. The latter type of trial, known as a *non-inferiority* trial, is a newer approach which offers a statistically valid way to establish that one treatment is not less effective than another, while avoiding the fallacy of using failure to achieve statistical superiority as a basis for claiming similarity.

Robert Temple of the US Food and Drug Administration[57] and Stuart Pocock, a statistician from the London School of Hygiene and Tropical Medicine,[58] presented the case for the appropriate use of placebo trials in the presence of proven treatments. Temple began by noting that a literal reading of article 29 of the October 2000 Helsinki Declaration revision would obviate all clinical trials – placebo controlled, active controls, no-treatment, or historically controlled – since patients given an experimental agent in a trial would be denied the best *proven* treatment. He did not believe that this was the intention of the writers of the Helsinki Declaration. He also reiterated that placebos should not be used in trials that involve serious morbidity or life-threatening conditions when doing so would deny patients a proven safe and effective therapy that would otherwise have been available to them. Conditions for which placebo trials could appropriately be used include those in which temporary deferral of treatment would pose no long-term threat to health or wellbeing, such as treatments for insomnia, headache, or allergic rhinitis.

That said, Temple compared clinical trials in terms of the evidence needed to support claims of superiority or non-inferiority. A well-designed clinical trial that shows superiority to an existing drug or placebo provides strong evidence of its effectiveness, within the limits of statistical inference. No prior studies or evidence external to the trial is necessary. In contrast, the finding that a new drug is no worse than an existing drug in a non-inferiority trial provides valid evidence of effectiveness only if there is good evidence that the existing drug would have demonstrated superiority to placebo if a placebo arm had been included in the trial. These are assumptions that rely on evidence external to the trial and Temple's point was that that evidence is often lacking or equivocal: "…for many types of effective drugs, studies of apparently adequate size and design do not regularly distinguish drugs from placebo". Technically, these studies lack "assay sensitivity", the ability of a study to distinguish between active and inactive treatments.

It is this issue of assay sensitivity that is the key to the need for placebo controls. Assay sensitivity cannot always be achieved simply by making a trial larger. A common way to show assay sensitivity is to show that the known active treatment in the trial has consistently beaten placebo in trials of similar design with similar kinds of patients. Temple and other conference speakers stated that the lack of assay sensitivity is a problem that particularly besets studies of antidepressant drugs, but also applies to trials of analgesics, antihypertensives, antihistamines, and many other classes of drugs in common use.[59] (As was emphasized throughout the conference, placebos can be powerful.) This does not mean that antidepressants or other prescription drugs in current use are ineffective, but it does cast doubt on the reliability of the evidence when these drugs are used as the active controls in non-inferiority trials without a placebo group. Temple concluded that the resolution of assay sensitivity problems, one which would restore confidence in the evidence found in non-inferiority trials, is to include a placebo arm in the design. Such designs are often used in circumstances where use of placebo is considered ethical.

## Use of placebo trials when effective agents exist: issues of risk to trial participants

Having established the need for assay sensitivity as a broad principle governing the use of placebo controls, Temple explored situations in which the condition under study raised particular ethical concerns that might preclude the use of placebos.[60] A case in point would be the study of antidepressants in which placebo subjects would be denied drugs over the period of the study, a factor which could potentially increase the risk for suicide. Studies of antipsychotic drugs in schizophrenia patients pose similar ethical concerns, with differing conclusions as to the appropriateness of placebo controls.[61,62,63] Careful selection and monitoring of patients in such studies should forestall adverse events, Temple suggested. Indeed, in a review of almost 20 000 patients in depression studies of drugs approved for marketing between 1981 and 1997 there was no difference found between placebo-treated and drug-treated groups in terms of suicides or suicide attempts. Such studies have raised questions about whether antidepressants do indeed prevent suicide.[64] Temple also remarked that in the case of non-inferiority trials unless the selection of patients is restricted to those newly diagnosed, patients in the experimental arm would have had to have undergone a withdrawal period from therapy prior to initiating new treatment.

Although the risks of delayed treatment may be small in other medical situations, such as short-term placebo controlled trials of anti-hypertensive agents in patients with mild-to-moderate hypertension, they may not be entirely absent, and must be taken into consideration by providers and patients in deciding to enter a clinical trial. When there appears to be a question about the safety of placebos in a given clinical setting, the safety should be documented, rather than assumed.[65] In some cases, meta-analyses of previous studies have been used to assess safety, insofar as they can show that there have been no increases in adverse events following short periods of withdrawal from therapy.[60,66]

The absolute ban posed by the *Declaration of Helsinki* on the use of placebos in clinical trials in the presence of effective agents avoids many difficult questions that clinical trial designers would otherwise have to address in deciding when placebo use is appropriate. Determining the evidence of safety needed to justify placebo use is clearly a key question. In addition, trialists must also determine the standards to be used in judging whether a non-inferiority trial provides adequate assay sensitivity to establish evidence of effectiveness. Ultimately it should be possible to balance the need to protect the public against the acceptance of an ineffective treatment into practice against the potential for harm to trial participants when a placebo control is used instead of an effective active control.

Pocock's presentation complemented and supported Temple's review of circumstances in which placebo controls are needed to strengthen the evidence from clinical trials. He underscored the need for assay sensitivity by noting that the safety and effectiveness of an active control which is "thought to be, hoped to be, believed to be, highly plausible to be, or in widespread use" did not equate to "known to be" safe and effective. He enumerated common pitfalls in trial design and provided formulas for estimating the sample size needed in order to meet desired confidence intervals for the outcome measures in a study. In particular he described how decisions of non-inferiority are critically dependent on the choice of $\delta$, defined as the smallest true magnitude of inferiority that would be regarded as *unacceptable* given a single primary outcome response for this purpose. Anything equal to or worse than δ would indicate that the experimental drug was inferior to the control.

### Issues of safety, tolerability, and cost

Non-inferiority trials have specific uses beyond establishing that a new drug has the same level of efficacy as an existing drug. If the new drug is of the same class, the manufacturer gains marketing approval for a "me, too" drug. Since no two drugs will have identical profiles, patients have more choices to determine which is best for them. Indeed, the notion that a new drug is merely a "me, too" drug unless it can be shown to be "better" than the "best" available therapy is an oversimplification that fails to take into consideration that better efficacy and better tolerability or safety are not always coincident. The first drug in a therapeutic category is often less well tolerated than subsequent entries, even though its efficacy may be the same or greater.

Other reasons for conducting non-inferiority trials are to determine if the experimental intervention can provide the same or some acceptable level of reduced efficacy in comparison to the active control, but offers other advantages. These trade-offs include increased safety, less invasiveness, and lower cost. Examples Pocock cited were the use of aspirin vs anticoagulation following thrombolysis after a myocardial infarction (aspirin causes less bleeding); carotid stenting over carotid endarterectomy for patients at high risk for stroke (the former is less invasive); and coronary angioplasty versus coronary bypass surgery for angina patients, where cost is an issue in addition to other considerations.

### Why placebo controls should not be used when effective measures exist

Countering the positions of Temple, Pocock, and others was Kenneth Rothman, an epidemiologist at Boston University School of Public Health,[67] who asserted that it is unethical to conduct a trial that deprives participants of the level of care for their condition that they would have received if they were not participants in a trial. His position is in accord with the Helsinki Declaration, which he quoted in two places: "The potential benefits, hazards and discomfort of a new method should be weighed against the advantages of the best current diagnostic and therapeutic methods," and "In any medical study, every patient – including those of a control group, if any – should be assured of the best proven diagnostic and therapeutic method."

In the absence of any effective treatment, Rothman (and the Helsinki Declaration) affirms that clinical trials with placebo controls are appropriate and provide essential scientific evidence. However, given that an effective intervention exists, Rothman asserted that unless a state of genuine uncertainty regarding which of two or more treatments is preferable – called the principle of equipoise – existed no trial should be conducted. "Doing so violates a basic maxim embodied in the *Declaration of Helsinki*, which states that in research on man, the interest of science and society should never take precedence over considerations related to the wellbeing of the subject."* How proponents banning the use of placebos would apply the principle of equipoise in trials of the trade-off kind, when there is evidence that an experimental intervention may not be as effective as the standard treatment, but may offer advantages in terms of safety, tolerability, or cost, is not clear.

Rothman made the important ethical distinction between a patient who comes to a provider expecting treatment and a patient who is not actively seeking treatment. In the former case it would be unethical for the patient to be enrolled in a placebo controlled clinical trial, given the possibility of assignment to the placebo control group. If the patient is not seeking treatment, however, participation in a placebo controlled trial would be ethical.

Rothman concluded his critique of placebo controls when safe and effective treatments exist by questioning the need for placebos on strictly scientific grounds. While it might be useful to add a placebo arm as a reference point in a non-inferiority trial, it is not necessary, he says, because the active control could serve as well as a reference. He said that the resolution of uncertainty because of lack of assay sensitivity for the active control should be addressed by conducting large studies in the first place to ensure better precision and better measures of effectiveness in later non-inferiority trials. However, as noted by Temple, assay sensitivity cannot always be achieved by making trials larger.

## Large-scale multi-site trials: ethical and research issues

The issue of the *ethical* use of placebo controls in large-scale clinical trials has been catalyzed by reports in the media and professional journals highly critical of trials sponsored by organizations in industrialized countries, but conducted in developing countries, primarily in sub-Saharan Africa and South-east Asia. Accusations of exploitation of vulnerable populations, inadequate informed consent, and failure to provide standards of care in the host country that are equivalent to the sponsoring country have been voiced.

The centerpiece of Yale University Professor Robert J Levine's presentation[68] was the use of placebo controls in trials in Africa to evaluate whether the short-term use of oral zidovudine would reduce the risk of perinatal transmission of HIV. Trial designers were faced with profound cultural differences and a lack of basic resources which would make it impossible to instigate the standard of care available in the US for the

* There are cases in which the protection of society overrides individual rights, as in the need to impose quarantine or mandatory vaccination in the case of infectious disease.

prevention of perinatal transmission of HIV. Not only is it not the custom for pregnant women in sub-Saharan Africa to seek early prenatal care, Levine observed, but there are generally no facilities for intravenous infusion of zidovudine during delivery. Thus the testing of a short-term regimen of zidovudine was sought as a practical means of preventing transmission of the AIDS virus, one that would be within reasonable grasp of the host countries, with assistance from international agencies in procuring the drug.

The requirement in the *Declaration of Helsinki* that new methods should only be tested against "the best current" methods regardless of whether these could be made available on a sustained basis in the country where the trial is conducted provides a high absolute standard of protection for trial participants. However, it makes it more difficult for developing countries to obtain clinical trial evidence to improve their standard of care. Instead of a trial comparing a new treatment to the best available in the country where the trial is conducted, the new treatment would need to be compared to the best available anywhere in the world, even if locally unfeasible and unavailable. Rather than follow the absolute standards of the Helsinki resolution, Levine and investigators designing trials in developing countries have proposed that principles stated in the *International Ethical Guidelines for Biomedical Research Involving Human Subjects* be followed.* These guidelines state that in conducting research in a developing country an agency from an industrialized country must be responsive to the health needs and priorities of the host country. In addition, the principles require that any product developed in the research be made reasonably available to the host country citizens. These precepts have been further articulated into an ethical standard called the "highest attainable and sustainable therapeutic method." Put simply, this means that a level of therapy be provided to subjects in a trial that can be practically handled in the host country and that can be maintained after cessation of the trial and withdrawal of sponsor resources. As one proponent notes, such a standard "tends to facilitate the efforts of resource-poor countries to develop needed therapies and prevention methods that are within financial reach".

## Placebo-control vs non-blinding (open-label) designs in large clinical effectiveness trials

Once clinical trials have been scaled up to embody large numbers of patients studied at a variety of national and/or international sites, the problems of research design and analysis, not to mention the cost of the trial, increase dramatically. Robert M. Califf of Duke University[66] commented that considering that such trials are growing in number and that they are often aimed at improving treatments for leading causes of

* This document was prepared by the Council of International Organizations of Medical Sciences in collaboration with the World Health Organization.

Table 1.1 Criteria for use of placebo in large clinical effectiveness trials.

| Less likely to use placebo | Criteria | More likely to use placebo |
|---|---|---|
| Objective, particularly mortality | Type of endpoint | Subjective |
| Different ancillary therapy required in each arm of trial | Medical and behavioral context | No interactions with other complex regimens |
| No concerns about strong investigator preference | – | Charged environment regarding treatment |
| Alternative treatment already proven effective | Ethical context | No proven effective treatment for the disease |
| Placebo use would make study too expensive | Cost to the study | Intolerable |
| Allow alternative design | Attitude of regulator | Placebo required |

death and disability, it is surprising that there has been so little research on the value of using placebo controls. Under what conditions are placebo controls likely to improve the odds of obtaining definitive results? When can they be waived? To what extent do placebos affect objective endpoints? It has been argued that the use of independent and blinded observers in trials with objective, irreversible endpoints such as a stroke, may make placebo controls unnecessary. This would have the advantage of greatly reducing trial costs, while allowing for an increase in the size of the study population for statistical analysis. On the other hand, it is not known, and would be worth studying to what degree placebo effects extend beyond subjective endpoints, such as reports of reduced angina pain in a study of acute coronary syndromes, to influence objectively measured endpoints, such as mortality or evidence of a non-fatal myocardial infarction (see Table 1.1). The work of the International Conference on Harmonization has been helpful in examining methodological issues of trial design, issuing guidelines allowing greater flexibility in the construction of control groups.[69]

He presented a number of case studies in coronary disease discussing endpoints, cost, the role of regulators, and how these variables affect decision-making with regard to the use of placebos. Randomized open-label designs are being increasingly used to compare active treatments requiring different administration schedules or to evaluate the effectiveness of adding a supplement to standard therapy. Traditionally, such trials would have used a "double blind, double dummy" design in which each patient receives a matching placebo for each active treatment, so that the patient receives four treatments (each active treatment and its placebo), a procedure that allows masking of each assigned treatment. The comparison would be between the two active treatments or between those who did or did not receive the supplement to standard therapy. This use of placebo to mask assignments is still considered necessary to avoid observer bias when the outcome measures involve either patient-reported outcomes or investigator judgments. However, in many clinical effectiveness trials, the outcome measures are counts of objective endpoints (for example, myocardial infarctions, fractures) whose classification is made by an independent expert panel blinded to therapy. In such settings the potential for observer bias may be minimal and the added cost and complexity of a double blind placebo control may not be justifiable, especially since this can easily turn a five million dollar trial into a fifteen million dollar trial. The added value of blinding needs to be judged against its added cost and complexity. Often the cost savings from a randomized open-label design can be used to greatly increase study size, yielding power to detect small, yet clinically important improvements in effectiveness.

The debate over use of placebo in such settings is typically not about ethics, since placebo would not be used in place of standard therapy. Rather the debate is over validity, study size, power to detect clinically important differences, and cost. Obviously, the decision about when treatment group blinding with placebo is necessary for validity would depend on how much observer bias could enter into the assessment of endpoints. Any suspicion about the integrity of the random allocation to treatment, any element of judgment in the selection of potential endpoints presented to the independent adjudication committee or any between-group difference in the evaluation or treatment of patients would require masking and placebo. Yet these issues can and have been faced with large effectiveness trials including the Second International Study of Infarct Survival (ISIS-2), which was a randomized trial of intravenous streptokinase, oral aspirin, both, or neither in cases of suspected acute myocardial infarction[70] and the Global Use of Strategies to Open Occluded Coronary Arteries, a comparison of reteplase with alteplase for acute myocardial infarction (GUSTO III).[71] So the use of very large randomized, open-label trials – without placebo – may come into wider use to compare small but clinically important differences in effectiveness between active therapies.

## Conclusion

The rich and varied perspectives on the placebo presented at the conference indicate a work in progress, one that resonates with changes in American society and in the culture of medicine. The idea that there could be a physiological basis for an inert pill, sham procedure, or symbolic meaning to allay a patient's symptoms or cure illness was all but unthinkable in orthodox medicine 50 years ago. In the interim, advances in genetics and molecular biology and in the behavioral and social sciences, in concert with ever-improving analytic and imaging techniques, are providing clues to the interactions between mind and body that operate in response to illness and therapy. By recasting placebo responses in terms of the meanings patients and providers ascribe to elements of their encounters, reasonable hypotheses can be constructed and experiments conducted to elucidate placebo phenomena. Not only can such research shed light on mediating factors such as conditioning, suggestion, and expectancy, but underlying cell and molecular mechanisms may be revealed. This is already happening in pain research where placebo analgesia and its reversal by selected antagonist molecules has been shown to be linked to specific pain-modulating pathways. Research on nervous–endocrine–immune system interactions can be expected to yield additional explanatory mechanisms.

The new look at the placebo has had repercussions in the conduct and analysis of clinical trials. The advent of randomized double blind placebo controlled clinical trials in the 1930s, when few effective drugs were available, marked the beginning of the movement to establish evidence-based medicine. The placebo control was deemed essential to establish a baseline by which to judge the worth of the experimental intervention. Subsequently, thousands of medications have come on the market, raising ethical questions about the necessity of placebo controls in studies where an effective treatment already exists. Such trials were expressly proscribed in the October 2000 revision of the World Medical Association's *Declaration of Helsinki*. Both sides of these controversial issues were addressed at the conference, with those arguing for the necessity for placebo controls invoking the need for assay sensitivity, but also indicating exceptions and refinements in design to mitigate against any harm to placebo subjects. Arguments on the issue of differing standards of care in trials conducted in developing countries appropriately contrasted an ideal world with present reality. Public health experts and clinical researchers at the conference emphasized that one must be pragmatic about the applications of ethical guidelines and should explicitly state that any biomedical research conducted in a host country should be aimed at addressing the priority health needs of that country. Some argued further that any product forthcoming from the research should be made available in the form of an attainable and sustainable therapy. Without this qualification, they argue that ethical principles that are held to be universal would seem to have little relevance for people living in poverty in the developing world. Others, however, noted that translating these ideals into practice remains a formidable challenge. As one speaker noted, "…the ethical issues are nowhere near resolved and … the urgent need to arrive at answers with respect to epidemics such as that of HIV-AIDS leads many to worry about ethical research standards they take to obstruct and impede progress".

The conference made clear that there are no easy answers to a number of ethical issues in medical practice and research. Rather, it provided a forum for the open discussion of differences, pointing to the urgency to address these issues, both in the conduct of clinical research and in the application of research findings to benefit all peoples of the world.

## Research agenda summary

Following the formal presentations at the conference, participants met in six breakout groups to develop research recommendations, which are presented in detail in Section 5 of this volume. In brief, the groups proposed:

**To advance the *science of placebo effects* research is needed to:**

- elucidate the role of psychosocial moderators of placebo effects (for example, qualities of the contextual setting, and characteristics of patient–provider interactions that enhance or diminish beneficial effects on health and wellbeing). Such research should include studies of classical conditioning and the role of suggestion/expectancy and other cognitive, emotional, and perceptual features of the therapeutic encounter. It should also examine meaning and related socio-cultural aspects of interpersonal relationships, using ethnographic studies
- identify the biological mechanisms/pathways/molecules/genes through which placebo effects occur
- develop investigational tools (for example, neuroimaging, genomic and proteomic analyses, animal models) to facilitate delineation of physiological pathways associated with placebo effects
- develop conceptual and research tools that enable the integration of biological, psychological, and social findings into the study of mechanisms of mind-body effects.

In all of these research efforts attention should be paid to principles of research design which would permit distinguishing actual biological effects of placebo from measurement artifacts, such as the natural history of disease, spontaneous remission, patient or investigator bias, and regression to the mean.

**To enhance *applications of placebo effects in clinical practice* research should determine:**

- the means of optimizing positive placebo effects and minimizing nocebo effects in clinical practice
- the potential for self-induced placebo effects
- characteristics of providers in relation to the placebo process and responses
- the dynamics of patient–provider interactions, including the roles each plays and the various props, costumes, communications, and settings, and how these affect placebo responses
- barriers to the eliciting of placebo effects.

**To address issues on the *use of placebos in clinical trials of drugs, procedural, and behavioral interventions*, research is needed to:**

- evaluate the empirical underpinnings of the ethical principles in the use of placebos in clinical trials, using both ethnography and quantitative methods
- conduct analyses of the attitudes and beliefs of trial subjects and characteristics that distinguish trial participants from non-participants
- assess attitudes and beliefs of clinicians and other research investigators
- develop new methods or new applications of existing methods of study design and analysis to address ethical and statistical issues of both placebo controlled and active trials
- study the process of informed consent and the participation of vulnerable populations such as children, in clinical trials.

## References

1 Hrobjartsson A, Gotzsche PC. Is the placebo powerless? An analysis of clinical trials comparing placebo with no treatment. *N Engl J Med* 2001;**344**:1594–602.
2 Harrington A. "Seeing" the placebo effect: historical legacies and present opportunities. This volume, chapter 2.
3 Moerman DE. Explanatory mechanisms for placebo effects: cultural influences and the meaning response. This volume, chapter 4.
4 Blackell B, Bloomfield SS, Buncher CR. Demonstration to medical students of placebo responses and non-drug factors. *Lancet* 1972;**1**(763):1279–82.
5 Branthwaite A, Cooper P. Analgesic effects of branding in treatment of headaches. *BMJ (Clin Res Ed)* 1981;**282**(6276):1576–8.
6 Desharmais R, Jobin J, Cote C, Levesque L, Godin G. Aerobic exercise and the placebo effect: a controlled study. *Psychosom Med* 1993;**55**:149–54.
7 Phillips DP, Ruth TE, Wagner LM. Psychology and survival. *Lancet* 1993;**342**(8880):112–15.
8 Gracely RH, Dubner R, Deeter WR, Wolskee PJ. Clinicians' expectations influence placebo analgesia. *Lancet* 1985;**1**:43.
9 Beecher HK. The powerful placebo. *JAMA* 1955;**159**:1602–6.
10 Moerman DE. Cultural variations in the placebo effect: ulcers, anxiety, and blood pressure. *Med Anthropol Q* 2000;**14**:1–22.
11 Bootzin RR, Caspi O. Explanatory mechanisms for placebo effects: cognition, personality, and social learning. This volume, chapter 5.
12 Shapiro AK, Shapiro, E. *The powerful placebo. From ancient priest to modern physician.* Baltimore, Maryland: The Johns Hopkins University Press 1997:39–40.
13 Thomas KB. The placebo in general practice. *Lancet* 1994:**344**:1066–7.
14 Barfod TS. Placebo therapy in dermatology. *Clin Dermatol* 1999;**17**:69–76.
15 Evans FJ. The placebo response in pain reduction. In: Bonica JJ, ed. *Advances in Neurology 1974; Pain*. New York: Raven Press, 1974:289–96.
16 Benson H, Epstein MD. The placebo effect: a neglected asset in the care of patients. *JAMA* 1975;**232**:1225–7.
17 Thomas KB. General practice consultations: is there any point in being positive? *BMJ* 1987;**294**:1200–2.
18 Bernstein CN. Placebos in medicine. *Semin Gastrointest Dis* 1999;**10**:3–7.
19 Andrews G, Harvey R. Does psychotherapy benefit neurotic patients?: a reanalysis of the Smith, Glass, and Miller data. *Arch Gen Psychiatry* 1981;**38**:1203–8.
20 Miller WR, Brown JM, Simpson TL, *et al.* What works? A methodological analysis of the alcohol treatment outcome literature. In: Hester RK, Miller WR, eds. *Handbooks of alcoholism treatment approaches: Effective alternatives, 2nd ed.* Boston: Allyn & Bacon 1995, pp 12–44.

21 Miller WR, Andrews NR, Wilbourne P, Bennett ME. A wealth of alternatives: effective treatments for alcohol problems. In: Miller WR, Heather N, eds. *Treating Addictive Behaviors, 2nd ed.* New York: Plenum Press 1998, pp 203–16.
22 Frank JD. Therapeutic components shared by all psychotherapies. In: Hawey JH, Parks MA, eds. *Psychotherapy Research and Behavior Change.* Washington DC: American Psychological Association 1981, pp 9–37.
23 Kirsch I, Weixel LJ. Double blind versus deceptive administration of a placebo. *Biomedical Therapy* 1998;**XVI**(3):242–6.
24 Kirsch I, Sapirstein G. Listening to Prozac but hearing placebo: a meta-analysis of antidepressant medication. In: Kirsch I, ed. *How Expectancies Shape Experience.* Washington: American Psychological Association 1999, pp 303–20.
25 Siegel S. Explanatory mechanisms for placebo effects: Pavlovian conditioning. This volume, chapter 6.
26 Collins KH, Tatum AL. A conditioned reflex established by chronic morphine poisoning. *Am J Physiol* 1925;**74**:14–15.
27 Pavlov IP. *Conditioned Reflexes* (Anrep GV, trans.). London: Oxford University Press, 1927.
28 Alarie Y. Irritating properties of airborne materials to the upper respiratory tract. *Arch Environ Health* 1966;**13**:433–49.
29 Wood RJ, Coleman JB. Behavioral evaluation of the irritant properties of formaldehyde. *Toxicol Appl Pharmacol* 1995;**130**:67–72.
30 Swyghuizen-Doorenbos A, Roehrs TA, Lipschutz L, Timms V, Roth T. Effects of caffeine on alertness. *Psychopharmacology* 1990;**100**:36–9.
31 Giang DW, Goodman AD, Schiffer RB, *et al.* Conditioning of cyclophosphamide-induced leukopenia in humans. *Neuropsychiatry* 1996;**8**:194–201.
32 Ader R, Cohen N. Behaviorally conditioned immunosuppression and murine systemic lupus erythematosus. *Science* 1982;**8**:379–94.
33 Pihl RO, Altman J. An experimental analysis of the placebo effect. *J Clin Pharmacol* 1971;**11**:91–5.
34 Siegel S. Conditioning of insulin-induced glycemia. *J Comp Physiol Psychol* 1972;**78**:233–41.
35 Siegel S. Conditioning insulin effects. *J Comp Physiol Psychol* 1975;**89**:189–99.
36 Woods SC, Shogren Jr RE. Glycemic responses following conditioning with different doses of insulin in rats. *J Comp Physiol Psychol* 1972;**81**:220–5.
37 Grisel JE, Wiertelak EP, Watkins LR, Maier SF. Route of morphine administration modulates conditioned analgesic tolerance and hyperalgesia. *Pharmacol Biochem Behav* 1994;**49**:1029–35.
38 Kim JA, Siegel S, Patenall VRA. Drug-onset cues as signals: intra-administration associations and tolerance. *J Exp Psychol: Anim Behav Process* 1999;**25**:491–504.
39 Krank MD. Conditioned hyperalgesia depends on the pain sensitivity measure. *Behav Neurosci* 1987;**101**:854–7.
40 Siegel S. Evidence from rats that morphine tolerance is a learned response. *J Comp Physiol Psychol* 1975;**89**:498–506.
41 Obál F. The fundamentals of the central nervous control of vegetative homeostasis. *Acta Physiol Acad Sci Hung* 1966;**30**:15–29.
42 Eskandari F, Sternberg EM. Neuroendocrine mediators of placebo effects on immunity. This volume, chapter 8.
43 Price DD, Soerensen LV. Endogenous opioid and non-opioid pathways as mediators of placebo analgesia. This volume, chapter 9.
44 Watkins LR, Cobelli DA, Mayer DJ. Opiate vs non-opiate footshock induced analgesia (FSIA): descending and intraspinal components. *Brain Res* 1982;**245**:97–106.
45 Voudouris NJ, Peck CL, Coleman G. Conditioned placebo responses. *J Per Soc Psychol* 1985;**48**:47–53.
46 Voudouris NJ, Peck CL, Coleman G. Conditioned response models of placebo phenomena: further support. *Pain* 1989;**38**:109–16.
47 Montgomery GH, Kirsch I. Classical conditioning and the placebo effect. *Pain* 1997;**72**: 107–13.
48 Amanzio M, Benedetti F. Neuropharmacological dissection of placebo analgesia: expectation-activated opioid systems versus conditioning-activated specific subsystems. *J Neurosci* 1999;**19**:484–94.
49 Price DD, Milling LS, Kirsch I, Duff A, Montgomery GH, Nicholls SS. An analysis of factors that contribute to the magnitude of placebo analgesia in an experimental paradigm. *Pain* 1999;**83**:147–56.

50 Kleinman A. *Patients and Healers in the Context of Culture*. Berkeley and Los Angeles: University of California Press 1980, pp 50–3.
51 Kleinman A, Becker A. "Sociosomatics": The contributions of anthropology to psychosomatic medicine. *Psychosom Med* 1998;**60**(4):389–93.
52 Davis CE, Regression to the mean or placebo effect? This volume, chapter 7.
53 McDonald CJ, Mazzuca SA, McCabe GP. How much of the placebo 'effect' is really statistical regression? *Stat Med* 1983;**2**:417–27.
54 Bok S. Ethical issues in use of placebo in medical practice and clinical trials. This volume, chapter 3.
55 Principles of Medical Ethics of the American Medical Association; Principle II.
56 Cassidy CM. Social science theory and methods in the study of alternative and complementary medicine. *J Altern Complement Med* 1995;**1**:19–40.
57 Temple RJ. Placebo controlled trials and active controlled trials: ethics and inference. This volume, chapter 10.
58 Pocock SJ. The pros and cons of non-inferiority (equivalence) trials. This volume, chapter 12.
59 Temple RJ, Ellenberg SS. Placebo controlled trials and active-control trials in the evaluation of new treatments. Part 1: Ethical and scientific issues. *Ann Intern Med* 2000; **133**:455–63.
60 Ellenberg SS, Temple R. Placebo controlled trials and active-control trials in the evaluation of new treatments. Part 2: Practical issues and specific cases. *Ann Intern Med* 2000;**133**:464–70.
61 Weijer C. Placebo controlled trials in schizophrenia: Are they ethical? Are they necessary? *Schizophr Res* 1999;**35**(3):211–8, discussion 227–36.
62 Streiner DL. Placebo controlled trials: when are they needed? *Schizophr Res* 1999;**35**(3):201–10.
63 Storosum JG, Elferink AJ, van Zwieten BJ. Schizophrenia: do we really need placebo controlled studies? *Eur Neuropsychopharmacol* 1998;**8**(4):279–86.
64 Khan A, Warner HA, Brown WA. Symptom reduction and suicide risk in patients treated with placebo in antidepressant clinical trials: an analysis of the Food and Drug Administration database. *Arch Gen Psychiatry*. 2000;**57**:311–17.
65 Lavori PW. Placebo control groups in randomized treatment trials: a statistician's perspective. *Biol Psychiatry* 2000;**47**:717–23.
66 Califf RM, Al-Khatib SM. Use of placebo in large-scale, pragmatic trials. This volume, chapter 13.
67 Rothman KJ, Michels KB. When is it appropriate to use a placebo arm in a trial? This volume, chapter 11.
68 Levine RJ. Placebo controls in clinical trials of new therapies for conditions for which there are known effective treatments. This volume, chapter 14.
69 Dixon JR Jr. The International Conference on Harmonization good clinical practice guideline. *Qual Assur* 1998;**6**:65–74.
70 ISIS-2 (Second International Study of Infarct Survival) Collaborative Group. Randomised trial of intravenous streptokinase, oral aspirin, both, or neither among 17 187 cases of suspected acute myocardial infarction: ISIS-2. *Lancet* 1988;**2**:349–60.
71 The Global Use of Strategies to Open Occluded Coronary Arteries (GUSTO III) Investigators. A comparison of reteplase with alteplase for acute myocardial infarction *N Engl J Med* 1997;**333**:1118–23.

# *Section 1:* Historical and ethical perspectives

# 2: "Seeing" the placebo effect: historical legacies and present opportunities

ANNE HARRINGTON


## Summary

Introduction: undigested perspectives

Reviewing legacies

- The legacy of "seeing" the placebo effect as sham
- The legacy of "seeing" the placebo effect as confound

"Seeing" the placebo effect as real and informative: an historian's perspective

- Interrogating fifty years of stockpiled data
- The idea of "sightings", or not confusing the finger with the moon
- Distinguishing maps from territory

A call to a radical encounter with one's legacies


## Introduction: undigested perspectives

In January 2000, a cover headline of the *New York Times Magazine* declared: "Astonishing Medical Fact: Placebos Work! So Why Not Use Them as Medicine?".[1] Six months later, the following email was forwarded to me from the public relations office of Harvard University Press, (I have deleted the author's name to protect his privacy):

> My name is...., I live in Cali, Colombia. A few days ago I listened about placebo effect. My father has cancer, and I believe a placebo can help him.
>
> I need to know where I can get the sugars pills or saline injections, and how I must to give him.
>
> My father's doctors have said that his cancer is very bad, and it's so difficult to treat. He has been following a treatment since 8 years, but he always fall ill again. I think the placebo effect is his last hope.
>
> If you can help me, I'll be grateful all my life.

We are at a moment in our cultural history when our faith in the placebo effect would seem to be at an all time high. Never have we come as close as we seem to be today to blurring the distinction between whatever we think this phenomenon is and the *materia medica* – the pills, syrups and injections – of medicine. When not only prominent US newspapers but lay people in the far-western corners of South America are asking us to add sugar pills to the arsenal of interventions doctors include in their archetypal black bag, it is a good bet that something culturally significant is afoot.

A lot of the current enthusiasm for this idea of "placebos as medicine" comes within the context of a belief that we may now be in a position to elucidate mechanisms underlying the placebo effect within the framework of increasingly sophisticated understandings of brain–endocrine–immune interactions. From this perspective, integrating the placebo effect into our workaday lives may in principle seem relatively straightforward – we figure out the mechanisms, and we take advantage of the practical applications. I want to suggest, however, that we might be more conflicted, less sure-footed in our views on how to move forward on harnessing the healing potential in sugar pills than we might think. Consider this.

- In the current rhetorical wars between mainstream and so-called alternative medicine, reference to "the placebo effect" is not seen as a way of celebrating the mind–body connection in all its power, but rather works as an accusation: a kiss of death for any therapy impugned by this effect. To say that homeopathy (for example) gains its efficacy through the placebo effect is to say that it does not "really" work at all – that it is effectively a sham treatment. Why this understanding?
- We are participating in a Trans-Division conference on the therapeutic potential of the placebo effect at the National Institutes of Health. Yet one of the larger divisions of the NIH, the National Institute of Allergy and Infectious Diseases, maintains a "clinical trials recruitment" website that explains that "a placebo is an inactive pill, liquid, or powder that *has no treatment value*" (italics added), and is used in clinical trials merely as a comparative reference point for assessing the efficacy of an experimental treatment.[2] Clearly, not everyone in the NIH sees the placebo effect as even in principle capable of functioning as

therapy. Why this difference among us, even within the same institution?

## Reviewing legacies

The argument of this chapter is rather simple. It is that history can help us see our way through to some answers to these questions. It can help because at least some of the tensions we see in the present have their sources in different agendas in the past that have not always collaborated or even agreed on common starting premises. Given this, the conclusion to be drawn is also rather simple: it would be better for all our efforts if our different inherited frames of reference could be made visible and explicit, rather than not. Only then might we (1) start to get clearer on the high stakes involved in our effort now to re-imagine the placebo effect as a therapeutic intervention, and (2) move forward in a more self-conscious way than we might otherwise have done.

### The legacy of seeing the placebo effect as sham

To this end, I begin with an historical narrative that has been largely forgotten in its details by the medical profession, but that left behind a legacy of shame and scandal from which medical practice and theorizing has yet to recover. This is a narrative that unfolded in Paris in the late 19th century, and features the leading neurologist of Europe at that time, Jean Martin Charcot (1825–1893). Charcot was a neurologist who had achieved international fame for his identification and analysis of various neurological disorders (for example, multiple sclerosis and tabetic arthropathy). In the 1870s, he turned his sights on a particularly elusive nervous disorder that was very common in the great hospitals of Paris. This disorder was called hysteria. It seemed that hysteria could really use the disciplining, discerning eye and mind of a great medical scientist like Charcot. For generations, its protean symptoms – convulsions, paralyses, tunnel vision, color blindness, patches of anesthesia, incessant coughing, tics, and feelings of choking – had been the frustration of clinicians. These symptoms had the infuriating tendency to shift around the body and replace one another. In addition, the disorder was often marked by periodic "crises" in which patients would convulse and hallucinate.

For most 19th century neurologists, this profile of symptoms, notwithstanding their elusiveness, made hysteria look like a brain disorder of some sort, perhaps related to epilepsy. Charcot's idea was to take the same analytic approach that had brought him such success with other brain disorders, and use it now to penetrate behind the baroque and bewildering world of hysteria's symptomatology. He would make hysteria lie down and reveal its secrets. And, to everyone's amazement, in his hands, it suddenly did. Underlying patterns for the permanent symptoms began to emerge. The convulsive crises associated with the disorder turned out to be far less chaotic than people had previously thought, unfolding with complete predictability in four stages that – as he put it – followed one another with "the regularity of a mechanism". In fact, the fits were so reliably linked to underlying mechanism that the doctors in Charcot's hospital noted that they could bring one on by squeezing particularly sensitive spots near the ovaries of these patients, called "hysterogenic" zones.

All of this was pursued within a frame of reference that involved little, if any attention to these women's subjective experiences: their memories and feelings, i.e., things that we today have learned to wonder about. For Charcot, progress in understanding hysteria would come by first elucidating its objective symptoms. This was where the foundations of clinical medicine lay, this is where you knew you would not be led astray.[3] In the Salpêtrière, Charcot's assistants were set to work sketching extensive pictures of the hysterics in action. Soon after, a photograph studio was installed in the hospital (a major innovation at the time) and photographic records of the patients were made. People said that the camera was as crucial to the study of hysteria as the microscope had been to the study of histology. The camera, it was said, did not lie, and therefore it provided the evidence Charcot wanted and needed to prove – as he put it – that the laws of hysteria which he had discovered were "valid for all countries, all times, all races", and "consequently universal".

Except he had not and they were not. In fact, as things unfolded, this turned out to be a physiology whose laws, far from being "universal", were in the end so local that they basically only unfolded inside the walls of Charcot's Salpêtrière. It turned out that the "subjective experiences" of Charcot's patients had had the upper hand after all, and had hoodwinked the great master by masquerading themselves as "objective" displays of universal significance. Using hypnosis (which Charcot had also helped rehabilitate during this time), a rival of Charcot, a man named Hippolyte Bernheim, showed that one could reproduce all the symptoms of hysteria, and one could also change them, or make them disappear. All the symptoms of hysteria, he said, were not due to anything "real" – that is, grounded in biology – but were a kind of sham: nothing more than the effects of a psychological process he called "suggestion".[4]

The idea of "suggestion" murdered Charcot's neurobiological program. Charcot became a growing target of ridicule, someone who was now perceived as having been duped by his own patients, and done in by his own psychological naiveté. His disciples, looking to rescue their own careers, scattered. The final blow came in 1901 when one of Charcot's previously most loyal students, Joseph Babinski, read a terse paper on hysteria before the Neurological Society of Paris. The paper was a *mea culpa* both on behalf of himself and of the whole approach of the school he had once defended: they had been wrong, he said, hysteria had nothing to do with organic dysfunctions of brain and biology. It was a "made-up" entity, nothing more than the sum total of symptoms that could be created by suggestion and removed by suggestion. A biologically-oriented medicine need pay no more attention to it.*[5]

The consequences of this moment, certainly in terms of our subsequent ability to bring the placebo effect into focus for ourselves, were momentous. It led to the conclusion that bodily symptoms that were "created" by the suggestive power of the mind were something akin to a physiological lie. It led to the suspicion that patients whose symptoms responded to interventions of this sort were not suffering from anything that could be considered a real disease. An irony in all this is that Bernheim's work on suggestion was not intended by him simply as a debunking project. He also offered it as a foundation for a new kind of therapeutics in medicine, that he called "suggestive therapeutics".[4] In the framework of that program, he increasingly emphasized that the effects of suggestion might include modifications in somatic processes associated with "real" diseases, i.e., not just diseases that were "hysterical" in origin. His school also increasingly emphasized that a patient did not inevitably have to be hypnotized for suggestion to work its effects: suggestion could be effective when it was just practiced in the context of a waking interaction between a doctor and a patient.

But this other face of Bernheim's program failed to take hold in the institutionalized memory of medicine the way that Charcot's disgrace would. While there were some efforts here and there to develop the ideas of suggestive therapeutics, these ideas found their real impact, not so much in professional medical practice, but more in various lay "mind cure" movements of the time: Christian Science, spearheaded by Mary Baker Eddy, the New Thought movements of the early decades of the century, the self-help "power of positive thinking" teachings of charismatics like Norman Vincent Peale, and so on.[6,7] In mainstream medicine, it was mostly a different story: the private practice offices and hospitals saw rather fewer examples of the dramatic displays of hysteria that had been the hallmark of Charcot's work. However, a tendency to dismiss a certain kind of patient as "hysterical" (or "neurotic" or "hypochondriacal") became increasingly widespread. "Hysterical" patients were now less individuals suffering from a series of puzzling but definite physical disabilities, and more individuals whose physical symptoms were vague, implausible, or elusive of both diagnosis and treatment. Doctors, wiser now to the gullible ways of the suggestible mind than before, thus tended to see these symptoms as "really"

* Babinski in fact went so far as to propose that medicine abandon the word "hysteria" to describe the syndrome in question, and instead to adopt a new term that would canonize a much narrower understanding: "pithiatism." This was a word derived from the Greek word for "persuasion." After some years of deliberation, the Society voted to adopt this new neologism (again, see Babinksi 1909).[5]

psychological; an interpretation which now had come to mean that they were basically a kind of sham.

At the same time, such patients with their sham symptoms were insistent in demanding satisfaction from their doctors. And many doctors found a way to mollify them: they gave them sham pills, pills whose efficacy, such as it was, was presumed to lie (drawing on the lessons of the 19th century) in "the power of suggestion". If such patients responded, this was sometimes seen as confirmation that the doctor had been right; there had been nothing "really" wrong. Incurable patients also sometimes came in for such ministrations, though the motives then were rather different. Here it was not that there was nothing "really" wrong, but rather that too much was wrong, and there was nothing more "really" that the doctor could do: "The human mind is still open to suggestion, even in these modern and disillusioned days. The sympathetic physician will want to use every help for these pathetic patients and if the placebo can help, he will not neglect it. It cannot harm and may comfort and avoid the too quick extinction of opiate efficacy".[8]

As we see above, by the 1940s, the general word used for these little packages of unreality was "placebo." Widely practiced to either strategic or compassionate ends, placebos were still not something that most doctors spent a great deal of time discussing in public forums.* Still, their differentiated use was generally accepted as part of the craft knowledge of the profession – a necessary bit of "humble humbug", as one frequently quoted editorial from the 1950s put it.[10,11,12,13]

## The legacy of seeing the placebo effect as confound

Then, by the mid-1950s, we see something happening within medicine that would have the effect of changing, at least in part, how people would "see" the placebo effect. The 1930s and 1940s had seen the development of new sulfa drugs capable of arresting the growth of bacteria; this was then followed by one of the great triumphs of medical science in the first half of the century: the discovery and development of the so-called

* Thus Pepper (1945) noted the almost total silence in the literature of his time on the topic. Clearly this silence was not due simply to lack of interest in the placebo effect, but to ambivalence about it. Most people remembered that people such as medical doyen Richard Cabot had early on pointed to the relationship between placebo giving and the deceptions of the so-called "patent medicine" salesmen that the American medical profession had recently fought to close down. For Cabot, placebo giving was "quackery", and had to be bad for the profession.

Parenthetically, the medical profession was not as successful as it had expected to be in its campaign to close down the patent medicine industry; and, ironically enough, one of the reasons offered for this was that the medicines evoked such a placebogenic effect in patients. Even after federal legislation required open labeling of ingredients and forbade false promises, people remained loyal to the products that they "knew" worked.[9]

antibiotics, with penicillin of course leading the way in 1941. It was becoming clear that medicine had some weapons in its arsenal that could pack a therapeutic punch of an order that had never been seen before. It was also clear to people of the time that the rational methodologies of the laboratory, not the quaint arts of the clinic, were providing these new weapons. Large profits were now in play as well. The stakes were high all around.

Within this new frame of concern, the placebo effect began to look like a potentially serious hindrance to the rational progress of medicine. These developments have been ably analyzed by Ted Kaptchuk,[10,14] whose argument I partly follow here. Kaptchuk sees the 1955 paper by Henry Beecher, "The Powerful Placebo"[15] as marking a sea change in medicine's attitude towards the placebo effect.* Beecher's paper, perhaps the most influential in the modern history of research on the placebo effect, had several goals. On the one hand, it wanted to demonstrate what its title said: that the placebo effect was powerful – and pervasive. Using recently-developed meta-analytic statistical methods, Beecher reviewed patient responses to placebo medications across 15 clinical trials. He claimed that roughly one third showed a therapeutic response to a dummy treatment (this idea of there being a consistent one third patient response to placebo medications would later be challenged, and the accuracy of Beecher's own reading of the data from these other studies would later be criticized, but nevertheless the idea has persisted into our own time). In making this claim for pervasiveness, Beecher was also very definite that earlier generations had been wrong to see the placebo effect as merely a psychological prop. New research was showing that the placebo effect was a phenomenon that could produce objectively measurable changes in a patient's physiology – some of which rivaled the effects of the active agent against which a placebo was being compared.

This took Beecher to the second goal of his paper. Because the placebo effect was so powerful, he argued, medicine had to protect itself against its obfuscating effects. The way for it to do this was by systematically adopting the newly-developing, randomized, placebo controlled clinical trials methodology. After all, if certain patients could have a powerful reaction to a sham pill, there was also a chance that they would respond to the merely symbolic or suggestive powers of a treatment that was being tested for its specific efficacy. By requiring all patients to be randomized

* Even as Kaptchuk rightly draws our attention to a new era in thinking about the placebo effect, the sea change he identifies was not monolithic. One can also track a further development into the 1960s and beyond of the view of placebo-giving as part of the art of medicine, the point being that this art was also not wholly supplanted by the rise of a more laboratory-based medical science.[16] And of course the ongoing tendency to use references to the placebo effect as a means of debunking unproven therapies also traces its roots to this earlier understanding of that effect.

into an experimental treatment group and a placebo control group, you would then have, on average, an even distribution of "placebo reactors" in both groups. Any hidden placebo effects operating in an active treatment arm could then be unmasked by measuring the magnitude of the effect in the placebo control arm – and could then be subtracted from your active treatment data. As one of Beecher's colleagues, Louis Lasagna, put it: "... the higher the incidence of placebo responses, the greater the dilution of the desired data ...".[17] It was crucial, then, to use a control group to reclaim the desired data – the data on specific efficacy – in as undiluted or pure form as possible.

The eventual enshrining of the randomized, placebo-control trial as the methodological "gold standard" of clinical research is of course well known, and is seen as one of the great accomplishments of medicine in the second half of the 20th century. Certainly, there is much about it that has been enormously productive and important. That said, there is also something problematic about this "powerful placebo" that was enshrined along with this new method, something that is worth noticing. The placebo had been identified as physiologically potent, yet apparently this was a physiology that worked a bit like oil on water; a kind of second-order physiology that floated on top of the physiological changes associated with the active treatment, without ever dissolving into or modulating them. If things were otherwise, if the physiological processes triggered by a placebo effect could actually modulate the physiological processes triggered by an active treatment, then you could not use the placebo effect seen in a control group as a necessary or reliable guide to assessing the nature of the placebo effect in the active treatment group. This is because, in the one case, you would have a biological treatment that has been modulated in some unclear fashion by a placebo effect, and in the other case you would have a placebo effect working on its own.

So this two-tiered vision of physiology was necessary to the logic of placebo controlled trials, but even at the time, there were some hints in the literature that it was problematic. In the 1950s, for example, Stewart Wolf's work on the "pharmacology of placebos" showed that if you gave patients a known active drug but misled them about what they were taking, the effects of the false belief could sometimes countermand the effects of the pharmacological agent itself (for example, Wolf deceptively – and successfully – gave ipecac to patients to cure their nausea). Wolf also argued that emotional states – anger, hostility, resentment – were also capable of measurably modifying the effects of a pharmaceutical agent like atropine on the motor and secretory activities of the stomach or colon. In short, his work suggested that the physiological processes associated with a placebo effect did have the capacity to subdue, divert, and otherwise alter the direct action of the somatic treatment in question.[18]

Maybe cases in which a placebo effect modified the pharmacology of a drug were rare; maybe they depended on the disease, the drug, the patient, or all three. An alternate history might now have seen a research program in which efforts were undertaken systematically to probe these questions, with a view to assessing the need for one or another modification to the clinical trials methodology in consequence. As things were, research of this sort seems not to have happened. The placebo effect had been named a powerful entity, but an entity that worked as "noise" in the system that masked but did not actually alter the information. An elegant and consistent method for subtracting out the noise had been developed, and most people involved in the heady early years of pharmaceutical research were now keen to get on with things.

There is another important legacy to come out of this way of seeing the placebo effect. It became clear in this time that patient suggestibility or expectation was not the only confound researchers needed to worry about. There was also the possible problem of researcher bias, measurement error, statistical regression to the mean, and spontaneous remission. The placebo control group thus became increasingly seen as a useful all-purpose filter that could "catch" all these confounds, and in the end let through only data about the direct effects of the treatment itself. As Sir Austin Bradford Hill, one of the architects of the modern clinical trial methodology, reviewed matters in 1971:

> The object [of including placebo controls in clinical trials] is two-fold. On the one hand, we hope to be able to discount any bias in patient or doctor in their judgments of the treatment under study. For example, a new treatment is often given a more favorable judgment than its value actually warrants. The effects of suggestibility, anticipation and so on must thus be allowed for. In addition, the placebo effect provides a vital control for the frequency of spontaneous changes that may take place in the course of a disease and are independent of the treatment under study.
>
> In these two ways the placebo aids us to distinguish between (a) the pharmacological effect of the drug and (b) the psychological effects of treatment and the fortuitous changes that can take place in the course of time.[19]

The recognition of these other confounds had at least one important further effect: it seemed to many of the designers of the clinical trial that some of these were likely to be at least as powerful as any effects directly associated with the taking of a sugar pill as such. Indeed, theoretically, these other confounds might be able to explain all the variance one sees in control group data – raising doubt that the placebo effect, understood as some kind of psychobiological response to a dummy pill, really exists. These radical skeptics found confirmation for their suspicions early on, when some studies were published that included, not only an active treatment and a placebo-control arm, but a no-treatment arm as well – and found no differences in magnitude of effect between the no-treatment and the placebo-control arms.[20,21] At this point, an alternative history might have seen the rise of a systematic research program in which efforts were made to isolate a change in a patient's condition caused by taking a placebo from changes caused in other ways. But, again, most people were interested in other things, and that research failed to happen in any systematic way.

## "Seeing" the placebo effect as real and informative: an historian's perspective

Instead we continued to sweep all our dirt into the same bin. We now begin to see that strategy as a problem only because we imagine that there might be some gold in that dirt. My argument so far has been that legacies of earlier ways of seeing the placebo effect – as sham, as noise – still condition our thinking, and will need to be reckoned with before we can move forward with any new reckoning of the positive therapeutic value of the placebo effect on its own terms. To this end, I have not provided a starting definition for the placebo effect, but have preferred instead to allow the implicit and explicit definitions that have existed at different times for this phenomenon to emerge as comprehensible products of specific and changing historical circumstances.*

In moving forward, I want now to suggest that the past offers us, not only challenges, but resources. Resources that may in fact help us begin to rise to our inherited challenges. I see these as consisting of two types: (1) ones that give us fuller insights into the phenomenological nature of the beast we are stalking here; and (2) ones that give us some perspective on the kinds of intellectual principles we will likely want to adopt as a basis for our efforts to domesticate this beast.

### Interrogating fifty years of stockpiled data

To begin with phenomenology: it turns out that some fifty years of clinical trials research has meant that, in spite of medicine's claimed lack of interest in the placebo effect *per se*, the profession has actually stockpiled quite a lot of potentially valuable information about it. This stockpile provides an obvious starting point for our effort to get clear on a series of basic questions. These are some of the things we should want to know.

---

* That said, there are certainly several influential definitions of the placebo effect in the literature: the Shapiros have defined the placebo effect as "any therapy (or that component of therapy) that is intentionally or knowingly used for its nonspecific, psychological, or psychophysiological therapeutic effect, or that is used for a presumed specific therapeutic effect on a patient, symptom, or illness but is without specific activity for the condition being treated".[22]

Philosopher Adolf Grünbaum has offered an influential definition of the placebo effect, that relativizes it to both the target disorder and the treatment type, working with an index of symbols: viz: V = victim; D = target of a disorder, P = treating practitioner; t = specific treatment modality employed; F = characteristic factors of t; C = incidental factors of t; TT = therapeutic theory specifying t as a treatment for D, and all its Fs.[23]

- What is the scope of the placebo effect?
- With what disorders does it work best?
- With what disorders doesn't it work?
- How long does it last?
- When the same disorder is paired with a new treatment, is the placebo effect seen the same or different?
- When the same disorder and treatment are tested in different kinds of groups of patients – women, men, people from different cultural backgrounds – is the placebo effect the same or different?

Of course, if we agree that fifty years of stockpiled data can help us with these questions, we will still have to grapple with the fact that much of the data will be quite "noisy". This is not only because there has been a frequent lack of methodological standardization across studies, but also because – as already discussed – most placebo control data do not let one distinguish between effects caused directly by taking a sugar pill, and effects that may be caused by other factors. Still, questions raised by patterns whose meaning is ambiguous might then act as strategic catalysts for new investigations, and that alone would be a contribution.

**What can placebos do?**
**Range of claims in the literature, 1950s through 1990s**

Inhibition of asthma attacks
Inhibition of hay fever
Suppression of coughs
Alleviation of tension and anxiety
Reduction of pain (cardiac pain, headache, menstrual pain, postoperative pain)
Alteration of blood cell counts
Alleviation of nausea, including sea sickness
Alleviation of insomnia
Alteration of state of alertness
Prevention of colds and alleviation of symptoms
Curing of ulcers
Reduction of fever
Inhibition of symptoms of withdrawal from narcotics
Altering of gastric functions
Controlling of blood sugar level of diabetes
Reduction of enuresis
Lessening of symptoms of arthritis
Disappearance of warts
Reduction in frequency/severity of angina attacks
Inhibition/reversal in growth of malignant tumors

## The idea of "sightings": or not confusing the finger with the moon

At the same time, if we are trying to get as comprehensive a handle as possible on the phenomenology of this beast, we would not want to limit our investigation to what is documented inside the literature of clinical trials. We would like to know something too about placebo effects that occur in various uncontrolled clinical settings, where patients are suffering and the stakes are high. We would like to see how such effects compare to placebo effects that, in more recent years, have been deliberately evoked for experimental purposes, and where the stakes generally are not high (for the subjects at least).*

Finally, we might want to pay some attention to what I call "sightings": phenomena that do not generally get catalogued as examples of the placebo effect, but that we might all agree have "something to do with it". "Sightings", in other words, are fauna that live in the same larger territory of human psychobiological functioning where the placebo effect makes its home as well. By expanding our vision to make room for at least some near-relations of that effect, we may find ourselves inspired to ask questions about that larger territory that otherwise might not have occurred to us.

An historical perspective, again, can help us to understand why it is so important to make this intellectual move. It is an historical fact that our ways of "seeing" the placebo effect have been conditioned by changing agendas within clinical medicine over time. These agendas need to be made a visible part of our consciousness in part so that we are not inappropriately hijacked by them. If clinical medicine has taught us to think of the placebo effect as a response to a sugar pill, our strategy must be to ask what larger human capacity is revealed through this historically specific ritual of ours that classically involves doctors, white coats and pills.

In no particular order, then, here are just a handful of some of the candidate "sightings" that I believe are worthy of our consideration.

### "Sightings" from outside the frame of current placebo research

*A room with a view* – lessons from hospital recovery rooms[25]
*Psychosocial dwarfism* – lessons from children in orphanages[26]
*Postponement of death* – lessons from family holidays[27]
*They cried until they could not see* – lessons from refugees[28]
*Voodoo death* – lessons from the social stigmatization of AIDS[29]

* Our elders in this field made their own suggestions about differences we might find here: "Great wounds with greater significance and presumably greater reaction are made painless by small doses of morphine, whereas fleeting experimental pains with no serious significance are not blocked by morphine … Morphine acts on the significant pain, not on the other …[24]

*A room with a view*

In a simple, elegant study, matched pairs of patients recovering from gall bladder surgery were housed in opposing wings of a hospital. Part of the larger research field of so-called "life enhancing" design, the study gave half (23) of the patients access to a window view overlooking a natural scene, while the other half of the patients were in rooms that looked out at a parking lot with a brick wall. The study found that patients with a natural window view had shorter postoperative hospital stays, made fewer complaints to nurses, tended to have lower scores for minor postsurgical complications, and required significantly weaker painkillers than patients whose window overlooked the brick wall.[25]

*Psychosocial dwarfism*

In the field of nutrition research and child development, observations of orphans in institutional care undertaken in the context of World War II first called attention to the phenomenon of children whose material needs are all met, but who nevertheless are markedly stunted physically. A widely drawn conclusion is that this biological disorder has its ultimate roots in the fact that the children in question lack a stable bond with a loving caretaker. Known technically as reversible somatotropin deficiency, and more informally as psychosocial dwarfism, the standard "treatment" for this syndrome is to remove the child from the toxic environment and put him or her into a home setting that is loving and secure.[26]

*Postponement of death*

A number of epidemiological studies have shown that mortality in coherent groups dips below expected levels just before a symbolically meaningful occasion, such as a major cultural or religious holiday, and then peaks in the weeks just afterward. The finding has been established for a large population of Chinese before the Harvest Moon Festival; and in a large population of Jewish males (but not females) before the Jewish Passover holiday. Other studies have looked at birthdays, particularly among famous people, and shown that there is a statistically significant tendency for such people to survive through a last birthday. And of course the clinical world is filled with anecdotal reports of dying patients who "hang on" until they can be reconciled with an absent child, or complete some other "unfinished business".[27]

*They cried until they could not see*

In California, some 200 cases of so-called psychogenic blindness have been independently reported among Cambodian refugee women who were forced by the Khmer Rouge to witness the torture and slaughter of those close to them, particularly their men-folk. Examination of these women has repeatedly confirmed that there is nothing organically wrong with their visual systems. In the culturally stylized language of the sufferers, it is explained that – having been made to bear witness to the unbearable – they "cried until they could not see".[28]

*Voodoo death*

In the field of "social support", various kinds of data – especially epidemiological – have long suggested that a person's capacity on average both to resist and to rally in the face of illness is connected to that person's perception of connection to loved ones and often the community as a whole.[30]

The phenomenon of "voodoo death", however, offers what is arguably the most extreme case-based window into some of the dynamics of this phenomenon: a rare form of death that is not simply connected with "hexing" but equally or more is linked to the feeling of community isolation that results from feeling "hexed". In the words of the physiologist Walter Bradford Cannon, who wrote a widely-cited paper on this phenomenon in the 1940s: "All people who stand in kinship relation with him withdraw their sustaining support. ... The organization of his social life has collapsed and, no longer a member of a group, he is alone and isolated. The doomed man is in a situation from which the only escape is by death".[31]

Still, for a long time, voodoo death seemed like an exotic phenomenon that we associated with "primitives" and did not see as relevant to "us". In the late 1980s, an article by Sanford Cohen called "Voodoo death, the stress response and AIDS", brought the phenomenon squarely into our own world. Cohen was interested in a range of situations in which death seemed to be hastened by experiences of extreme hopelessness and isolation – for example, displaced refugees trying to come to terms with an isolating and alienating new culture.

Perhaps the most poignant of the evidence that Cohen explored came from the clinical literature on the apparent physiological effects of familial rejection and social stigma associated with AIDS. Cohen told the story of a mother who "learned on the same day that her son was gay and had AIDS. She reacted to this with hostility and openly maintained a prayer vigil outside the intensive care unit, praying that her son would die because of the shame he had caused her. The patient could hear his mother praying. One hour later the patient died, much to the surprise of his physician, since he did not appear to be terminal".[29]

Such "sightings" clearly could be multiplied, but the point by now should be clear. There is an old Chinese saying that speaks of a finger pointing to the moon and then exhorts us to avoid a common human error of confusing the pointer with the target: "Look at the moon, not the finger that points." What we begin to learn when we engage with our historical legacies is that sugar pills are not themselves the point: they are instead themselves pointers to an arena of human functioning bigger than themselves.

And "sightings" are one way for us to begin to "see" how we might ultimately need to map the topography of that bigger arena.

### Distinguishing maps from territory

My last suggestion for how best to see our way forward out of our current undigested ways of thinking about the placebo effect concerns the difference between maps and territories – between a phenomenon we describe and the explanatory models we develop to account for the phenomenon. Again, some stock-taking of the major efforts to explain the placebo effect undertaken over the years should make clear why holding a clear distinction between maps and territory is likely to be so important.

**Dominant explanatory approaches to the placebo effect, 1950 through 2000**

1 Individual differences: the "placebo reactor" idea[32,33]
2 Interpersonal dynamics: the doctor-patient relationship[34,35,36,37]
3 Perceptual filtering: "attribution theory"[38,39]
4 Emotional processes: anxiety reduction/hope[40,41]
5 Brain biochemistry: for example, endorphins[42,43]
6 Conditioning, classical and otherwise[44,45]
7 Expectancy[46]
8 Individual/collective beliefs ("meaning-making")[47,*]

* Moerman D. Meaningful dimensions of medical care. (Paper prepared for the NIH conference on the placebo effect, Nov. 18–20, 2000.)

Looking over these contenders for our intellectual allegiance, as they have developed and jostled against one another over half a century, we may notice several things.

- Even though some approaches are currently more in favor than others, none has wholly disappeared from our radar screen; this suggests that the questions motivating each still have not been fully resolved.
- No consensus has yet emerged that would enthrone one explanatory approach as definitive and encompassing of all the others; this suggests that we have not yet developed a set of common goals for explaining the placebo effect, or clarified our procedures for adjudicating among different approaches.
- There is also no integrating conceptual frame available for distilling and integrating the diverse insights provided by each of the strongest explanatory approaches developed so far; this suggests that we still have to tackle the larger questions this phenomenon raises for us about the

logic of our diverse sciences of human functioning, and the reasons this phenomenon still sits so uneasily at the fault lines of so many different academic disciplines. The map is not the territory, and given how apparently fragmentary our maps still are, we would do well, as we develop our research strategies, to keep interrogating the phenomenon as such: how it looks, when it happens, under what conditions it happens. If theory is at odds with presenting phenomenon, so much the worse for theory.

## A call to a radical encounter with one's legacies

And what happens if we succeed? If we really do our work well? Will we end up where the reporter for the *New York Times Magazine* and my email correspondent from Colombia hoped – with a series of understandings of how to use sugar pills as medicine, alongside aspirins and antibiotics, and a strategy for training future doctors in the scientific basis for their use? One of my chief goals in this paper has been to suggest that there are indeed exciting prospects ahead, but that things are unlikely to be so straightforward.

Let me explain. I carry inside my head a certain image of the recent history of modern medicine. It is an image of a road that had its first stones laid down, somewhat unsystematically, in the middle years of the 19th century. By the early 20th century, large segments of it had been laid to asphalt, and the road was increasingly divided into separate lanes of traffic. The successes of this construction project have been, on many measures, nothing short of fantastic. Nevertheless, all alongside this road that, over the years, has gradually turned into a superhighway, I imagine a series of *trash cans*. These trash cans have been the places where the builders of this road have tossed the bits and pieces of human functioning that could not quite be ground down, that people kept tripping over as they went about their work. These bits of trash have been given a series of names over the years: "*hysteria*", "*suggestion*", "*psychosomatic*", and of course "*the placebo effect*". It is clear that some of the more thoughtful workers over the years have felt uneasy about needing to toss out these things – some even promised themselves that they would go back someday and properly sort through the trash, but by and large, medicine as a whole has not made good on this promise.

The reasons are understandable. A lot of the logic that has helped build our present superhighway of biomedicine has depended on maintaining a boundary between the kinds of things that sit in those trash cans and the kinds of things that have seemed like good material for the road. This means that, if we now want to encourage the placebo effect to "go mainstream", we probably will not just be able to lay down a little side artery off the superhighway and do the project there. We may well have to take a look at the entire superhighway itself, and see ways in which it might now need to be widened, maybe even partially reconstructed. In this way, something that started out as a humble humbug in medicine just could end up being an impetus both for a foundational rethinking of legacies that no longer work, and for the imaginative development of new research programs that have more room for all of what we are as human beings, inside and outside, mind and body, meaning and mechanism.

## References


1 Talbot M. The Placebo Prescription. *New York Times Magazine*, January 9, 2000.
2 *http://www.niaid.nih.gov/clintrials/clinictrial.htm*
3 Janet P. *Psychological Healing: A Historical and Clinical Study*, trans. Eden Paul. London: George Allen & Unwin Ltd/NY: The Macmillan Company, 1925.
4 Bernheim H. *Suggestive Therapeutics; A Treatise on the Nature and Uses of Hypnotism*, trans. CA Herter. New York ; London : GP Putnam's Sons, the Knickerbocker Press, 1890.
5 Babinski J. Démembrement de l'hystérie traditionelle: Pithiatisme. *Semaine médicale* 1909;**29**(1[January 6, 1909]):3–8.
6 James W. *The Varieties of Human Experience: A Study in Human Nature.* NY: Penguin Books, 1987.
7 Parker GT. *Mind-Cure in New England: from the Civil War to World War I.* Hanover, New Hampshire: University Press of New England, 1973.
8 Pepper OH. A Note on the Placebo. *Am J Pharm* 1945;**117**:409–12.
9 Young JH. *Medical Messiahs: A Social History of Health Quackery in Twentieth-Century America.* Princeton, NJ: Princeton University Press, 1969 (reprinted, with a new introduction by the author in 1992).
10 Kaptchuk TJ. Powerful placebo: the dark side of the randomised controlled trial. *Lancet* 1998;**351**:1722–5.
11 White S. Medicine's Humble Humbug: Four Periods in the Understanding of the Placebo. *Pharm Hist* 1985;**27**(2):51–60.
12 Leslie A. Ethics and Practice of Placebo Therapy. *Am J Med* 1954;**16**:854–62.
13 Handfield-Jones RPC. A Bottle of Medicine from the Doctor. *Lancet* 1953;**2**:823–5.
14 Kaptchuk TJ. Intentional ignorance: a history of blind assessment and placebo controls in medicine. *Bull Hist Med* 1998;**72**:389–433.
15 Beecher HK. The powerful placebo. *JAMA* 1955;**159**(17):1602–6.
16 Spiro H. *The Power of Hope: A Doctor's Perspective.* New Haven: Yale University Press, 1999.
17 Lasagna L, Mosteller F, von Felsinger JM, Beecher H. A study of the placebo response, *Am J Med* 1954;**16**:770–9.
18 Wolf S. Effects of suggestion and conditioning on the action of chemical agents in the human – the pharmacology of placebos. *J Clin Invest* 1950;**29**:703–9.
19 Shephard M. The placebo: from specificity to the non-specific and back. *Psychol Med* 1993;**23**:1–10.
20 Kienle GS, Kiene H. The powerful placebo effect: Fact or fiction? *J Clin Epidemiol* 1997; **50**:1311–18.
21 McDonald CJ, Mazzuca SA, McCabe GP. How much of the placebo 'effect' is really statistical regression. *Stat Med* 1983;**2**:417–27.
22 Shapiro AK, Shapiro E. *The Powerful Placebo: From Ancient Priest to Modern Physician.* Baltimore, Maryland: The Johns Hopkins University Press, 1997.
23 Grünbaum A. Explication and implication of the placebo concept. In: White L, Tursky B, Schwartz GE, eds. *Placebo: Theory, Research, and Mechanisms.* New York: The Guilford Press, 1985.
24 Beecher HK. The subjective response and reaction to sensation: the reaction phase as the site of effective drug action. *Am J Med* 1956;**20**:107–13.
25 Ulrich RS. View through a window may influence recovery from surgery. *Science* 1984;**224**(4647):420–1.
26 Mouridsen SE, Nielsen S. Reversible somatotropin deficiency (psychosocial dwarfism) presenting as conduct disorder and growth hormone deficiency. *Dev Med Child Neurol* 1990;**32**(12):1093–8.
27 Phillips DP, Smith DG. Postponement of death until symbolically meaningful occasions. *JAMA* 1990;**263**:1947–51.

28 Cooke P. They cried until they could not see. *New York Times Magazine* June 23, 1991.
29 Cohen S. Voodoo death, the stress response, and AIDs. In: Bridge TP, Mirsky AF, Goodwin FK, eds. *Psychological, neuropsychiatric, and substance abuse aspects of AIDS*. New York: Raven Press, 1988.
30 House JS, Landis KR, *et al.* Social relationships and health. *Science* 1988;**241**:540–5.
31 Cannon WB. Voodoo death. *Am Anthropol* 1942;**44**:169–81.
32 Klopfer B. Psychological Variables in Human Cancer *J Proj Tech* 1957;**21**:331–40.
33 Crowe McCann C, Goldfarb B, Frisk M, Quera-Salva MA, Meyer P. The role of personality factors and suggestion in placebo effect during mental stress test. *Br J Clin Pharmacol* 1992;**33**:107–10.
34 Honigfeld G. Physician and patient attitudes as factors influencing the placebo response in depression. *Dis Nerv Syst* 1963;**24**:343–7.
35 Shapiro AK. Iatroplacebogenics. *Int Pharmacopsychiatry* 1969;**2**:215–48.
36 Frank JD. *Persuasion and healing: a comparative study of psychotherapy*. Baltimore: Johns Hopkins Press, 1973.
37 Brody H. The Doctor as Placebo. In: Harrington A, ed. *The Placebo Effect: An Interdisciplinary Exploration*. Cambridge, MA: Harvard University Press, 1997.
38 Zanna MP, Cooper J. Dissonance and the pill: An attribution approach to studying the arousal properties of dissonance. *J Per Soc Psychol* 1974;**29**:703–9.
39 Ross M, Olson JM. An expectancy-attribution model of the effects of placebos. *Psychol Rev* 1981;**88**:408–37.
40 McGlashan TH, Evans FJ, Orne MT. The nature of hypnotic analgesia and placebo response to experimental pain. *Psychosom Med* 1969;**31**:227–46.
41 Siegel, B. 1986 *Love, Medicine, Miracles*. Reissue edition (June 1990). New York: Harper Perennial Library; 1983.
42 Levine JD, Gordon NC, Fields HL. The mechanism of placebo analgesia. *Lancet* 1978; **2**:654–7.
43 Benedetti F. The opposite effects of the opiate antagonist naloxone and the cholecystokinin antagonist proglumide on placebo analgesia. *Pain* 1996;**64**:535–43.
44 Herrnstein RJ. Placebo effect in the rat. *Science* 1962;**138**:677–8.
45 Ader R. The Role of Conditioning in Pharmacotherapy. In: Harrington A, ed. *The Placebo Effect: An Interdisciplinary Exploration*. Cambridge, MA: Harvard University Press, 1997.
46 Kirsch I. Specifying Nonspecifics: Psychological Mechanisms of Placebo Effects. In: Harrington A, ed. *The Placebo Effect: An Interdisciplinary Exploration*. Cambridge: Harvard University Press, 1997.
47 Hahn A, Kleinman A. Belief as pathogen, belief as medicine: "voodoo death" and the "placebo phenomenon" in anthropological perspective. *Med Anthropol Q* 1983;**14**:3–19.

# 3: Ethical issues in use of placebo in medical practice and clinical trials

SISSELA BOK


## Summary

This chapter takes up the ethical issues raised by intentional uses of placebos in therapy and research, leaving to one side the many uses throughout history of remedies in which physicians and patients may have had what turned out to be misplaced faith. The ethical issues of placebo use arise in a manner that cuts across the various interpretations of how placebos act and of the nature of placebo effects, so long as the persons prescribing or giving out what they take to constitute a placebo aim to facilitate or to test its effects in the recipients.*

The central ethical problem for intentional placebo use in patient care is that of the recourse to deception by caregivers, whether through outright lying or through distortions or omissions intended to mislead recipients. Such deception is often thought to be so innocuous and so clearly altruistic as to warrant little or no moral justification. The chapter weighs the intended benefits for individual patients from placebo use against possible risks, not only for the patients but also for other patients, health professionals, and society. It posits as the central moral challenge for placebo use in patient care that of finding ways for caregivers and patients to collaborate in seeking to achieve the benefits of the placebo effect without recourse to deception; and suggests ways in which additional research might clarify the risks and benefits of placebo use and shed light on non-deceptive means of enlisting the placebo effect.

In the conduct of clinical trials, placebo use is more strictly regulated than in patient care; and deception is largely ruled out in principle, though by no means unknown in practice. The central ethical problem for placebo use in clinical trials is that of the perceived dilemma between fully respecting the rights of human participants in research, on the one hand, and, on the other, seeking


* I thank Howard Brody, Robert Levine, Kenneth Rothman, Robert Temple, and the editors for valuable comments.

knowledge that might benefit others: whether they be populations afflicted with illnesses such as AIDS or Parkinson's Disease, communities, investigators, or commercial firms. The chapter examines this perceived dilemma as it arises in debates about informed consent and the protection against harm, about whether many or all trials using placebos are unethical, and about when, if ever, investigators from developed societies doing research in third world countries may engage in placebo research not permitted in their own societies. A final section suggests areas where additional research is needed to shed light on placebo use in clinical trials and to explore methods and research designs that overcome the perceived dilemma by granting full respect both for the rights of human subjects of research care and for the needs of larger populations.

## Placebo use in patient care

### Definitions

Arthur K Shapiro and Elaine Shapiro define a placebo as "any therapy prescribed knowingly or unknowingly by a healer, or used by laymen, for its therapeutic effect on a symptom or a disease, but which actually is ineffective or not specifically effective for the symptom or disorder being treated". Such a placebo "may be an inert sugar pill, an active drug, or any treatment no matter how potentially specific or by whom administered".[1]

The ethical conflicts regarding placebo use arise in what the Shapiros point to as therapies prescribed knowingly, rather than in the numerous treatments provided throughout history in which caregivers and patients have placed what is now seen as unwarranted faith. True, ethical questions of caregiver negligence and patient gullibility may come up even in the latter cases; but the moral problems with placebo usage arise most clearly in cases of intentional recourse to placebos.

For the purpose of considering these ethical conflicts, many standard definitions of "placebo" and "placebo effect" will do, so long as they delimit cases in which a placebo is knowingly prescribed and a placebo effect is intended or hoped for, and so long as they do not mistakenly limit the definition of "placebos" to inert substances. Likewise, many explanations of the mechanisms thought to underlie placebo effects will do for this purpose, whether psychosocial mechanisms, such as those of expectancies or conditioning effects or the "meaning response", or neurobiological/neuroendocrine biomarkers, again so long as placebos are knowingly given to elicit or test such effects.

Intentional uses of placebos have long been thought to offer sometimes powerful means of relieving pain, at times of reversing disease processes. Yet a dilemma is often perceived with respect to such uses: the very process by which the placebo appears capable of relieving anxiety and suffering seems to depend upon keeping the recipient in the dark, and upon conveying confidence in its medicinal properties. Deception, whether through outright lies or other means of misleading patients, has traditionally been thought necessary to achieve the hoped-for beneficial effect. What becomes, in that case, of patients' rights to give or refuse informed consent to all forms of treatment?

**Deception**

*Mentiris ut medicus.* "Lie like a doctor", the 17th century British Bishop Jeremy Taylor counseled, when doing so can help patients. This injunction, he wrote, had grown to become a proverb, so common was the practice of deceiving the sick; but it was always "to be understood in the way of charity and with honour to the profession". Just as it is right, he held, for anyone to lie to children and madmen, so physicians should not hesitate to do so whenever they see the need "to abuse the fancies of hypochondriacal and disordered persons into a will of being cured".[2]

Over the centuries, very few codes enjoined doctors to truthfulness toward patients.[3] Surveying the recent shift in physicians' attitudes in this regard, Eric Cassell pointed out that doctors withheld the truth from patients who had life-threatening diseases until the 1970s, and did not tell patients, earlier, about the facts of their illnesses even when they were not serious.[4] It was not until 1980 that the American Medical Association added the stipulation to "deal honestly with patients and colleagues" to its Principles of Medical Ethics.[5]

There is no evidence, however, that this stipulation has been thought to apply to the use of placebos in patient care, a practice less examined and less carefully regulated than placebo use in clinical trials. Paternalistic deception of patients "for their own good", with the intention of enlisting in them what Jeremy Taylor called "the will of being cured", is seen by many as unproblematic by comparison to deceiving research subjects, and as less problematic than, say, lying to insurance companies or to relatives on behalf of patients. The reason? Such paternalistic deception is not only thought altruistic and benevolent in general but also aimed to help the very persons being deceived. Why consign sick persons to needless suffering or anxiety in such cases out of misguided scruples concerning honesty? Placebos have been considered so innocuous, and so purely beneficial when they work, that prescribing them for therapeutic purposes to patients has been regarded as falling squarely in the category of harmless but altruistic white lies. Thinking through ethical pros and cons in such cases has seemed unnecessary and insisting on procedures of informed consent still more so.

What about statements that are not outright lies but that simply withhold information from patients about their condition and the placebic nature of the treatment provided to them? Statements such as "Take these pills and let me know how they work" or "These pills have helped a number of people"? In medicine as in other professions, both lying and failure to offer information count as deceptive so long as the information distorted or withheld is regarded as due those who are being misled. Yet the history of medicine reveals the strength of the belief, among doctors, that both forms of deception are needed whenever full truthfulness will not serve their patients' best interests. The Code of Ethics of the American Medical Association of 1847 went so far as to insist that the physician has a sacred duty "to avoid all things which have a tendency to discourage the patient and to depress his spirits".[6]

Both outright lies and the silent or evasive withholding of information due to patients leave them in ignorance of what physicians take their condition to be and what they are aiming to achieve. In principle, both forms of deception go, therefore, against the stipulation introduced by the AMA in its 1980 Principles of Medical Ethics, that physicians deal honestly with their patients; as well as against the stress on informed consent.

### Bypassing informed consent

Just as deception in prescribing or giving placebos is often thought of as not rising above the threshold of what matters from a moral point of view, given the presumed altruism of the physician and the innocuousness of what is prescribed, so placebo use remains fluid territory when it comes to bypassing informed consent. According to the doctrine of informed consent, patients have the right to receive sufficient information regarding the diagnosis, prognosis, and proposed treatment so that they can make an informed choice, including that of refusing treatment, on the basis of what they learn. Stressing such a right is in part a safeguard against health professionals engaging in deceit, no matter how benevolent in intent, and in part also a safeguard against being manipulated by caregivers who may be less than altruistic, less than competent in evaluating patients.

The failure to examine the ethics of placebo use for therapeutic purposes through outright lies or omissions rests on largely unexamined premises regarding the kindly intentions of the caregiver and the harmlessness yet potential beneficial nature of the placebo. How could the act of giving placebos meant to help, yet in their own right so innocuous, be worth challenging on grounds of informed consent?

The philosopher Onora O'Neill goes further and argues that such acts may be not only permissible but indispensable. Although deception wrongfully violates informed consent, "some non-fundamental aspects of treatment to which consent has been given may have to include elements of deception … Use of placebos or of reassuring but inaccurate accounts of expected pain might sometimes be non-fundamental but indispensable and so permissible deceptions".[7]

Such conclusions as to permissible or indispensable "non-fundamental" deceptions are more easily drawn in the abstract, without considering the possibility that, in practice, caregivers might be in error, impaired, or acting not in patients' but in their own interest. These are the very circumstances under which the importance of informed consent is obvious.

Failure to examine the underlying premises about when innocuousness and benevolent intent permit the bypassing of informed consent leaves out of account risks to patients, caregivers, and medicine that together contribute to a heavy burden for societies.

### Risks from therapeutic placebo usage

"I didn't know there could be pain so great", a man once wrote me from prison. He had repeatedly complained to the staff physician of strong pain in his left kidney area and had tried to explain that the shots prescribed for his pain had brought no relief. When he tried once again to ask for help, the physician, who said he was in a hurry to go home for the evening, prescribed yet another injection. "I looked to see what medication he ordered and it was water". The prisoner's protests and mounting distress finally convinced those in charge to send him to a hospital. He was found to have an unusually painful kidney stone and was given immediate care and pain relief. "But to realize that the doctor was prescribing water for this will always leave a memory", he wrote "and I don't think I would ever trust a doctor again".[8]

This case illustrates the risk from casual reliance on placebos by physicians in a hurry aiming to placate patients – risks never greater than when placebos take the place of appropriate treatment after a faulty diagnosis. The injection of a few milliliters of saline solution or, for that matter, the provision of sugar pills or other common placebos, was hardly what this patient needed. This may seem an extreme case, hardly consonant with the risks from erroneous placebo prescriptions to the great majority of patients. But in the light of the mounting documentation of the human costs of medical error, it is no longer possible to brush aside cases such as that of this prisoner as extreme. An Institute of Medicine report has characterized medical error as a leading cause of death and disability in the US, estimating that deaths from such error each year exceed those from highway accidents, breast cancer, or AIDS; and that the 7000 deaths resulting from medication errors exceed those from workplace injuries.[9] The interaction of the different factors of computer errors, provider incompetence and impairment needs to be sorted out with care to try to cut back on the resulting devastation; but from the point of view of the person injured by such errors, it is already too late to benefit from such risk analysis.[10]

The case also illustrates a risk for patients who find that they have been duped that is rarely obvious at the time a physician prescribes a placebo; it is that some among them may lose confidence in *bona fide* medication given to them at some later time, possibly at a time when it would be very important for them to take such medication. This is the danger with all deception – that its discovery can lead to a failure of trust when trust is most needed. In this way, even the many health professionals who do not mislead their patients are harmed by those who do. Physicians can ill afford to undermine the trust that is their most precious asset by trading on it through recourse to manipulation.

Regardless of how innocuous the substances prescribed may be in their own right, there is also growing documentation of the role played by undesirable, sometimes dangerous, side effects of placebos, such as nausea, dermatitis, or migraines. An especially dangerous side effect, even from a harmless substance, is that of addiction for patients who become dependent on prescriptions, especially if they have come to believe them to be indispensable to avoid relapsing. (Such side effects are sometimes called "nocebo effects". It is important to distinguish two senses of this expression: some use it to designate undesirable side effects of a placebic treatment that are not intended by the caregiver who is providing it in the hope of its bringing about positive effects; others limit the term to conditions where the subject expects a negative outcome, as in the extreme case of "voodoo death".[11])

In today's medical climate, moreover, the image of the placebo as inert, as a harmless sugar pill or saline solution hardly corresponds to the many treatments knowingly prescribed as placebos to the population at large, such as antibiotics, *x* ray films, forms of psychotherapy, at times even surgery. This shift away from inert placebos results in part from consumer demand for active medications, in part from the advertising directly to consumers now undertaken by drug companies. In the US, with drug expenditures rising by 17–20 per cent every year and contributing more than any other factor to rising health costs, the consequences are anything but minor.[12]

For health professionals under constraints to see patients for shorter amounts of time than in the past, with the length of average office visits shrinking, the temptation may be especially great to terminate a visit with a placebo prescription. With more time and careful attention on the part of the physician, it would be possible to limit unintentional side effects from placebos considerably. This is not only true when the placebo administered is simply given in error, but in the many cases where antibiotics and other potent medications are provided as placebos – to "placate" demanding patients or parents, simply to terminate a consultation.

When Jeremy Taylor draws an analogy between deceiving children and madmen on the one hand, and "hypochondriacal and disordered persons" on the other, he adds that no lies should be told to those who are wise enough to be able to choose for themselves.[2] Placebos are still often seen as especially useful for when it comes to pleasing or "placating" patients that caregivers see as "anxious or insatiable".[13] The very term "placebo", with its meaning "I shall please", helps to lend the practice of giving out placebos a benevolent aura that masks such human and societal costs. The practice then acts as a placebo upon physicians, not patients alone. Just as placebo-giving is meant to please patients and to improve their health, so it pleases some physicians and gives them a comforting sense of competence and kindness at little personal cost. And just as there can be unintended deleterious side effects for patients from the practice of prescribing placebos, so there can be such effects upon physicians and health professionals more generally.

Such a poorly scrutinized practice offers room to maneuver for the hurried, the impaired, and the incompetent. Deceptive practices, by their very nature, bypass the normal requirements for feedback and, in turn for accountability. So long as the placebic nature of prescriptions remains undocumented, the resulting costs are hard to pinpoint. The casual attitude of health professionals to deceit that they take to be benevolent and harmless, moreover, can carry over to other forms of deception. There are no watertight barriers between such deception and the concealment of risks associated with an operation, the failure to deal honestly with patients at the end of life, or false statements to insurance companies.

True, many in the public press for more medication even when they are fully informed that it is not what they need. In this way they contribute to the overuse of medication. But this pressure from patients offers no justification for physicians to add to that societal burden. They must consider not only the possible side effects on patients from such inappropriate prescriptions, but the consequences for other patients and for society as a whole. Patients, Richard Cabot suggested in a seminal article on truth and deception in medicine published almost a century ago, are not born with the expectation of a medicine for every symptom: "It is we physicians who are responsible for perpetuating false ideas about disease and its cure ... With every placebo that we give we do our part in perpetuating error, and harmful error at that".[14]

Looking at each act of giving placebos in isolation blinds individual physicians who prescribe them to the billions of dollars expended upon useless therapies with transient placebo effects. Such uses are the prototype of the quick fix. They bypass any genuine search with the patient for ways to heal and to prevent future complaints, future needs for more placebos.

To forestall the individual and societal costs of such uses of placebos in patient care, deceptive prescription of placebos should be sharply curtailed. It should be undertaken only after careful diagnosis and consultation with colleagues in cases where there appears to be no other way out to attempt self-healing on the part of the patient. No active placebos should be prescribed, only ones known to be inert; and no protracted use should be undertaken, given the risks of addiction and untoward side effects even from sugar pills. Most important, placebos should only be given out after careful consideration of non-deceptive ways to seek to stimulate the "will of being cured". Finally, as a protection for patients, any deceptive placebo prescription should be fully documented as such in the patient's records. As with all deception by health professionals, such documentation, were it required, would change practices considerably. A British physician put it this way in a 1992 letter to the Editor of the *Journal of Medical Ethics*: "Perhaps a doctor who believes himself justified in lying or slanting the truth should be required to make a written record at the time, and subsequently be obliged to show it to the patient or his next of kin. I suspect that if this was done, there would be a lot less 'benevolent deception'".[15]

## Non-deceptive therapeutic approaches

For most patients, it is in their best interests to seek to achieve the benefits of placebo effects without running the risks inherent when health professionals resort to deception. But to what extent is it possible to achieve such benefits without misleading patients? The dilemma many have sensed in the past, between honesty and doing what is best for patients when it comes to placebos, may dissipate as we learn more about factors that contribute to placebo effects quite apart from what a physician may say in providing a sugar pill or other placebo. Among these factors are the expectations aroused in some simply by the fact of being in a doctor's office and receiving the attention of health professionals. If the latter explain that patients' fears about what is causing their symptoms are unfounded when this is the case – say, the fear that cancer or heart disease or Alzheimer's Disease might be causing the symptoms, sheer relief can change expectations regarding whether or not symptoms are going to disappear on their own or can be treated without prescriptions of any kind.

Physicians themselves are increasingly seen to be capable of serving as placebos.[16,17,18] Once they recognize that they can exercise this power by conveying compassion and sympathy and providing comforting assistance, they should feel no pressure to add needless prescriptions with all the expenses and risks they entail. Jay Katz points out that, "if physicians were to provide hope and reassurance in a more honest fashion, then the placebo effect of doctors would augment faith in new ways, and the need to resort to placebo-pills and placebo-treatment would be markedly reduced, if not eliminated". Physicians, he holds, should learn to use their inherent placebo effect to render their scientific treatments more effective: "To attain this objective, placebos must not be employed to satisfy patients' demands for treatment, to hide diagnostic or therapeutic ignorance, to save doctors' time or to make money".[19]

From the point of view of health care consumers, however, the need to do what they can to guard against the risks from medical error and physician impairment, mentioned above, remains, whether or not they are at the receiving end of placebos given for therapeutic purposes. For these consumers, it is important to go beyond the traditional model of informed consent, with the physician doing the informing and the patient only deciding whether or not to consent. Given the risks consumers run in the present health care system, caution and self-protection are as important when it comes to health concerns as in defensive driving. The preventive measures and the risk assessments involved include, but are far from limited to, guarding against the risks from misuses of placebos: either from accepting them with needless gullibility or from pressing health professionals for inappropriate forms of treatments and thus inviting the recourse to placebos. This is not to say that people should set aside all the measures that could possibly turn out to be serving as placebos in their lives. Many people invest certain objects and rituals with comforting, sometimes healing properties even when they recognize that these may have primarily placebic functions. Life would be barren indeed without them; and dismissing them as "mere placebos" leaves out of account the powerful beneficial role that placebo effects can play.

Above all, health care consumers and health professionals can learn to work together in enlisting the benefits of the placebo effect without placebo prescriptions – the more so as knowledge about the placebo effect increases. It is urgent, as prescriptive drugs drive up health care costs the world over, to study the ways in which the healing powers of the placebo effect can be achieved in such ways as to cut back on the need for drugs and other treatments. This will, in turn, allow people a more active role in preventive health and self-healing, and thus in reducing the need for "being" a patient.

**Research opportunities regarding placebos in patient care**

Remarkably little is known about how placebos are actually used in patient care. Health care professionals who prescribe them for therapeutic purposes rarely do so openly. As a result, what is known about the forms this usage takes, the frequency with which it occurs, the time periods for which placebos are prescribed, and the limitations and safeguards that are observed, is largely of an anecdotal nature. It will be important to survey textbooks and course materials in medical schools, to inquire with medical students, physicians, and other health care professionals prescribing placebos, and to examine the growing literature regarding placebo use, in order to come to greater clarity about current practices.

A simple first step, in examining actual uses of placebos in patient care, would be to look at instruction materials in the different medical specialties. For comparative purposes, reference might be made to a survey, in 1973, at a time when debates about ethical issues in placebo use were rare.[20] This survey found that, of 19 popular textbooks in medicine, pediatrics, surgery, anesthesia, obstetrics and gynecology, only three mentioned placebos, and none dealt with either the medical or the ethical problems placebos present; while four out of five textbooks on pharmacology mentioned them, all but one considered only the experimental role of placebos and were silent on ethical issues; and four out of eight standard texts on psychiatry referred to placebos without mention of any ethical issues.

To what extent has the coverage changed today?

- How, if at all, do current instructional materials define "placebo" and "placebo effect"?
- Do these texts discuss *types* of substances most commonly used as placebos?
- Is reference made to quantities to be used, lengths of time, and costs of placebos?
- What proportion of the texts raise ethical issues?
- What proportion, if any, suggest entering placebo prescriptions as such in patient records?
- How frequently do the materials warn against prescribing antibiotics and other non-inert substances as placebos?
- Do they take up kinds of side effects? Has the concept of "nocebos" entered the discussion in these materials?
- Are distinctions made between types of patients when it comes to placebo response, and to patients more likely than others to be disturbed at learning they have been misled regarding the medicinal properties of placebos prescribed to them?

A second step would be to survey medical students and recent MDs, to find out what they learned informally about placebo use in patient care, regardless of how little they came across in written documents.

- What kind of statements were they taught to make, in accompanying placebo prescriptions?
- Were they instructed in alternative ways of seeking to achieve placebo effects among patients?
- How often did they prescribe placebos?
- What proportion of the time did they consult with colleagues regarding such a practice?
- Did they enter placebo prescriptions *as* placebos in patient records?

A third step would be to undertake a thorough study of the health care literature generally for debates concerning the ethics of placebo use in patient care. Increasingly, the media carry articles about the marvels and powers of placebos: the cover of a recent *New York Times Magazine* issue, for example, announced as an "Astonishing Medical Fact" in fat, bold type that "Placebos Work!"[21] Both the popular and the professional literature should be surveyed, comparing the changing coverage over the course of the past century.

- What roles are now seen for placebos in patient care?
- And in preventive self-help?
- To what extent is new information regarding non-deceptive ways to elicit the placebo effect taken into consideration?

- What about studies finding that when physicians prescribe a placebo while explaining to patients that it is a placebo, what its functions are, and indicating that some people find it helpful, it turns out to be helpful in about the same proportion of cases as when deception is employed?

## Placebo use in clinical trials

### Placebo use in larger contexts of research ethics

"Placebos have doubtless been used for centuries by wise physicians as well as by quacks", Henry K Beecher wrote in his classic 1955 article, "The Powerful Placebo"; but it was only recently that two clinical functions for this tool have been recognized: "to distinguish pharmacological effects from the effects of suggestion, and … to obtain an unbiased assessment of the result of experiment".[22] A decade later, Beecher shocked the medical world by detailing severe ethical shortcomings in clinical research, including growing numbers of studies using placebos for such purposes, in which patients were entered without their knowledge much less their freely given, informed consent.[23]

The casual research climate to which Beecher drew attention is hardly conceivable today. But debates about placebo use in clinical trials still give urgency to ethical questions about human experimentation more generally. Since so many federally funded studies involving human subjects are randomized double blind studies in which a group of individuals receive placebos, the moral requirements for how these individuals should be treated clearly ought to have high priority; and to the extent that these requirements are slighted or violated in any one trial, the trial as a whole is open to criticism. This is the case not only with respect to the adequacy of informed consent procedures but also with respect to conflicts of interest for investigators, the scientific validity of studies, the recruitment of subjects, risks for vulnerable populations, and the role of Institutional Review Boards (IRBs) in protecting human subjects.

In recent years, the scope of potential ethical problems in clinical trials has expanded, and doubts are mounting as to whether existing regulations concerning informed consent and institutional oversight provide adequate protection.[24,25,26] In earlier decades, there were far fewer trials under way, and most investigators responsible for them worked in a single institution with a discrete cohort of subjects. By now, there has been a vast influx of money for research purposes, much of it going to growing numbers of randomized double blind trials. Concern is mounting about inducements offered to potential research subjects in the process of recruiting them and about financial and other incentives for investigators/physicians to enroll their patients as research subjects. Many studies are now multisite, often international undertakings less easily monitored by IRBs – themselves stretched and overburdened as never before. Pressures from pharmaceutical companies and academic centers to expedite institutional review place at risk the timely consideration both of the scientific validity and of the ethical adequacy of proposals. In some cases, there are also mounting pressures from patients suffering from illnesses such as AIDS to be participants in ongoing studies.

I shall focus, in what follows, on two sets of ethical issues concerning placebo use that bear on the perceived dilemma between fully respecting the rights of human subjects of research, on the one hand, and, on the other, seeking knowledge that might benefit others: first, questions about the adequacy of informed consent procedures regarding the role of placebos; second, the question of whether it is ethical to conduct trials involving placebos whenever it would be possible to compare, instead, a drug or treatment to an existing drug or treatment rather than to placebos. I shall then discuss recent challenges on both grounds to placebo trials in less developed, often poor, societies, and conclude with a section stressing the need for documentation and further research regarding the uses and misuses of placebos in clinical trials.

## Informed consent

Earlier in this century, deceptive placebo use was nearly as common in experimentation on human beings as in patient care.[20,23] In many cases, participants were not even told that they had been included in a study; it stands to reason that they did not find out, either, that they might receive either placebos or active medication. For example, a 1967 study entitled "An Analysis of the Placebo Effect in Hospitalized Hypertensive Patients" reports that six patients were asked to "accept hospitalization for approximately six weeks ... to have their hypertension evaluated and to undertake a treatment with a new blood pressure drug", only to be given placebos instead.[27]

Such out-and-out deception is ruled out in today's randomized double blind clinical trials, through the requirement that investigators adhere to strict provisions for informed consent.[28,29] Prospective participants must be asked to give voluntary consent only after they have been adequately informed about the purposes of the study, the research design requiring placebos to be given to some among them, the possible benefits and risks from participation in a study thus designed, and different forms of treatment that might be beneficial to them.

Participants must also be asked for voluntary consent to the double blind nature of the study, requiring that they not be told whether or not they are in the group receiving the treatment under study or a control group; if members of the control group are to receive placebo, this, too, should be explained to the potential participants. Because the placebos offered to members of control groups are usually pharmacologically inert (unlike many placebos provided in patient care for therapeutic purposes), it has not been customary to inform participants about possible risks from the placebos themselves, only about risks from receiving or not receiving the treatment being studied. Given all that is coming to be known about the powerful effects placebos may have, however, it would be important to inform participants, as well, of the possible benefits and risks to them from the placebos in their own right.

Might there be a moral conflict for investigators in providing such information about placebos? Some might fear that doing so could produce expectancies about the role of placebos among participants that could skew the comparison between the effects of placebos and those of the drug being tested; or else that the most suggestible among subjects could differ in their responses in ways that would be hard to anticipate beforehand and account for after the completion of the study.

A more general conflict for investigators arises when the research design and/or purposes are such that informing participants might well skew their responses, sometimes leading them to decline participation. The study may address a troubling issue such as substance abuse or domestic violence, or be designed to test, surreptitiously, subject reliability.[30] In psychological research, deception is common, not only in such cases but, more generally, when investigators "have determined that the use of deceptive techniques is justified by the study's prospective scientific, educational, or applied value and that equally effective alternative procedures that do not use deception are not feasible".[31,32]

In biomedical research, by contrast, deception in securing informed consent is generally ruled out. But there appear to be exceptions. A "commentary" on investigator obligations regarding informed consent in the *International Ethical Guideline for Biomedical Research Involving Human Subjects* leaves the door open to certain kinds of "justified" deception. According to this commentary, investigators have a duty to "exclude the possibility of unjustified deception" in securing informed consent from subjects; they may, however, seek to have an ethical review committee allow them to engage in deception held to be "indispensable to the methods of an experiment", provided that "nothing has been withheld that, if divulged, would cause a reasonable person to refuse to participate".[33] It is not clear from this commentary, however, whether the deception involved could concern the nature or the role of placebos in such permissible experiments. What does seem clear is that allowing deception regarding any aspect of clinical trials represents a denial of informed consent and therefore goes against the best interests of prospective subjects.

Individuals differ in levels of risk aversion and in the concerns they bring to decisions about whether or not to take part in research. Some of their concerns may appear idiosyncratic to investigators and review boards but must nevertheless be respected, in order to serve basic functions of informed consent such as those of protecting individual autonomy and of avoiding fraud and duress.[34] It is not enough for investigators and IRBs to conclude, without consulting participants in studies, that minimal risks to the latter justify bypassing informed consent requirements.

Apart from actual deception, ethical issues abound when it comes to the nature of the consent obtained in a number of clinical trials involving placebos.

- How freely is the consent given?
- How carefully are the alternatives, including that of not participating, explained to prospective subjects?
- How clearly have investigators explained the difference between therapy and research in the particular investigation, and pointed out that participants are unlikely to benefit directly, when this is the case?

Of special concern in these regards are psychiatric patients, children, and other persons with undeveloped or impaired capacity to provide fully informed consent. When can parents or other proxies legitimately provide consent on their behalf? What about cases where there are no prospects that participants themselves will benefit from the results of the study in which they are asked to take part? In such cases of problematic consent capacity, a different moral conflict arises than the one mentioned above with respect to informing subjects – one that opposes considerations of what might be best for particular children, for example, to the desire to pursue research that benefits unspecified children in the future. Even as much clinical research balances risks for individual participants in studies against potential benefits to larger groups and to society, there are special moral problems with entertaining such risks for persons not fully able to consent to them. Yet there are also problems in excluding such persons from all research so long as there is inadequate knowledge about risks and benefits to these populations from existing treatments and from possible new ones. While children, for example, require special protections against exploitative use as research subjects, ruling them out as research subjects could, in the eyes of many investigators, delay progress in establishing the proper dosages of drugs that could help them.

The perception of how best to balance the needs of individuals not able to give fully informed consent against those of society is bound to differ, depending on the perspective of investigators or of persons asked to consider whether or not to give surrogate consent. Anyone in a fiduciary position such as a parent or a court-appointed guardian has an obligation to give priority to the best interests of the person in their charge. For this reason, they must protect that person against all invitations to take part in placebo research posing serious risks of death or disability. No one disagrees on this score. Likewise, many agree with the guideline offered in 1995 by the American Academy of Pediatrics, holding that "Placebo or untreated observational control groups can be used in pediatric studies if their use does not place children at additional risk", and setting forth conditions under which placebos may be ethically employed.[35] But what about placebo research presenting some risk? Should proxies decline participation in all cases of placebo research on conditions such as clinical depression or asthma? On this score, opinions diverge; but there is growing pressure on parents and physicians, at times accompanied by financial and other inducements, to enter children into clinical studies in which some among those receiving placebos might be at more than minimal risk.[36]

The pressure stems in part from the felt need to locate significant numbers of children for studies of many treatments never tested on them in earlier decades. The pace and scale of research on children has escalated in the United States in recent years, with the numbers of children enrolled in such research tripling between 1997 and 2000 according to one study.[37] The Federal Government has pushed to have more medicines tested on children, culminating with the regulation issued by the Food and Drug Administration in December 2000, requiring pharmaceutical companies to test almost all new medicines on children.[38] Understandably, given such sharply accelerating research on children and the mentally ill, debates have intensified about the moral questions concerning proxy consent to placebo studies, levels of acceptable risk, and research with no prospect of direct benefit to participating children.[39–42]

The World Medical Association's (WMA) most recently revised version of the *Declaration of Helsinki*, setting forth "Ethical Principles for Medical Research Involving Human Subjects", repeatedly stresses the requirement for researchers to disclose any possible conflicts of interest to IRBs and participants.[43] But there is, at present, little evidence that such disclosures – regarding, for instance, financial incentives for physicians or investigators – are regularly made either to participants more generally or to persons asked to give consent for those unable to do so themselves. Nor is there sufficient oversight of how well IRBs deal with new types of issues involving conflicts of interest or ensure the adequacy of existing informed consent procedures. Awareness of these problems intensifies concern about the conditions under which there may be inherent problems with using placebos in drug trials, regardless of whether prospective subjects or their proxies have consented to their participation in such trials.

## Can placebo use in research be inherently unethical?

After heated debate regarding revisions in the *Declaration of Helsinki*, the WMA reaffirmed certain fundamental positions in October 2000, including one holding that "In medical research on human subjects, considerations related to the wellbeing of the human subject should take precedence over the interests of science and society".[44] Not included in the revised version was a suggested article, holding that "When the outcome measures are neither death nor disability, placebo or other no-treatment controls may be justified on the basis of their efficiency".[45] Instead, the revised version reiterated that, for medical research combined with medical care, "The benefits, risks, burdens, and effectiveness should be tested against those of the best current prophylactic, diagnostic, and therapeutic methods. This does not exclude the use of placebo, or no treatment, in studies where no proven prophylactic, diagnostic or therapeutic method exists".[46]

According to this clause, placebo studies involving as participants persons seeking medical care would be acceptable so long as there is equipoise, or genuine uncertainty about which treatment is preferable, but not studies in which placebos are given to persons suffering from conditions for which effective treatments already exist. It is not clear how this position taken by the WMA will be squared with research practices, especially common in the US, that conflict with it. The disagreement is primarily an ethical one weighing claims regarding the rights and interests of existing subjects of research against claims that scientific progress intended to benefit society requires more general testing against placebo controls; but it is also a disagreement concerning research design and possible alternatives to placebo research that might, if developed, bypass such ethical conflicts.[47–49]

Two papers in the present volume reflect the disagreement on the ethics of placebo research expressed at the October 2000 NIH workshop. Robert Temple, restricting his remarks to "the fully-informed subject" and to protocols presenting no serious risks to subjects, argues that it would be paternalistic to prevent such subjects from freely choosing to take part in clinical trials, and highly damaging to the scientific enterprise.[50] Kenneth Rothman, emphasizing that he is talking about research participants who are not healthy volunteers but rather patients seeking treatment, maintains that "It is unethical to conduct a trial that deprives participants of the level of care for their condition that they would have received if they were not participants in a trial". Informed consent is not an adequate protection, Rothman holds, since true informed consent is a legal fiction, never achieved in actuality. Nor do IRBs as presently constituted offer sufficient protection for the rights of patients.[51]

While the disagreement between Rothman and Temple is sharp, they may have some ground in common, given that they are focusing on different, though partially overlapping groups of research participants. Temple would clearly agree to exclude or delay placebo trials where there are serious doubts about the adequacy of the consent process. He also agrees "that where there are serious doubts about the risks placebo patients would be exposed to, placebo controlled trials may not be possible".* And Rothman, in turn, would agree that there is less reason to worry about placebo trials enrolling healthy and thoroughly informed volunteers who have freely agreed to participate in research presenting minimal or no risk.

* Temple R. Memorandum, April 9, 2001. Temple adds that "Those doubts, however, should bear some relation to what is actually known about the benefits of therapy and the risks of placebo exposure."

Agreement on these scores offers a basis from which to examine the ethical appropriateness of other types of placebo research and to consider safeguards and procedures to protect participants. Such an examination will require attention to particular studies and to the nature of the consent sought from participants, to accountability and possible conflicts of interest for physicians and researchers, to the adequacy of IRB oversight, and to practical issues of line-drawing and education and formulation of best practices when it comes to placebo research.

## Placebo use in trials in less developed societies

The controversies concerning consent procedures, levels of risk, IRB oversight, and conflicts of interest have arisen in still sharper form in recent years with regard to placebo controlled clinical trials in developing societies, and in particular to those increasingly conducted in South-east Asia and in Sub-Saharan Africa.[†] Concern is rising about shoddy or non-existent consent procedures, levels of risk poorly explained to participants, IRB oversight at great distance from sponsoring institutions in the US, and conflicts of interest exacerbated when physicians and co-investigators in poor societies receive more compensation for entering patients into clinical trials than for their professional activities. Such practices have come under growing scholarly and media scrutiny in the past five years, as commercial organizations in the US and other industrial states sponsor more numerous trials in developing societies and as the sense of urgency grows about the scourges of AIDS and other infectious diseases besetting them.[52]

- Should research subjects in poor societies receive the same protection when it comes to consent procedures, levels of risk, IRB oversight, and conflicts of interest as is mandated in trials in developed societies?
- Or are the benefits to be derived from lowering these standards of protection so great and so urgent that placebo controlled trials should be allowed in poor countries that would never pass muster in rich ones?
- Is it paternalistic to seek to impose "Western" standards on investigators abroad, or, rather, paternalistic to assume that if the purpose of trials is to benefit populations in poor societies then this altruistic aim justifies treating subjects in ways that would otherwise not pass muster?
- Can informed consent requirements be bypassed, shortened, or made less strict when investigators conclude that participants are illiterate or unable to understand the information provided?
- What about the monitoring of risks imposed on participants in studies in far-flung regions by review boards in the home country?

---

[†] For a recent statement concerning such trials, see the National Bioethics Commission's draft report, September 29, 2000 "Ethical and policy issues in international research".

It was inevitable that different proposals should be made for revising the Helsinki Declaration with a view to international research. In the end, the World Medical Association modified its stance somewhat on the subject of vulnerable research populations, mandating "special attention" rather than "additional standards" for research subjects "who cannot give or refuse consent for themselves, for those who may be subject to giving consent under duress, for those who will not benefit personally from the research and for those for whom the research is combined with care".[53] The WMA also insisted that, in international research, "no national ethical, legal, or regulatory requirement should be allowed to reduce or eliminate any of the protections of human subjects set forth in this Declaration".

As investigators, regulating agencies, and IRBs consider the ethics of international research, it is important to counter one specious argument, to the effect that the most fundamental protections for the rights of research participants in some societies can be lowered on "cultural" grounds. Such an argument assumes that although one set of minimal research standards for informed consent and protection against harm can be shared by developed societies even as culturally different as those of Japan, the US, and Sweden, cultural differences in developing countries may call for less demanding standards. But such dichotomies between standards for developed and developing societies are harder to maintain once one inquires with those most at risk from exploitative or incompetent research – potential study participants in, say, South Africa or Indonesia. Indeed, even if one looks only at a developed society such as that of the US, it is clear that there are immense religious, ethnic, and other cultural differences among its people; the poorest parts of its cities are often expressly compared to developing societies. But whereas US investigators once took such cultural differences to grant them greater leeway in lowering the standards of protection in doing research involving poor or illiterate or impaired populations, this is no longer the case. Members of vulnerable populations are now seen to require special protection, not a lowering of ethical standards. There should be a heavy burden of proof for anyone maintaining that the case should be different when it comes to international research.

A separate set of questions, often confused with those regarding equal access to informed consent and protection against harm, concerns comparisons of standards of medical care in rich and poor societies and the responsibilities of investigators.

- Does an altruistic purpose obviate the necessity of providing individuals in placebo groups with existing remedies for conditions such as HIV-AIDS, which can hardly be claimed not to be life-threatening?
- Is it right to carry out placebo studies in societies that do not possess the means to make use of any beneficial result, once achieved?
- Are there different requirements, in this regard, for research in rich and poor societies?

A set of placebo controlled trials that brought out the differences of opinion on this score concerned perinatal transmission of HIV infection and involved over 12 000 women in seven countries. Would a short course of AZT given to mothers cut the rate of HIV transmission? After preliminary results in Thailand, showing a reduction of 51 per cent in mothers given such a short course of AZT compared to others receiving placebo, similar trials under way in Africa and the Dominican Republic were suspended.[54] As Carol Levine points out, "Both enthusiastic proponents of the trials and their vociferous opponents asserted that their views had been vindicated. The proponents declared that such significant results could only have been achieved with placebo arms; the opponents saw the results as evidence that placebos were never needed in the first place".[55]

It is unclear how the debates over international placebo controlled research will affect ongoing and future research in less developed societies. What is clear is that the ethical issues are nowhere near resolved, and that the urgent need to find remedies for epidemics such as that of HIV-AIDS leads many to worry about ethical research standards they take to obstruct and impede progress.

Those on different sides of these debates might find a common basis from which to pursue deliberations about these ethical issues if they could agree on the need to ensure that there should be common standards for informed consent and protection against harm in research conducted in all societies, rich or poor. It would make a difference, for instance, if standard consent procedures required investigators to make sure that participants understood the difference between therapy and research in trials where that difference is relevant; and if they were fully informed about risks from the research, including risks from possibly being in the control group receiving placebo.

Given all that is at stake in clinical trials conducted in developing countries and the rate at which new trials are launched, however, such agreement is unlikely to provide anything near adequate protection for the rights of many participants in such trials. What is urgently needed, to ensure their protection, is an international body capable of regulating what are at present poorly regulated international research practices, of ensuring accountability and transparency with respect to ongoing trials, and of encouraging research proposals capable of meeting high scientific as well as moral standards.

## Research opportunities on placebo use in clinical trials

Some aspects of the actual use of placebos are more carefully documented in randomized double blind clinical trials than in either patient care or in the types of research with human beings beyond the reach of Federal regulations. The kinds and amounts of placebos given to subjects in such clinical trials, for example, can be documented, as can the length of time during which subjects are given placebos. But there is considerably more variation when it comes to what information regarding placebos is provided to subjects in clinical trials and to members of IRBs. For this reason, it would be important to examine the conduct of past and ongoing clinical trials to determine what subjects are actually told in the process of the informed consent procedures about the role of the placebos that they may be given. While the regulations regarding such procedures stipulate that participants should be told that they may be given placebos, depending on the group they are assigned to, it matters to document just what different investigators communicate about exceptions to informed consent obligations held to constitute "justifiable deception" and the frequency with which IRBs permit such exceptions.

There may be variations, as well, when it comes to information provided about possible side effects of receiving the placebos instead of the drug being studied, and, for some, of receiving the placebos in their own right. Failure to provide adequate explanation in this regard may be especially problematic for participants with conditions rendering them especially vulnerable to those side effects. For instance, persons who are clinically depressed may need to know more than those who are not about headaches, depressive symptoms, and nausea that may result from placebos. In turn, however, persons who are especially suggestible may also be at risk from developing the very symptoms which are presented to them as possible, from the placebos.

Members of IRBs, likewise, may receive quite different levels of information in different clinical trials, as they examine the informed consent forms and procedures for seeking subject consent. Different IRBs, moreover, may give different levels of scrutiny to these forms, especially if they are hard pressed to review a large number of proposals. The same is true of the care with which they consider how informed consent is sought from vulnerable populations, how thoroughly they provide information about possible risks and about whether or not participants stand to benefit from taking part, and the nature of possible conflicts of interest for researchers and physicians.

The debates regarding placebo use in studies where accepted remedies exist, are not only about ethical priorities but also about research design and validity. The same is true of the debates concerning such research in less developed societies. Much remains to be done in examining possible alternative designs to clinical trials presenting moral problems of both kinds; and thus to "go between the horns" of the central ethical dilemma in clinical research – of how to ensure full respect for the dignity and rights of individual participants while seeking knowledge to benefit communities and society at large.

Media and scholarly attention to the shortfalls and abuses of clinical research on populations in poor societies now contributes to much-needed public debates in rich and poor societies alike about the moral responsibilities of investigators and their sponsors and the rights of participants in clinical trials. But debates alone cannot bring about reform, any more than codes of ethics or law suits. It is high time that national and international agencies, pharmaceutical companies, universities, investigators, and advocacy organizations co-operate in shaping strong international supervision and regulations governing research wherever it is undertaken.

## References


1 Shapiro AK, Shapiro E. The placebo: is it much ado about nothing? In: Harrington A, ed. *The placebo effect: an interdisciplinary exploration.* Cambridge: Harvard University Press, 1997.

2 Taylor J. *Ductor dubitandum or the rule of conscience.* London: 1660. Book III:84.

3 Bok S. *Lying: moral choice in public and private life, 3rd ed.* New York: Vintage, 1999:223–4.

4 Cassell EJ. The principles of the Belmont report revisited: how have respect for persons, beneficence, and justice been applied to clinical medicine? *Hastings Center Report* Jul–Aug 2000;**30**:17.

5 Principles of Medical Ethics of the American Medical Association, Principle II.

6 Code of Ethics of the American Medical Association, 1847, Ch. I, Art. I, Par. 4.

7 O'Neill O. Paternalism and partial autonomy. In: Windt PY, Appleby PC, Battin MP, *et al. Ethical issues in the professions.* Englewood Cliffs: Prentice-Hall, 1989.

8 Bok S. MDs' delusion: placebos do no harm. *Am Med News* July 1/8 1983:96.

9 Kohn LT, Corrigan JM, Donaldson MS, eds. *To err is human: building a safer health system.* Committee on Quality of Health Care in America, Institute of Medicine, Washington, DC: National Academy Press, 1999:1–16.

10 Bok S. Impaired physicians: what should patients know? *Camb Q Healthcare Ethics* 1993;**2**:331–40.

11 Hahn RA. The nocebo phenomenon: scope and foundations. In: Harrington A, ed. *The placebo effect: an interdisciplinary exploration.* Cambridge: Harvard University Press, 1997.

12 *Washington Post*, June 17, 2000:21.

13 Harrington A. Introduction. In: Harrington A, ed. *The placebo effect: an interdisciplinary exploration.* Cambridge: Harvard University Press, 1997:1.

14 Cabot R. The use of truth and falsehood in medicine: an experimental study. *Am Med* 1903;**5**:344–9. Reprinted in: Reiser SJ, Dyck AJ, Curran WJ, eds. *Ethics in medicine.* Cambridge: MIT Press, 1977:219.

15 Kessel RW. Doctors who lie. *J Med Ethics* 1992;**18**:49.

16 Shapiro AK. Iatroplacebogenics. *Int Pharmacopsychiatry* 1969;**2**:215–48.

17 Katz J. *The silent world of doctor and patient.* New York: Free Press, 1986:189–95.

18 Brody H. The doctor as therapeutic agent: a placebo effect research agenda. In: Harrington A, ed. *The placebo effect: an interdisciplinary exploration.* Cambridge: Harvard University Press, 1997:77–92.

19 Katz J. *The silent world of doctor and patient.* New York: Free Press, 1986:194.

20 Bok S. The ethics of giving placebos. *Scientific American* 1974;**231**(5):17–23.

21 Talbot M. The placebo prescription. *New York Times Magazine* January 9, 2000.

22 Beecher HK. The powerful placebo. *JAMA* 1955;**159**:1602–8.

23 Beecher HK. Ethics and clinical research. *N Engl J Med* 1966;**274**:1354–60.

24 Dresser R. Time for new rules on human subjects research? *Hastings Center Report* Nov/Dec, 1998:35–36.

25 Moreno J, Caplan AL, Wolpe PR. Updating protections for human subjects involved in research. Project on Informed Consent, Human Research Ethics Group. *JAMA* 1998;**280**:1951–8.

26 Rothman DJ. The shame of medical research. *New York Review of Books* Nov 30, 2000:60–4.

27 Moutsos SE, Sapira JD, Scheib ET, Shapiro AP. An analysis of the placebo effect in hospitalized hypertensive patients. *Clin Pharmacol Ther* 1967;**8**:676–83.
28 Department of Health and Human Services. *Federal Register* 56, June 18, 1991. 45 CFR:46:101–46.
29 National Institutes of Health. *Informed consent in research involving human participants.* RFA OD-97-001. NIH Guide 25. No 32. 199:1–18.
30 Bok S. Informed consent in tests of patient reliability. *JAMA* 1992;**267**:1118–19.
31 American Psychological Association. *Ethical principles of psychologists and code of conduct.* 1992, 3.03.
32 Bok S. Shading the truth in seeking informed consent for research purposes. *Kennedy Institute of Ethics Journal* 1995;**5**(1):1–17.
33 Council for International Organizations of Medical Sciences, World Health Organization. *International ethical guidelines for biomedical research involving human subjects.* Geneva, 1993:16–17.
34 Capron AM. Informed consent in catastrophic disease research and treatment. *Univ Pa Law Rev* December 1974;**123**:364–76.
35 American Academy of Pediatrics, Committee on Drugs. Guidelines for the ethical conduct of studies to evaluate drugs in pediatric populations (RE9503). *Pediatrics* 1995:**95**:286–94.
36 Jetter A. Efforts to test drugs on children hasten drive for research guidelines. *New York Times* September 12, 2000: D7.
37 Dembner A. Dangerous dosage. *Boston Globe* February 18, 2001:1.
38 Stolberg G. Children test new medicines despite doubts. *New York Times* February 11, 2001:1,24.
39 Alderson P. Did children change, or the guidelines? *Bull Med Ethics* August 1999;**150**:38–44.
40 Jetter A. Trying to end guesswork in dosing children. *New York Times* September 12, 2000: D7.
41 Michels R. Are research ethics bad for our mental health? *N Engl J Med* 1999;**340**:1427–30.
42 Capron AM. Ethical and human-rights issues in research on mental disorders that may affect decision-making capacity. *N Engl J Med* 1999;**340**:1430–4.
43 World Medical Association. *Declaration of Helsinki.* Edinburgh, October 2000. Articles 13, 22.
44 World Medical Association. *Declaration of Helsinki.* Edinburgh, October 2000. Article 5.
45 Proposed revision, article 19, cited in: Brennan TA. Proposed revisions to the Declaration of Helsinki – will they weaken the ethical principles underlying human research? *N Engl J Med* 1999;**341**:529.
46 World Medical Association. *Declaration of Helsinki.* Edinburgh, October 2000. Article 29.
47 Brennan TA. Proposed revisions to the Declaration of Helsinki – will they weaken the ethical principles underlying human research? *N Engl J Med* 1999;**341**:527–30.
48 Levine RJ. The need to revise the Declaration of Helsinki *N Engl J Med* 1999;**341**:531–4.
49 Rothman KJ, Michels KB, Baum M. For and against: The Declaration of Helsinki should be strengthened. BMJ 2000;**321**:442–5.
50 Temple RJ. Placebo controlled trials and active controlled trials: ethics and inference. This volume, chapter 10.
51 Rothman KJ, Michels KB. When is it appropriate to use a placebo arm in a trial? This volume, chapter 11.
52 See *Washington Post* six-part series: The body hunters. December 17–22, 2000, and the responses to the series including by pharmaceutical companies; for example by Pfizer at *http://www.pfizer.com*.
53 World Medical Association. *Declaration of Helsinki.* Edinburgh, October 2000. Article 8.
54 Levine CA. A world of research subjects: placebos and HIV: lessons learned. *Hastings Center Report* Nov–Dec, 1998:43–8.
55 *Ibid.* For debate regarding the ethical aspects involved, see also Angell M. The ethics of clinical research in the third world. *N Engl J Med* 1997;**337**:847–9; Varmus H, Satcher D. Ethical complexities of conducting research in developing countries. *N Engl J Med* 1997;**337**:1003–5; Brennan TA. Proposed revisions to the Declaration of Helsinki – will they weaken the ethical principles underlying human research? *N Engl J Med* 1999;**341**:527–30; Levine RJ. The need to revise the Declaration of Helsinki. *N Engl J Med* 1999;**341**:531–4.

# *Section 2:*
# Elucidating placebo effects: explanatory mechanisms

# 4: Explanatory mechanisms for placebo effects: cultural influences and the meaning response

DANIEL E MOERMAN

**Summary**

In this chapter, I reconceptualize elements of the "placebo effect" as the *meaning response*. The meaning response is defined as *the physiological or psychological effects of meaning in the treatment of illness*. Much of what is called the placebo effect – meaning responses elicited with inert medications – is a special case of the meaning response, as is the "nocebo effect". Several implications of this reconceptualization are described, and emphasis is placed on the idea that meaning effects accompany *any* effective medical treatment.

## Introduction

A few years ago, Anne Harrington wrote that there was a tension in studies of placebos, a tension between the cultural or hermeneutic sciences, those concerned with "meaning", and the natural sciences, roughly committed, she said, to explanations in terms of "mechanisms". "Because placebos as a phenomenon seem to hover ambiguously at the crossroads between these two perspectives, they are at once a frustration and wonderful challenge".[1] In this chapter, I plan to "hover at the crossroad", trying to connect meaning with mechanism.

## Definitions

Placebo effects are, today, most commonly recognized in research medicine where they are among the reasons for the requirement for the randomized controlled trial (RCTs). It is commonly the case that patients who are given inert medications ("dummies", "placebos") in RCTs get well just as do the patients given the drug under study (the "verum"). For this reason, the "placebo effect" is often defined as the response of patients to inert treatments. This definition leads quickly to paradox and ambiguity,[2] largely because it involves a confusion of correlation with cause. All the control group patients had inert tablets, therefore the inert tablets caused their improvement; and similarly, in the experimental group, all the patients had active treatments, therefore the drug caused their improvement. Neither, of course, is a valid claim. I take an alternate approach and define the *meaning response* as *the physiological or psychological effects of meaning in the treatment of illness*; when these responses are elicited after the use of inert or sham treatment, these responses, although still meaning responses, can be called the "placebo effect" when they are desirable and the "nocebo effect" when undesirable. Note that this definition excludes several elements that might help to account for the improvement of some patients in either arm of an RCT that might include "natural history" (some things might "go away by themselves") or regression to the mean, experimenter or subject bias, systematic error in measurement or reporting, and the like; under certain very special and unusual circumstances some improvement may be attributable to "conditioning". Notice that this definition is not phrased in terms of "non-specific" effects; while many elements of the meaning response or placebo effect may seem to be non-specific, they are often quite specific in principle once they are understood. Several examples may make clear what this definition entails.

## Medical treatments are meaningful

### One, two; pink, blue

A group of medical students was asked to participate in a study of two new drugs, one a sedative and the other a stimulant.[3] Each student was given a packet containing either one or two blue or pink tablets; the tablets were inert. Later, the students' responses to a questionnaire indicated that the red tablets tended to act as stimulants while the blue ones acted as depressants; and, two tablets had more effect than one. The response of these students was not to the inertness of the tablets, and cannot easily be accounted for by natural history, conditioning or regression to the mean. Rather, they can be accounted for by the "meanings" in the experiment: pink or red means "up", "hot", "danger", while blue means "down", "cool", "quiet". And, two means more than one.

### Branding

In a British study, 835 women who used analgesics for headache were randomly assigned to one of four groups.[4] One group (D) received aspirin labeled with a widely advertised brand name ("one of the most popular … analgesics in the United Kingdom widely available for many years and supported by extensive advertising"). The other groups received the same aspirin in a plain package (group C), or placebo marked with the same widely advertised brand name (group B), or unmarked placebo (group A). The women took the pills when they had headaches, then reported how they felt an hour later on a 6-point scale (from $-1$ for "Worse" to $+4$ for "Completely better"). "Mean pain relief after one hour for each group ... was: group A (unbranded placebo) 1·78, group B (branded placebo) 2·18, group C (unbranded active) 2·48, and group D (branded active) 2·7". These differences were statistically significant; the active treatment groups reported more pain relief than placebo groups ($F = 40{\cdot}96$, $p < 0{\cdot}001$), and branded preparations provided more pain relief than did non-branded ones ($F = 18{\cdot}84$, $p < 0{\cdot}001$).

In particular, for 435 headaches reported by branded placebo users, 55% were reported as improved after an hour (rated two, three or four on the scale) while only 45% of 410 headaches were reported to be that much better by unbranded placebo users ($\chi^2 = 6{\cdot}76$, $p < 0{\cdot}01$). Aspirin relieves headaches. But so does the knowledge that the pills you are taking are good ones, which you learned on TV.

## Aerobic exercise

In a study of the benefits of aerobic exercise, two groups carried out a 10-week exercise program. One group was told the exercise would enhance their aerobic capacity while another was told the exercise would enhance aerobic capacity and psychological wellbeing. Both groups improved their aerobic capacity; but only the second improved in psychological wellbeing (actually "self-esteem"). The researchers call this "strong evidence ... that exercise may enhance psychological wellbeing via a strong placebo effect".[5]

In the red versus blue pill study, we can correctly (if not very helpfully) classify the responses of the students as "placebo effects". But in the second study, the presence of the brand name enhanced the action of both the inert and the active treatments. It does not seem reasonable to classify the "brand name effect" as a "placebo effect" since there need not be any placebos involved. And calling the consequences of authoritative instruction to the exercisers a "placebo effect" could only come from someone who believes that words are inert, and do not affect the world, someone who has never been told "I love you", or someone who has never read the reviews of a rejected grant proposal. It seems quite reasonable to label all these effects (except, of course, of the aspirin and the exercise) as "meaning responses".*

---

* As this was written during the fall of 2000, I saw a similar use of language in discussions of the effect of new "drag free" suits which might give an edge to Olympic swimmers. *US News and World Report* said "[S]wimming officials aren't convinced this is anything more than the placebo effect. Swimmers excel because they *think* they've got an edge" (Aug 21, 2000, p. 55). "Thinking", in my view, is not inert.

## Chinese astrology

Such fateful effects of meaning can occur in much broader and more diffuse contexts than simple experiments. A large study examined the cause of death of 28 169 adult Chinese Americans and nearly half a million randomly selected matched "white" controls, all from California. It was found that "Chinese Americans, but not whites, die significantly earlier than normal (1·3–4·9 yr) if they have a combination of disease and birth year which Chinese astrology and medicine consider ill fated".[6] For example, among the Chinese Americans whose deaths were attributed to lymphatic cancer (n = 3041), those who were born in "Earth years" – and consequently were deemed, by Chinese medical theory, especially susceptible to diseases involving lumps, nodules, or tumors – had an average age at death (AAD) of 59·7 years; among those born in other years, AAD of Chinese Americans also suffering from lymphatic cancer was 63·6 years, nearly four years longer. Similarly, for Chinese Americans who died of illnesses related to lung diseases (bronchitis, emphysema and asthma), those who were born in "Metal years" – "the Lung [is] the organ of Metal"[7] – had an average AAD of 66·9 years; among those born in other years, AAD of those dying from such lung diseases was 71·9 years, five years longer. Similar differences were found for other sorts of cancers, for heart attack, and for a series of other diseases. No such differences were evident in a large series of "whites" who died of similar causes in the same period; the difference in age of death, for example, from lung diseases for whites born in "metal years" and those born in other years was 0·07 years (26 days). The intensity of the effect was shown to be correlated with "the strength of commitment to traditional Chinese culture".

It is clear from this case that these significant differences in longevity among Chinese Americans (up to six or seven per cent of length of life) is not due to having Chinese genes, but to having Chinese ideas, to knowing the world in Chinese ways. The effects of meaning on health and disease are not restricted to placebos or brand names, but permeate life.

## Sociosomatics

I hope that by now my argument has indicated that the "placebo effect" is only a tiny portion of a much larger field linking social and meaningful processes with human biological ones. Arthur Kleinman has characterized an aspect of these relationships as "sociosomatics",[8] which he describes as "the fundamental dialectic between the body and the social world".[9] While the placebo effect is only a very small piece of that dialectic, it is an important one since it is subject to experimental observation. One can randomly give people inert pills or real drugs and see what happens; one cannot randomize half a group to be Chinese and the other half to be Tahitian.

## Dimensions of the effects of meaning in medicine

The meaning response has many dimensions in medical care.

### Meaning permeates medical treatment

Insofar as medicine is meaningful, it can affect patients, and it can affect the outcome of treatment. Most elements of medicine *are* meaningful, even if practitioners do not intend them to be so. The doctor's costume (the white coat with stethoscope hanging out of the pocket),[10] manner ("enthusiastic" or not), style ("therapeutic" or " experimental"), and language are all meaningful and can be shown to affect the outcome;[11] it has been argued that diagnosis itself is an important form of treatment.[12] Many of these factors have recently been reviewed by Gracely.[13]

Many studies can be cited to document aspects of the therapeutic quality of the practitioner's manner. Perhaps the best of these compared four different factors contributing to the placebo effect: status of the communicator of drug effects (dentist versus technician), attitude of the dentist and attitude of the technician ("warm" versus "neutral"), and message of drug effect ("oversell" versus "undersell"). By far the most significant of these effects was the last. A strong message of the effect of a drug (actually an inert capsule) substantially reduced the patients' reports of the pain of mandibular block injection compared with a weak message, and those who received the weak message reported less pain than a group that received no placebos and no message at all.[14]

In a more recent study of general practice consultation, Thomas showed the effect of a "positive" manner compared with a more matter-of-fact approach on the part of the physician. A series of 200 patients with symptoms but no abnormal physical signs (characteristic of roughly half of office visits to the general practitioner), were randomly assigned to a "positive" consultation with or without a prescription (of a generally neutral drug, 3 mg tablets of thiamine hydrochloride), or a "negative" consultation with or without the same prescription. In the positive consultations, "the patient was given a firm diagnosis and told confidently that he would be better in a few days". In the negative consultations, the doctor said "I cannot be certain of what is the matter with you". In a survey of patients two weeks later, 64% of positive consultation patients said they were better, while only 39% of those who had negative consultations thought they were better ($p < 0{\cdot}001$). Receiving a treatment in this study made no difference; physician attitude overrode any considerations of the pills patients might have received.[15] The physician had an effect but the placebos did not.

Such physician attitudes can be conveyed to patients in extremely subtle and delicate ways. Gracely has described a phased experiment in which dental patients were told they would receive either placebo (which might reduce the pain of third molar extraction, or might do nothing), naloxone

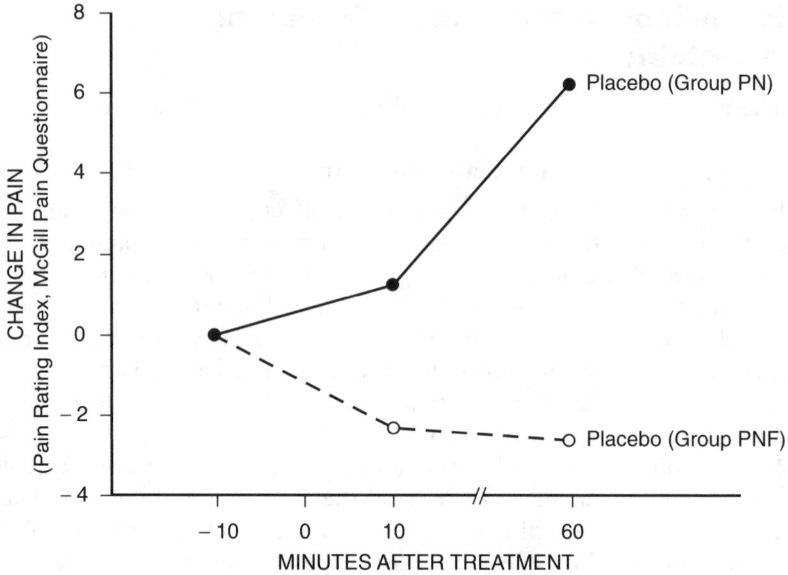


**Change in pain rating index between baseline (10 min before injection) and 10 and 60 min after administration of placebo.**

PN = group that could have either received placebo or naloxone.
PNF = group that could have received placebo, naloxone, or fentanyl (PNF).

Figure 4.1 Physician effects in placebo treatment can be very subtle.[16]

(which might increase their pain, or do nothing), fentanyl (which might reduce their pain, or do nothing), or no treatment at all. Subjects were all recruited from the same patient stream, with consistent selection criteria by the same staff. In the first phase of the study, clinicians (but not patients) were told fentanyl was not yet a possibility because of administrative problems with the study protocol, yielding the PN group. In the second phase, clinicians were told that patients might indeed receive fentanyl, yielding the PNF group; see Figure 4.1. Placebo treated patients during the second phase experienced significant pain reduction from their inert treatment while those in the first group did not.[16] The only apparent difference between the two groups was that the clinicians knew that the first would not get fentanyl and the second group might (although none represented in the figure actually did; they all received only placebo).

It is often suggested that one should use drugs quickly before they lose their effectiveness (this quip has been attributed to several people, among them the 19th century French physician Armand Trousseau[17] and William Osler[18]). In particular, there is evidence to suggest that the effectiveness of drugs declines as new drugs come along. In Figure 4.2, the results of a large series of studies of two different treatments for peptic ulcer disease are plotted by year of publication. It is, of course, research physicians, not patients, who are aware of the significance and possible value of new drugs.

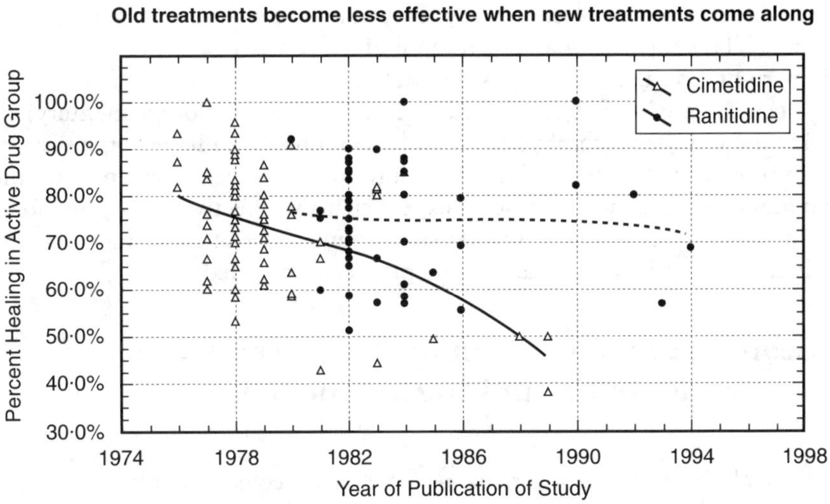


Figure 4.2 Two sets of trials of treatments of peptic ulcer disease.[44]

While there is strong evidence for such "physician effects", there is little to show that "patient effects" are very important. A mass of research in the 1970s designed to identify "placebo reactors" produced only inconsistent and contradictory findings.[19–21]

## Physician and patient need not share the same meanings

It is interesting that, in some of these cases, doctor and patient may not share the same system of meaning. Traditional Chinese Medicine is based in large part on the manipulation of *chi* using a combination of herbal treatments, acupuncture and so on.[7] Acupuncture, in particular, has become quite popular in the West.[22] Yet few Western patients know much about *chi* or its manipulation, and most would have difficulty fitting such knowledge into their school-based understanding of physiology – nerves, blood vessels, and so on. Their knowledge of oriental medicine in general and acupuncture in particular is probably based on their watching Bill Moyers on public television, where they may have learned that "acupuncture works" although for no evident reasons. Cassidy has found that, even after six months of acupuncture care, American patients still have a very sketchy understanding of the system, at least in terms authentic to oriental medicine, yet they are very enthusiastic about their care which they deem extremely effective.[23]

In conventional medicine, too, the conceptualization of illness is often quite distinct for patient and physician. The contrast of the physician's view of "hypertension" ("a disease of unknown origin, a risk factor for stroke") and the patient's view of "hypertension" ("a physical illness characterized by excessive nervousness caused by untoward social stress") is a case in point.[24] This suggests that the strength of a physician's convictions is more important than the convictions themselves.

Regardless of the style of medicine (conventional, complementary) or what the fit is between physician and patient understandings of the system, it is important to recognize that, until there is clear evidence to the contrary, it makes most sense to expect that the effectiveness of *any* form of medical treatment will include some component of meaning response, whether or not it is the meaning the physician intended.

## Meaning responses can be demonstrated in surgery as well as in internal medicine

### BIMAL

The classic example of surgical placebo effects comes from two studies of the bilateral internal mammary artery ligation (BIMAL) as a treatment for angina;[25,26] in this procedure, the idea was that ligating the mammary arteries would increase the amount of blood flow to the heart via a set of arteries postulated to exist for a variety of (rather obscure) reasons which were (none the less) easy to convey to patients. Combining these two studies, 24 of 33 patients (73%) showed substantial improvement on patient and physician assessment while nine did not. Patients in both studies showed increased exercise tolerance and reduced nitroglycerine consumption. Patients who received the sham surgery (local anesthesia, chest incision, and artery exposed but not ligated) did somewhat better overall as 10 of 12 (83%) showed substantial improvement. While the operation, which was becoming quite popular at the time, quickly disappeared from practice after publication of these two studies, it is worth noting that these effectiveness rates (and those reported by the proponents of the procedure at the time, for example, see Kitchell, *et al.*[27]) are much the same as those achieved by contemporary treatments like coronary artery bypass or beta blockers; to my knowledge, no double blind trials of the former have been carried out.

### TMR

Meaning responses may occur in the most contemporary forms of heart surgery:

> "PLC, The Heart Laser, opening new *bloodlines*: What are *bloodlines*? *Bloodlines* are conduits created by the Heart Laser through the wall of the left ventricle. These *bloodlines* allow oxygen rich blood to saturate the oxygen-starved heart tissue".

At least that is what it says on the website of the company that makes the laser, PLC Medical Systems, Inc.[28]

Transmyocardial laser revascularization (TMR) is the most recent surgical approach to angina. A company spokesperson told me that they estimate they were approaching a total of 6000 procedures worldwide (in Spring 2000) explaining that, after the procedure was covered by Medicare, it quickly gained widespread acceptance in the medical world (Floody P, personal communication).

**Elements of transmyocardial revascularization**

In TMR, an incision is made in the side of the chest between two ribs. The pericardium is removed, and the myocardium is exposed. A laser (several different types are used) is touched to the surface of the heart, and a laser beam is fired into the heart, presumably to make a channel thru the heart. Usually 30 to 50 such channels are made. The idea is that this will make a sort of substitute artery, a "bloodline" in the terms of one company, thru which blood will flow providing oxygen-rich blood directly to the heart muscle. The pericardium is replaced, and the chest is closed. More recently, a less invasive version of the surgery, using a catheterized version of the laser (percutaneous transmyocardial laser revascularization), has been developed, for example see Bortone, *et al.*[29]

By the mid '90s, a number of fairly large trials had been carried out. The procedure was reserved for people who were not healthy enough to be treated by the standard techniques (CABG, angiography), and who had very serious, unstable end-stage angina, that is, for very sick people. The results were quite remarkable: success rates were in the range of 75% to 90%. Successful improvement in these studies required a two stage improvement in the four stage Canadian Cardiovascular Society system; that is a lot of improvement for such very sick people.

For a history of the procedure, see Kantor B, *et al.*[30]

The interesting thing is that no one really knows how or why this operation "works". The "bloodlines" close up in a matter of hours, and there is no evidence that the myocardial blood flow actually increases by the best type of evidence, perfusion imaging.[31] But people do get better (see box). Why? Some say that the laser beams disrupt the nerves of the heart, and denervate the affected areas[32] but others seem to show quite clearly that this is not the case.[33,34] There is some reason to believe that the scarring process may lead to angiogenesis, but there is little evidence that this has any effect on angina.

A number of observers suggest that, by analogy with the bilateral internal mammary artery ligation, the improvements observed may be due to the meaning response (or in their terms, the placebo effect), for example see Kantor, *et al.*, Lange, *et al.*[30,35]

While surgeons remain enthusiastic about the procedure,[36] one interesting study showed that, in sheep, TMR led to angiogenesis in lased channels, but "failed to improve myocardial function";[37] one would not expect much of a meaning response from sheep.

And most recently, Dr Martin Leon and a group of colleagues from across the US have enrolled 300 patients in a placebo controlled trial of a related procedure similar in form to angioplasty. A laser catheter is inserted in the femoral artery and threaded up into the left ventricle; the laser pulses are administered from inside out; this requires much less invasive surgery. These patients were very sick:

- all were rated as class III or IV on the 4-stage Canadian scale
- 90% had previously had bypass surgery
- 65% had previously had heart attacks
- all had had angioplasty within the previous 4 months
- yet they were relatively young people, averaging about 62 years in age.

Patients were randomly assigned to one of three groups, a high-dose group (20–25 laser punctures), a low-dose group (10–15 laser punctures), or a mock procedure with only simulated laser treatment. All three groups displayed similar impressive improvement six months after surgery on all objective and subjective measures which were observed. Exercise tolerance was increased in all three groups. The percentage of patients who improved two or more classes on the Canadian scale ranged from 25% (high dose) to 33% (placebo) to 39% (low dose). Frequency of angina declined, and physical functioning and disease perception scores increased, in all three groups. None of the modest differences between the three groups was statistically significant.[38]

A few years ago, before the FDA approved this laser treatment, Dr Alan G Johnson, in an article titled "Surgery as a placebo" in the *Lancet* said (with notable prescience), "Electrical machines have great appeal to patients, and recently anything with the word 'laser' attached to it has caught the imagination".[39] It may be worth suggesting that doctors, as well as patients, find their imaginations fired by lasers.

## Other placebo surgery

Similar results – 70% improvement in objective and subjective measures in both surgical treatment and surgical sham groups – have been shown for Meniere's disease (an inner ear disturbance causing loss of balance where patients tend to fall towards the affected ear), with a three year follow up.[40]

In a review of 2504 diskectomies for lumbar disk disease, 346 patients were found to have no herniation (this might then be called a "diagnostic diskectomy"); regardless, many of these patients subsequently experienced partial (38·4%) or complete (37·0%) relief of sciatic pain (total = 75·4%) after their surgery.[41]

More recently, in a prospective, randomized placebo controlled trial, patients with osteoarthritis of the knee were given one of three arthroscopic procedures. The placebo patients were put to sleep, draped, examined, injected with local anesthetic, and given three stab wounds in the skin with a scalpel. No arthroscopic instruments were inserted, but "a standard arthroscopic debridement was simulated as closely as possible in the event the patient was not totally unaware during the event".[42] This surgery was compared to standard arthroscopic debridement and to arthroscopic lavage (a diagnostic arthroscopy). In this pilot study, the five patients receiving the sham procedure responded essentially the same as did those who received the full surgical treatment, and as do similar patients in normal clinical practice: they "reported decreased frequency, intensity and duration of knee pain" six months after surgery. A full scale study is currently underway with 180 patients.

While studies such as these are rare, their results are consistent with the notion that medical acts are meaningful, and that meaning has an effect on patients. Surgery is particularly meaningful: surgeons are among the elite of medical practitioners; the shedding of blood is inevitably meaningful in and of itself. In addition, surgical procedures usually have compelling rational explanations which drug treatments often do not. The logic of these procedures ("we'll clean up a messy joint", or "we'll get more blood to your heart") is much more sensible and understandable, especially for people in a culture rich in machines and tools, than is the logic of non-steroidal anti-inflammatory drugs ("which may block the production of prostaglandins which seem somehow to be involved in the inflammatory process").

## Meaning responses can be extremely variable

It is common for researchers to cite Beecher's famous paper of 1955 to the effect that placebos are effective 35% of the time.[43] House officers have been shown to estimate placebo effects as occurring less frequently than that, averaging about 20% while nurses estimate much lower still.[44] (My experience over the years teaching these issues suggests that nurses are among the very hardest to convince that inert medications, or meaningful interactions, can affect illness or disease.) Indeed, inert treatment can be effective far more often than either of those estimates, or, indeed, Beecher's estimate. In a series of 117 RCTs of cimetidine or ranitidine for treatment of endoscopically diagnosed ulcer, ulcer healing (also endoscopically confirmed) after four or six weeks of therapy with inert pills ranged from 0% to 100% with a mean of 35·5 and a standard deviation of 16%.[45] To say that "the placebo group healing rate is 35%" under these circumstances is rather like saying "American men are five feet ten inches tall" because that is the mean adult stature.

In these 117 studies, the drug group healing rate is also highly variable, from about 38% to 100%. The correlation between the placebo rate and the drug rate is 0·43 ($p < 0·0001$); the higher the placebo effectiveness, the higher the drug effectiveness.

## Formal factors account for some variation

What sorts of factors account for this variation? The research on this issue is in its infancy, and much remains to be learned. There are formal factors which seem to make a difference: capsule or tablet size or color can make a difference in the effect of drugs.

### *Color*

In addition to the study with medical students already mentioned, others have shown such variations. In one study, the tranquilizer oxazepam relieved symptoms of anxiety better when presented in a green tablet, while depressive symptoms were relieved better when the drug was presented in a yellow tablet.[46] A Czech study of patients with a variety of somatic and psychological problems showed that capsules with warm colors acted as stimulants and cool ones acted as sedatives.[47] This finding has been found generally; a systematic review "suggests that green and blue may have more sedative effects and red and orange may have more stimulant effects".[48]

But meaning can be more complex than this. In an Italian study of the sedative effect of inert tablets, while women preferred blue tablets (as is ordinarily the case), men did not; blue tablets prolonged their time until sleep.[49] In Italy, the color blue seems to have different meanings for men and women. For Italian women, blue is the color of the dress of the Virgin Mary; since the Mother of God is a very reassuring and protective figure for many Italian women, it seems reasonable that blue sleeping pills should be effective for them. By contrast, for Italian men, blue is the color of Azzurrii, the national Italian soccer team. Blue (or *azure*) means success, powerful movement, strength and grace on the field, and, generally, great excitement. So it is at least plausible that blue sleeping tablets would work less well for Italian men than for women. Another apparent exception to the notion of blue pills as tranquilizing is that of Viagra, marketed in a blue pill, prominently displayed in advertising, its lozenge shape usually pointing upward to the right. The Oxford English Dictionary, reflecting the racy aspect of the color blue notes that it can mean indecent or obscene, smutty or libidinous, as in a "blue movie".* Particular cultural details, like soccer team names, can disrupt otherwise widespread relationships of meaning; but the inherent polysemy of richly meaningful symbols also requires close attention to detail.

In any case, a recent Dutch study has shown that stimulant medications tend to be marketed in "hot" colors – red, yellow, or orange tablets – while depressants tend to be marketed in "cool" colors – blue, green, or purple tablets.[48] One can consider "one-a-day" vitamins to be among the most neutral of medications; they are not imagined to have immediate or dramatic effects. Observations suggest that vitamins are usually marketed

---

* Robert Hahn suggested this line of thought.

in tablets with pale pastel tones. Whether these marketing decisions are made consciously or otherwise, they are amenable to a rational analysis.

*Number and type*

In addition to the study with medical students, several others have shown that two pills work better than one.[50] One study showed that patients receiving three different placebos for two weeks each did better than patients receiving the same placebo for six weeks.[51] Similarly, a study of antacid treatment of ulcers had an interesting element.

> Seven patients were switched to a [randomly selected] second batch of medications because of continuing peptic discomfort of high intensity after three days of therapy. Due to lack of pain relief after the first switch, one patient was switched twice. The sequence of switching was from placebo to placebo to placebo again. On the third batch of placebos, the patient obtained pain relief and his ulceration healed after four weeks of therapy.[52]

The number of placebo tablets taken can have real clinical significance. In 71 RCTs of cimetidine or ranitidine for endoscopically diagnosed ulcer disease, control group patients took placebos for four weeks. In studies where they took two placebos a day, 249 of 751 patients (33%) were healed (endoscopically verified) while in studies where they took four placebos a day, 427 of 1129 (38%) were healed; this difference is statistically significant, $\chi^2 = 4{\cdot}26$, $p < 0{\cdot}05$.[45] This same proposition has been demonstrated for the same condition (four placebos per day: 44·2% healing rate; two per day: 36·2%) but with much more statistical precision in a formal meta-analysis.[53] In this study, the authors very carefully considered other variations between the studies which might have accounted for the differences; none of the adjustments they could make – given the published data – diminished the difference. For example, patients in the 4 per day trials were "slightly more often male, were somewhat younger, and were more often smokers. Male gender, younger age, and smoking have been associated with lower healing rates [for ulcer disease], so adjusting for these baseline characteristics would have resulted in a larger rather than smaller healing rate difference". The authors note that, although they adjusted for all possible confounding factors for which data were available, they could "not rule out that in this non-randomized comparison the observed difference was caused by some unrecognized confounding factor or factors". Regardless, given what is currently known about these differences, the Number Needed to Treat for a beneficial effect, the $NNT_B$, for four placebos a day versus two per day is 13.

In addition to the number of pills, other factors can modify efficacy. One study has shown capsules of chlordiazepoxide to be more effective against anxiety than tablets of the same drug,[54] and parenteral placebo has been shown to be more effective than oral placebo several times, for hypertension,[55] rheumatoid arthritis,[56] and migraine headache,[57] among others.

## Cultural factors account for some variation

Again looking at 117 ulcer trials, three studies from Brazil demonstrate that placebo healing rates there are much lower than in other countries. The placebo healing rate is seven per cent in Brazil versus 36% in the rest of the world ($t = 3{\cdot}13$, $p = 0{\cdot}0016$). Similarly, the placebo healing rate in six studies in Germany averages 59%, twice as high as in the rest of the world ($t = 3{\cdot}88$, $p = 0{\cdot}00018$) and three times that of two of its neighboring countries, Denmark and the Netherlands, where, in five studies, it averages 22% ($t = 3{\cdot}21$, $p = 0{\cdot}011$). For ulcer patients taking placebo, the $NNT_B$ for being German (not Danish or Dutch) is 3.*

The placebo effect is not always high in Germany. In a series of 32 comparable trials of treatment of moderate hypertension, active drug treatment reduced diastolic blood pressure (DBP) by an average of 10·9 mm Hg (range 7 to 21) while placebo treatment reduced DBP by 3·5 mm Hg (range –5 to 9; in two studies, placebo-treated patients had an increase in mean DBP). The clearest international variation in these data is opposite to the findings in the ulcer data. The mean placebo group change in DBP in four German trials is 0·25 mm Hg, while in the remaining 29 trials it is 3·9 ($t = 2{\cdot}6$, $p = 0{\cdot}013$); one study that showed an *increase* of 5 mm Hg in DBP with placebo treatment was done in Germany. The drug group change in the German studies is the same as in the remaining trials. Hence, Germany, with the highest placebo healing rates in ulcer disease, shows the least improvement in placebo treatment of hypertension. High rates of placebo effect seem to vary by medical condition within national cultures.[45]

That there should be such substantial differences in outcome with the same treatments for the same conditions in places with such deeply shared traditions of the life sciences and biomedicine seems surprising until one becomes more aware of the deep differences in understanding of illness between these closely related cultures. Thus the German experience of hypotensive drugs may be affected by their broad concern for a condition – *Herzinsuffienz* – which generally does not exist in the United States, France, Great Britain, and so on. This syndrome and its scope have been described in some detail;[58] suffice it to say that German physicians routinely treat low blood pressure and other symptoms of "heart insufficiency" in a very large proportion of older adults, treatment which, in the US, would probably be considered malpractice. The French have their *crise de foie*, *fatigué*, and *spasmophilie*,[59] while the Americans have their nearly unique infatuations

* Such differences found in different countries could have additional explanations. There could be systematic differences in study populations or disease characteristics. Ulcer disease is now known to be due in part to infection with *Helicobacter pylori*; if Brazilians had a much higher prevalence of such infection than Germans, it might account for some of these differences. When these studies were done, the role of *H. pylori* was unknown. While this might account for some differences, it seems unlikely that it would account for the differences between the Germans and the neighboring Dutch and Danes.

with "sinus", "low-grade viruses", and multiple personality (or dissociative identity) disorder.[60] These different understandings of illness and suffering can have as significant an effect on medical treatment as can the more familiar (and exotic) "culture bound syndromes" from around the world like *susto*, *amok*, and *latah*, all of which, Hahn reminds us, encourage a focus on the ways in which "culture, psychology and physiology [are] ... mutually relevant across cultural and nosological boundaries".[61]

## "Adherence" and placebos

One of the strangest examples of variation in the effect of inert medication comes from a series of studies which show significant difference in outcome depending on the amount of medication patients consume. Table 4.1 summarizes five such studies. The first row in the table gives the results from a very large study of the use of cholesterol-lowering drugs by individuals who had experienced myocardial infarction. After five years, there was no difference in the 5 year mortality rates for patients taking clofibrate and those taking placebo (20·0% v 20·9%; $z = -0{\cdot}60$, $p = 0{\cdot}55$). However, good adherers to the clofibrate regimen (those who took more than 80% of their drugs; three tablets three times per day) did much better than poor adherers (15·0% v 24·6% mortality). And, good adherers to the placebo regimen likewise did much better than poor adherers (15·1% v 28·2% mortality). The other cases – infection after chemotherapy for cancer patients, one year relapse for schizophrenia, and beta blocker treatment for men and women who had survived a serious myocardial infarction – show similar results.

These results are hard to interpret for a number of reasons. The most significant one is that patients can not be randomly assigned to good versus poor adherent groups; the groups are, somehow, self selected. And, interestingly, not much is known about how and why people do, or do not, adhere to drug regimens. In most of the studies reported, there were no apparent differences between the adherent and non-adherent segments of the samples; for all factors (except the study outcome) the groups looked as if they *had* been randomly assigned. In the case of the clofibrate trial, there was some evidence that the less adherent patients had "a somewhat higher prevalence of baseline factors [associated with mortality]".[62] Controlling for these factors with a multiple regression analysis adjusted the five year mortality for adherent placebo patients to 16·4% versus 25·8% for less-adherent patients; that is, it made practically no difference. The Canadian study of amiodarone for survivors of acute myocardial infarction, with similar outcome, considered a broad range of medical and social factors to attempt to account for the differences; no single factor predicted the difference in both placebo and drug groups.[63] This is a very compelling problem for which, at the moment, there is no reasonable explanation. Adherence may be associated with several other important factors in health and meaning, considered next.

Table 4.1 "Adherence" and response to drug and placebo.

| Drug tested | N | Outcome | Drug group | | Placebo group | | Source (ref. no.) |
|---|---|---|---|---|---|---|---|
| | | | Adherent* | Not adherent | Adherent* | Not adherent | |
| clofibrate | 3760 | 5 year mortality | 15·0% | 24·6% | 15·1% | 28·2% | 62 |
| antibiotics | 150 | infection after chemotherapy | 18·1% | 53·0% | 32·2% | 64·0% | 99 |
| chlorpromazine | 374 | 1 year relapse | 13·0% | 57·0% | 40·0% | 80·0% | 100 |
| propranolol (men) | 2175 | 1 year mortality | 1·4% | 4·2% | 3·0% | 7·0% | 101 |
| propranolol (women) | 602 | 1 year mortality | 4·5% | 8·7% | 6·8% | 19·0% | 102 |
| amiodarone | 1141 | 2 year all cause mortality | 7·4% | 14·8% | 8·8% | 18·7% | 63 |

*Adherent patients took more than 75% or 80% of medication (65% in amiodarone study); non adherent patients took less.

**Disclosure**

In the 1980s, James Pennebaker began a series of experiments with college students. He randomly assigned half of a group of them to write for about 20 minutes about their very deepest thoughts and feelings about the most traumatic experience of their whole lives. The other half of the group was asked to write about everyday, ordinary phenomena: to describe the laboratory, or the furniture in it, etc. The students in the first group took to the task with intensity and imagination, often writing long and complex stories, and displaying significant emotional responses; many students cried while writing. Even so, most reported that they enjoyed the experiment, and would readily do it again. It was psychologically positive. Pennebaker followed up on the students for the rest of the school year. He found that, among other things, the emotional writers were admitted to the student health service significantly less often than students who had written about everyday items.[64]

This experiment has subsequently been repeated many times around the world, with corporate executives, prison inmates, medical students, people with chronic pain, men laid off from their jobs, and Holocaust survivors. Almost always the results are the same: there is a positive health effect of some sort. In more recent work, Pennebaker has analyzed the content of such writing, and compared it to the outcomes (which are, inevitably, variable). Those with the most health improvement are writers who construct the most coherent stories and express most clearly their negative emotions.[65] In our terms, they are the ones who create the most meaningful story out of their pain, deciding most effectively what to leave out, and what to put in.

**Self-assessed health**

Nearly 7000 Californians over 60 were asked one question in 1965 "In general, would you say your health is: excellent, very good, good, fair, [or] poor?". Nine years later, adjusting for their ages, men who had rated their health as excellent were 2·33 times as likely to be alive as were men who rated their health as poor; women were 5·1 times as likely to be alive when they rated their health as excellent.[66] In a follow up study 17 years after the study began, the combined, age-adjusted advantage for those who had rated their health as excellent remained: those who professed excellent health were 2·3 times as likely to be alive as were those who rated it to be poor.[67]

The most subtle work on this issue has been done by Ellen Idler of Rutgers University and her colleagues. She has tried to tease out just what it is that causes this effect, trying to find what personal characteristics people have who report excellent health compared to those who do not. She had similar results in a study of 2800 men and women over 65 living in New Haven, Connecticut.[68] Men who rated their health as excellent were nearly seven times less likely to die within four years than those who rated it as poor; women with excellent self-rated health were 3·1 times as likely to die as those with poor self-rated health. Idler included a whole range of other factors in her analysis; among them were the subjects' disease history, age, smoking behavior, and weight; their medical history and health status: whether they had recently been hospitalized or in a nursing home, and the number and kind of medications they took; the support they had available, the number of friends and family, their religious activity and religiosity, their attitudes and moods. Several of these (age, smoking) predicted some portion of four year mortality, but none had as much effect as did global self-assessment of health. "Self-rated health", Idler writes,"appears to have a unique, predictive, and thus far inexplicable relationship with mortality". Other research like that by Maruta[69] shows that there is a general relationship between optimism and longevity; but Idler's work shows that there is only a modest relationship between the *specific* evaluation of one's health, and the *general* assessment of one's attitude to life.

Idler suggests two explanations for these observations, first, that the story people tell about themselves is a self-fulfilling prophesy, that the attitude itself is protective of health, and, second, that people simply know themselves better than anyone else does. These need not, of course, be mutually exclusive. And, as with Pennebaker's work, your answer to the question "What is the overall status of your health?" may just be one of the shortest, and most meaningful, stories you can tell.

A number of these factors – adherence, disclosure, self-rated health – may be related. It may be, for example, that those with lower self-rated health have lower levels of adherence than others; some studies might be interpreted as saying that "knowing" that their health is poor, patients may feel it is a waste of time to take medication.[70] This is obviously testable. It may be that medicine simply has less meaning for patients who take less of it. There may be cultural differences in compliance, or in self-rated health, or in the consequences of these matters. These and several other combinations offer a number of testable hypotheses.

## Meaning responses may be higher in clinical than experimental settings

There is little evidence available to indicate that what happens in clinical trials has much relationship to what happens in actual medical practice. There is some evidence to indicate that treatment may be more effective in practice than it is in research.

### Abandoned treatments of angina pectoris

Benson and McCallie reviewed the reports of a number of treatments for angina pectoris which, in the period before the widespread adoption of controlled trials, were widely utilized, but then later abandoned. They summarized the results of treatment of angina pectoris with methyl xanthines, khellin, vitamin E, ligation of the internal mammary arteries (mentioned above), and Vineberg's implantation of the internal mammary artery. Data from the 13 studies they cite "reveal that subjective improvement was seen in 82·4 ± 9·7 per cent (mean ± SD) ... In addition to subjective improvement, objective changes occurred: the placebo effect increased exercise tolerance [in four studies], reduced nitroglycerin usage [in three studies], and improved electrocardiographic results [in two studies] ... [and in seven studies] relief [lasted] for a year or more".[17]

## Other abandoned treatments

In a similar study of treatments "once considered to be efficacious by their proponents but no longer considered effective based upon later controlled trials", Roberts and co-workers looked at a series of reports on glomectomy for bronchial asthma, levamisole for herpes simplex virus (HSV) infection, photodynamic inactivation for HSV infection, organic solvents (ethyl ether and chloroform) for HSV infection, and gastric freezing for duodenal ulcer. "Despite our current understanding of the inadequacy of these five treatments, enthusiastic adherents reported good or better outcomes for patients ranging from 45% ... for gastric freezing (N = 598) to 89% for photodynamic inactivation (N = 169) ... For a total of 6931 patients treated by these five methods, 2784 (40%) were reported to have had excellent outcomes, 2049 (30%) good outcomes, and 2098 (30%) poor outcomes".[71]

In these cases, apparently inert treatments (but not "dummy pills") seem to have been satisfactory (that is, good or excellent) 70% or 80% of the time, not 35% of the time. The difference between the two circumstances is primarily the attitudes of the physicians. In the studies described by Benson and by Roberts, the providers of these treatments were enthusiastic about them; they had physiological theories they believed in, and treatments which made sense to them, which they could explain to their patients. In RCTs, the same is true, but only half the patients will benefit from this new improvement; and all the patients have had to provide informed consent.*

## Chiropractic and conventional treatment of low back pain

A somewhat different comparison yields a similar result which indicates how context can affect meaning responses. Kaptchuk and colleagues have reviewed the evidence for efficacy of a number of areas in complementary medicine including chiropractic medicine.[74] In nine studies of spinal manipulation therapy for low back pain "three show no difference between manipulation and a sham ..., two are positive for manipulation ..., one is clearly positive for manipulation plus injected drug ..., and ... three trials could be construed as showing some benefit for manipulation over sham

---

* Research on the effects of informed consent on active or inert treatments has had highly variable results; compare, for example Kirsch, *et al.*[72] with Sprafkin, *et al.*[73]

during some course of the complaint". It is, from this perspective, difficult to say that chiropractic manipulation is "better than a placebo". Another meta-analysis of eight studies of chiropractic manipulation comes to similar conclusions: "the available RCTs provided no convincing evidence of the effectiveness of chiropractic for acute or chronic low back pain".[75]

But other comparisons can be made. If there is little evidence that chiropractic is "better than placebo", there is ample evidence to indicate that it is better than conventional medicine for this complaint. In a survey of members of a HMO (Health Maintenance Organization) which provided both types of care, "chiropractic patients were three times as likely as patients of family physicians to report that they were very satisfied with the care they received for low back pain (66% [of 348] v 22%)".[76] In a half dozen such surveys, from 65% to 85% of chiropractic patients express such satisfaction.[74]

Similar results are seen in a Dutch study which randomly assigned patients with low back and neck pain to manual therapy, physiotherapy (exercise, massage, ultrasound, etc.), general medical care (analgesics, home exercise, bed rest), or placebo treatment (detuned shortwave diathermy and detuned ultrasound). At six week follow up, physiotherapy and manual therapy had very similar outcomes and were significantly better than general medical care. Placebo treatment was intermediate, somewhat less effective than the active treatments (only one of four measures was statistically significant), and somewhat better than treatment by general practitioners on two measures (one significant, one not).[77]

One might be able to show that the analgesics and muscle relaxants of general medical care are more effective than placebo for pain and muscle stiffness. So here the paradox is that care which cannot reliably be shown to be better than placebo seems to work better than care which can. Why?

Whatever the details of treatment may be, there is one huge difference between the care one typically receives for low back pain from an MD and from a chiropractor: its *meaningfulness*. Participant observation on my part suggests that the approaches of chiropractors and physicians vary dramatically for this condition; see also Oths.[78] The chiropractor immediately carries out a focused, pointed, attentive examination asking pertinent questions about history, injury, mobility and so on, asking you to bend this way and that, usually taking *x* ray films and showing them to you, pointing out misaligned vertebrae, explaining the course of treatment, its goals and likelihood of success. The walls in a chiropractor's office are frequently hung with large posters displaying the spine, explaining its function and workings; there are colorful brochures explaining the history and value of chiropractic treatment. Occasionally one finds articles, popular or scholarly, photocopied perhaps, showing the results of studies on the effectiveness of chiropractic. One may even see a model of an actual spine with simulated spinal nerves arrayed along it, hanging from a doorknob. The entire experience is validating, encouraging, supportive and positive. We have not yet had an adjustment and we feel better already. The adjustment, on an elaborate adjustable table, is itself replete with satisfying pops and snaps, rolling over, and just enough pain to suggest that something good may come from it.

Contrast this with the physician's attitude. No diagrams. No spine on the doorknob. The advice usually is of the order of "take aspirin, rest in bed, take it easy". Of course, the patient has been doing that for ten days before the appointment, and is there because those things have made no difference. *The Merck Manual* uses the word "malingering" twice: once in the phrase "pathologic malingering", a synonym for Munchausen syndrome, and once in its discussion of low back pain. While it is said to be uncommon, "Inconsistent historic and physical findings on sequential examinations may make one suspicious of this diagnosis". If your back problem is anything but linear and does not heal up quickly, you are suspect. "When suspected, [malingering] can only be established by garnering evidence that the patient is faking". Under these circumstances, the doctor's approach should become that of the lawyer, not the healer. "Direct evidence of malingering may best be acquired by someone other than the physician". The *Manual* does not say more, but one imagines a detective is in order to expose this fraudulent patient.[79]

It is striking that the same symptoms could elicit such varying responses. But surely it is clear which approach is likely to be more meaningful, and hence potentially effective, for the patient with back pain, regardless of what studies about the effectiveness of specific treatments may have found. In this way, the case of chiropractic is similar to the abandoned treatments discussed earlier: 70% or 80% of patients achieve satisfactory treatment outcomes marked by measurable subjective and objective improvement with enthusiastically employed techniques – rich in meaning – which seem not to be substantially more effective than sham treatments in blind trials.

## Meaning responses in other medical systems

It is sometimes suggested – as I suggest for chiropractic – that some medical systems have, over the generations, elaborated their meaningful elements in order to enhance the meaning response; it seems as if many of them do little research to extend the specifics of their systems, and most contemporary research is designed to demonstrate the effectiveness of existing treatments, not to develop new or better ones. (One may wish to say the reverse of conventional medicine, that it has enhanced the specific effectiveness of the system through persistent research in pharmacology and physiology at the same time as it has generally neglected the meaningful; that is not to say the meaningful is not there, but it is not there as the result of deliberate study.) While such a proposition seems plausible, it is hard to demonstrate convincingly in general terms.

### Navajo medicine

Consider an extreme case which points up the difficulties. One of the most complex forms of medical treatment is that developed by the Navajo of the American Southwest. There are a dozen or so major treatments known as Blessingway, Evilway, Holyway and so on, each with many variants. For an example, see Wyman's account of the Blessingway;[80] Sandner gives a rich account of Navajo medicine from a clinician's perspective,[81] and Silko gives the perspective of an artist.[82] Many family members and friends gather for such an event which can last for a week or ten days, and which involves the singing of dozens of complex chants by several highly trained medicine men who also create a series of beautiful drypaintings (or "sandpaintings") – which, in effect, concentrate beauty – on which the sufferer sits. Different herbal infusions are used several times, each containing 30 or 40 different plant medicines which are drunk and rubbed over both the sufferer and all the attending medicine men and other visitors, family and friends. The focus of the event is twofold: the intention is to banish evil, and then to re-establish the beauty (*hózhó*) which has somehow been lost from the sick person's life.[83] This form of healing is "likened to a spiritual osmosis in which the evil in man and the good of deity penetrate the ceremonial membrane in both directions, the former being neutralized by the latter";[84] it is, then, a powerful social experience suffused in meaning.

To determine just which elements of this rich treatment were "active" and how they interacted would require an extraordinary series of studies which compared this system with one lacking the meaningful elements (Placeboway?). Such a scheme would not be Navajo medicine, rather like psychoanalysis without talk, or surgery without the knife. But thinking about a medical system so different from the one we are immersed in – where the meaningful elements are so apparent – might allow us to gain a sense of the fullness of the meaningful dimensions of our own approach to healing.

## Mechanisms in the meaning response

It is, of course, very difficult to specify the mechanisms involved in these processes. This is often the case in internal medicine, and, while undesirable, is not generally a serious problem. For example, it seems plausible that non-steroidal anti-inflammatory agents have their effects by somehow interfering with prostaglandin production, but that this is not clear in detail does not reduce the effectiveness of drugs ranging from willow bark tea to naproxen. The mechanisms of action of the opiates were unclear until research in the 1970s uncovered the endogenous opiates; the drugs were as useful before as after those discoveries. One need not know how a treatment works in order to use it effectively.

## Pain

There is one area where 25 years of (intermittent) research has shown us something of the mechanisms involving meaning responses, namely in pain. Since the pioneering work of Levine and Fields in the late 1970s,[85–87] it has been reasonable to argue that some forms of placebo analgesia involved the production of endogenous opiates which could be blocked by the opiate antagonist naloxone. The matter was not a simple one, and Gracely showed that there may have been more complex mechanisms involved.[88]

More recently, Italian researcher Fabrizio Benedetti has carried out an elegant and ingenious series of experiments clearly showing that one can induce significant analgesia with inert substances, that these effects can be reliably blocked by naloxone, and that they can be enhanced by the cholecystokinin antagonist proglumide (as naloxone blocks opiate action, proglumide has been shown to enhance it); he has also shown that one can induce placebo hyperalgesia (a "nocebo" effect) which can be blocked by proglumide.[89,90] The clear inference here is that the symbolic and meaningful experience of a saline injection can somehow engage the production of endorphins in the brain.

In another study, this same team has shown very clearly that there need not be any placebos in order to evoke these responses. Surgical patients were either given pain medication openly by a physician, or by hidden injection from a pre-programmed infusion machine without any clinician in the room. Patients in the open injection groups (receiving four different analgesics) reported substantially less pain than patients receiving similar doses of hidden analgesic. "By eliminating the placebo component of analgesia by means of hidden injections, ... the effectiveness of ... these analgesics [was] significantly reduced".[91] In this study, since there were no placebos, it seems unwise to call these differences "placebo effects". In an editorial accompanying the paper, Donald Price notes that although the increases in analgesia were not huge – 1 to 1·5 units on a pain intensity scale, and might not be clinically significant taken alone, "both pain research scientists and the pharmaceutical industry go to the ends of the earth to make improvements of this magnitude. Adding one or two sentences to each pain treatment might help to produce them".[92] Those two sentences are not placebos, but are sources of meaning.

## Immune response

There is also evidence to show that several of these factors can influence the immune system. In one study, medical students were randomly assigned to write about personal traumatic events or control topics on four consecutive days. Following the writing, they were given vaccinations for hepatitis B. "Compared with the control group, participants in the emotional expression group showed significantly higher antibody levels against hepatitis at the four and six month follow up.[93] Similarly, it has been known for 25 years that death of a spouse depresses lymphocyte function in the elderly;[94] similar findings have been shown in suddenly bereaved parents.[95]

These studies of pain, disclosure and bereavement do not explain how experience can move biological systems. But they surely indicate that they *can* move them. Understanding how this happens is far off; it seems to me that, today, we know about as much about how information and experience are encoded in the brain as we knew of the genetic code in 1950. This seems to me a hopeful analogy.

## Thinking about causality

There is a clear relationship between these meaning responses and active drug effects; I hope I have made it clear that meaning responses adhere not only to inert treatments, but also to active ones. That was the take home message from one of the first studies mentioned in this paper which showed that branded placebo was more effective for headaches than unbranded placebo, and branded aspirin was more effective than unbranded aspirin. Kirsch and Sapirstein have shown an astonishingly high correlation between drug effects and placebo effects in treatments for depression; in 19 trials, the correlation was $r = 0{\cdot}90$ ($p < 0{\cdot}001$).[96] These results come from comparing group results, but they can also be shown for individuals. Amanzio and Benedetti have shown that under a half dozen different conditions in patients treated with either morphine or ketorolac and then treated with saline, that there is a strong correlation between the drug effect and placebo effect in individuals; the correlations under six different experimental conditions range from 0·554 to 0·855, with a mean of 0·679.[90]

I have shown a similar relationship in RCTs of peptic ulcer disease treated with cimetidine or ranitidine. In 83 studies of treatment of duodenal ulcer, the correlation between the endoscopically verified healing rate in the control group and in the inert treatment group was $r = 0{\cdot}49$* ($p < 0{\cdot}000003$; see Figure 4.3).[45]

While the relationship is clear, it is not so clear how to account for it. Several different approaches to this might be taken. It seems reasonable to infer that we cannot account for such variations by referring to conditioning theory. Ader has suggested that there is heuristic value in considering "a pharmacotherapeutic regimen as a series of conditioning trials".[97] But in these cases, the various individuals, or study groups, each had identical (or at least very similar) regimens, and yet the outcome

* In 37 comparable trials of treatment of generalized anxiety disorder, the correlation between drug and placebo group improvement rates is 0·39 ($p = 0{\cdot}017$). But this is not always the case. In 32 studies of treatment of hypertension, the correlations between drug and placebo improvement were 0·20 for systolic blood pressure, and 0·10 for diastolic blood pressure; neither was statistically significant.

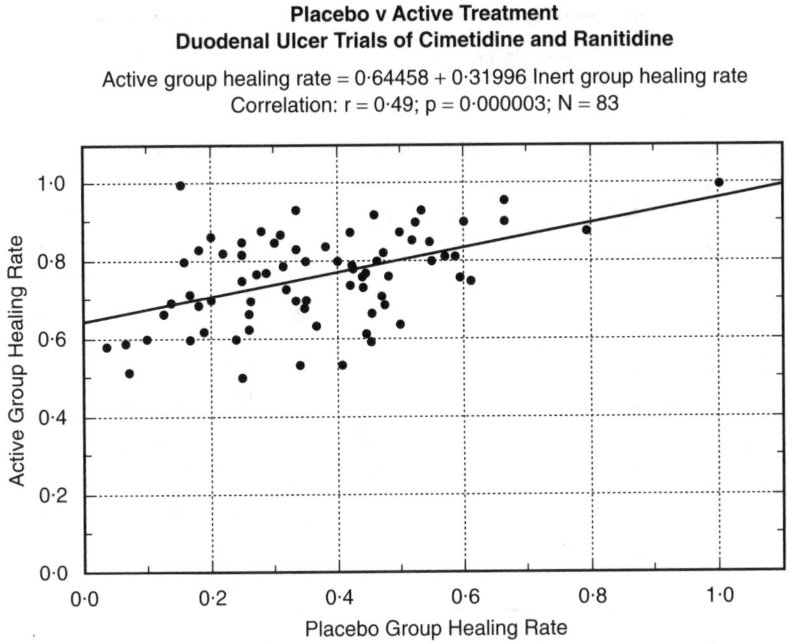


Figure 4.3 Relationship between active and inert treatments in duodenal ulcer disease.[45]

varied; patients, or study groups, with low responses to inert drugs had similarly low responses to active drugs, and vice versa.

In cases where drugs of differently appreciated "power" or "intensity" are at issue, one is drawn to an explanation based on the influence of the physician; it is s/he who best understands the varying powers of the pharmacopoeia. A similar argument may apply to the situation where older drugs seem to lose their power as newer ones come along.

But the most common approach to this issue seems to me to be somewhat more subtle and ambiguous. When these sorts of things are reported, the language usually is something like this: "the larger the active drug response, the larger the placebo response". And graphically, these things are usually represented so that the drug effect is displayed on the x-axis (usually conceived of as the "independent variable") while the drug effect is displayed on the y-axis, suggesting that y = f(x), that the placebo effect is dependent on, is a function of, the drug effect. Figure 4.4 serves as an example; the graph shows the relation between responses of individuals to morphine injections and then later to either saline (filled circles) or naloxone (open circles). The key here is not the data itself (interesting as it is), but the structure of the data, the way it is displayed, which, in standard scientific argot has the independent variable on the horizontal axis.

Since the 1980s, morphine has been considered an "exogenous opiate", in contrast to the "endorphins", or "endo[genous morph]ins". Proglumide

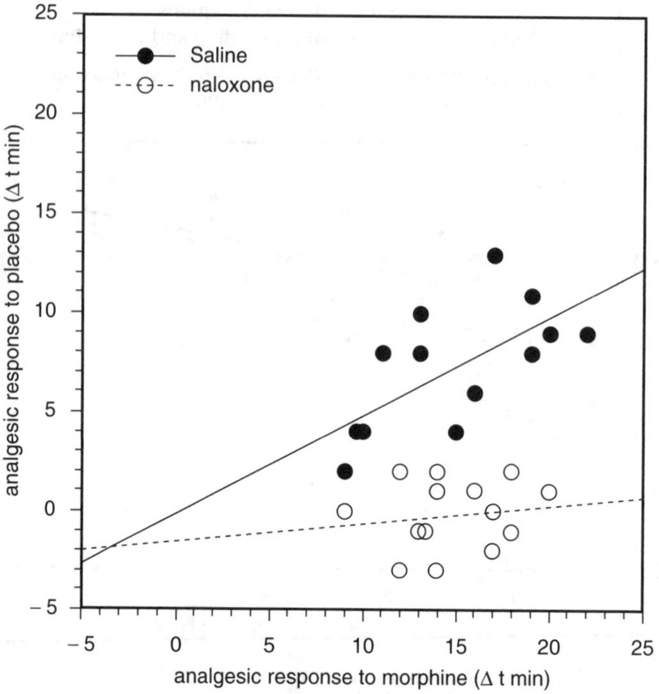


Figure 4.4 Relationship between active and inert treatments in pain. (Figure 5A from[90])

is, by contrast, considered an opiate agonist, while naloxone is considered an opiate antagonist. The data in Figure 4.4 might better be interpreted as showing that morphine is an endorphin agonist. Morphine is derived from phytochemicals which evolved in poppies to affect (negatively) the nervous systems of insect and vertebrate browsers; the endogenous opiate process preceded the exogenous one, and is the independent variable in the system (it seems clear that poppies evolved in response to the pre-existing nervous systems of browsers rather than vice-versa). From this perspective, it makes much more sense to say "the larger the placebo response, the larger the morphine response", and to reverse the axes on the graph (as was done on Figure 4.3). The enthusiasms of doctors are still real factors here, but from this perspective, it is clearer on what that enthusiasm is acting.

One implication which I intend here is that, at least on some occasions, the biology of the meaning response probably accounts for the effectiveness of some very common and very useful drugs. That we don't understand this biology very well does not change the fact that it happens, and ought only to be a challenge to understand better some of these human – that is, *meaningful* – dimensions of life. And this perspective brings to the fore one of the most important unresolved issues in this whole research area, one which has enormous potential to improve medical care around the world:

why is it that, in study after study, only a third to a half of patients are able to experience a meaning response? Why is a majority of the population (more often than not) unable to experience the benefits of a beneficial response to a meaningful interaction? Solving this problem would get my vote for a Nobel Prize.

## Conclusions

The application of a focused, meaningful theory to injury or disease – angina, back pain, peptic ulcer or bad knees – can make a huge difference for patients in the objective and subjective dimensions of their illness, regardless of the effectiveness of the specifics of the treatment. In all likelihood, highly effective specific treatment effects can be amplified (or damped down) by meaningfulness (this seems evident in the data on ulcers presented earlier, where a doubtless effective therapy is still highly variable in its outcome around the world). A magic bullet is useless (or worse) in the hands of someone who cannot shoot straight.

But the evidence also suggests that treatments do not need very powerful specific effects to energize highly effective therapeutic systems; the use of minor tranquilizers for generalized anxiety disorder may be such a case. Similarly, Kirsch, reporting a meta-analysis of the effects of antidepressant medication, state that the "data indicate that 27% of the response to medication was a pharmacologic effect, 50% was a placebo effect, and 23% was due to other 'nonspecific' factors".[96]

In general, the way meaningful and pharmacological effects interact is a very complex and difficult problem which requires substantial research.[98] If you are interested in characterizing the forces needed to smash a rock with a sledge hammer, a simple design will suffice. If you are interested in characterizing the forces which move the tides, more subtle experiments will be needed, not because the forces involved are smaller or less significant, but because there is nothing against which you can compare the forces. And when forces this different interact, extremely subtle work will be required to understand the matter.

It seems nonetheless undeniably the case that doctor and patient can establish a dynamic meaningful relationship which can often materially affect illness. The meaning response – the desirable effects of meaning in the treatment of illness – (of which the placebo effect is a small special case of treatment without active ingredients) is a crucial clinical and research issue, complementary to all forms of medicine.

## Acknowledgments

I wish to thank Wayne Jonas, Ted Kaptchuk, Claire Cassidy and Paul Zitzewitz for helpful discussion. Robert Hahn, Thomas Csordas, Harry Guess, Linda Engel and Arthur Kleinman commented on this paper when it was originally presented at the NIH conference "The Science of the Placebo"; their comments were extremely helpful in my preparation of the final version. Sincere thanks to Martin Leon, MD, who provided as yet unpublished data on PTMR. Work reported here was supported by NSF grant SBR-9421128. For Jennifer.

## References


1 Harrington A. *The Placebo Effect an Interdisciplinary Exploration*. Cambridge, Mass: Harvard University Press, 1997:1.
2 Gøtzsche PC. Is there logic in the placebo? *Lancet* 1994;**344**:925–6.
3 Blackwell B, Bloomfield SS, Buncher CR. Demonstration to medical students of placebo responses and non-drug factors. *Lancet* 1972;**1**:1279–82.
4 Branthwaite A, Cooper P. Analgesic effects of branding in treatment of headaches. *BMJ* 1981;**282**:1576–8.
5 Desharnais R, Jobin J, Cote C, *et al.* Aerobic exercise and the placebo effect: a controlled study. *Psychosom Med* 1993;**55**:149–54.
6 Phillips DP, Ruth TE, Wagner LM. Psychology and survival. *Lancet* 1993;**342**:1142–5.
7 Beinfield H, Korngold E. *Between Heaven and Earth: A Guide to Chinese Medicine*. New York: Ballantine Books, 1991.
8 Kleinman A. *Social Origins of Distress and Disease*. New Haven: Yale University Press, 1986.
9 Kleinman A, Becker AE. "Sociosomatics": the contributions of anthropology to psychosomatic medicine. *Psychosom Med* 1998;**60**:389–93.
10 Blumhagen DW. The doctor's white coat. The image of the physician in modern America. *Ann Intern Med* 1979;**91**:111–16.
11 Uhlenhuth EH, Rickels K, Fisher S, *et al.* Drug, doctor's verbal attitude and clinic setting in symptomatic response to pharmacotherapy. *Psychopharmacology (Berl)* 1966;**9**:392–418.
12 Brody H, Waters DB. Diagnosis is treatment. *J Fam Pract* 1980;**10**:445–9.
13 Gracely RH. Charisma and the art of healing: can nonspecific factors be enough? In: Devor M, Rowbotham MC, Wiesenfeld-Hallin Z, eds. *Proceedings of the 9th World Congress on Pain: Progress in Pain Research and Management*. Seattle: IASP Press, 2000, pp 1045–67.
14 Gryll SL, Katahn M. Situational factors contributing to the placebo effect. *Psychopharmacology (Berl)* 1978;**57**:253–61.
15 Thomas KB. General practice consultations: is there any point in being positive? *BMJ* 1987;**294**:1200–2.
16 Gracely RH, Dubner R, Deeter WR, *et al.* Clinicians' expectations influence placebo analgesia. *Lancet* 1985;**1**:43.
17 Benson H, McCallie DP Jr. Angina pectoris and the placebo effect. *N Engl J Med* 1979;**300**:1424–9.
18 Taylor GR. *The Natural History of the Mind*. New York: Dutton, 1979.
19 Moerman DE. Edible symbols: the effectiveness of placebos. *Ann NY Acad Sci* 1981; **364**:256–68.
20 Fisher S. The placebo reactor: thesis, antithesis, synthesis, and hypothesis. *Dis Nerv Syst* 1967;**28**:510–15.
21 Liberman RP. The Elusive Placebo Reactor. In: Brill H, ed. *Neuro-Psycho-Pharmacology: Proceedings of the Fifth International Congress of the Collegium Internationale Neuro-Psycho-Pharmacologicum*. Amsterdam, Excerpta Medica Foundation, 1967, 57–66.
22 Eisenberg DM, Davis RB, Ettner SL, *et al.* Trends in alternative medicine use in the United States, 1990–1997: results of a follow-up national survey. *JAMA* 1998;**280**:1569–75.
23 Cassidy CM. Chinese medicine users in the United States. Part II: Preferred aspects of care. *J Altern Complement Med* 1998;**4**:189–202.
24 Blumhagen DW. Hyper-tension: a folk illness with a medical name. *Cult Med Psychiatry* 1980;**4**:197–224.
25 Dimond EG, Kittle CF, Crockett JE. Comparison of internal mammary ligation and sham operation for angina pectoris. *Am J Cardiol* 1960;**5**:483–6.
26 Cobb L, Thomas GI, Dillard DH, *et al.* An evaluation of internal-mammary artery ligation by a double blind technic. *N Engl J Med* 1959;**260**:1115–18.

27 Kitchell JR, Glover RP, Kyle RH. Bilateral internal mammary artery ligation for angina pectoris: preliminary clinical considerations. *Am J Cardiol* 1958;**1**:46–50.

28 PLC Medical Systems. The Heart Laser: How TMR Works. (*http://www.plcmed.com/laser/tmr.htm*) Accessed 20 June 2000.

29 Bortone AS, D'Agostino D, Schena S, *et al.* Inflammatory response and angiogenesis after percutaneous transmyocardial laser revascularization. *Ann Thorac Surg* 2000;**70**: 1134–8.

30 Kantor B, McKenna CJ, Caccitolo JA, *et al.* Transmyocardial and percutaneous myocardial revascularization: current and future role in the treatment of coronary artery disease. *Mayo Clin Proc* 1999;**74**:585–92.

31 Landolfo CK, Landolfo KP, Hughes GC, *et al.* Intermediate-term clinical outcome following transmyocardial laser revascularization in patients with refractory angina pectoris. *Circulation* 1999;**100**:II128–33.

32 Al-Sheikh T, Allen KB, Straka SP, *et al.* Cardiac sympathetic denervation after transmyocardial laser revascularization. *Circulation* 1999;**100**:135–40.

33 Hirsch GM, Thompson GW, Arora RC, *et al.* Transmyocardial laser revascularization does not denervate the canine heart. *Ann Thorac Surg* 1999;**68**:460–8; discussion 468–9.

34 Chiang BB, Roberts AM, Kashem AM, *et al.* Chemoreflexes: an experimental study. *Arch Surg* 2000;**135**:577–81.

35 Lange RA, Hillis LD. Transmyocardial laser revascularization. *N Engl J Med* 1999;**341**: 1075–6.

36 Kornowski R, Baim DS, Moses JW, *et al.* Short- and intermediate-term clinical outcomes from direct myocardial laser revascularization guided by biosense left ventricular electromechanical mapping. *Circulation* 2000;**102**:1120–5.

37 Ozaki S, Meyns B, Racz R, *et al.* Effect of transmyocardial laser revascularization on chronic ischemic hearts in sheep. *Eur J Cardiothorac Surg* 2000;**18**:404–10.

38 Leon MB, Baim DS, Moses JW, *et al.* A Randomized Blinded Clinical Trial Comparing Percutaneous Laser Myocardial Revascularization (Using Biosense LV Mapping) vs. Placebo in Patients With Refractory Coronary Ischemia. *Paper presented at American Heart Association*, 2000.

39 Johnson AG. Surgery as a placebo. *Lancet* 1994;**344**:1140–2.

40 Thomsen J, Bretlau P, Tos M, *et al.* Placebo effect in surgery for Meniere's disease: three-year follow-up. *Otolaryngol Head Neck Surg* 1983;**91**:183–6.

41 Spangfort EV. The lumbar disc herniation. a computer-aided analysis of 2,504 operations. *Acta Orthop Scand Suppl* 1972;**142**:1–95.

42 Moseley JB Jr, Wray NP, Kuykendall D, *et al.* Arthroscopic treatment of osteoarthritis of the knee: a prospective, randomized, placebo-controlled trial. Results of a pilot study. *Am J Sports Med* 1996;**24**:28–34.

43 Beecher HK. The powerful placebo. *JAMA* 1955;**159**:1602–6.

44 Goodwin JS, Goodwin JM, Vogel AV. Knowledge and use of placebos by house officers and nurses. *Ann Intern Med* 1979;**91**:106–10.

45 Moerman DE. Cultural variations in the placebo effect: ulcers, anxiety, and blood pressure. *Med Anthropol Q* 2000;**14**:1–22.

46 Schapira K, McClelland HA, Griffiths NR, *et al.* Study on the effects of tablet colour in the treatment of anxiety states. *BMJ* 1970;**1**:446–9.

47 Honzak R, Horackova E, Culik A. Our experience with the effect of placebo in some functional and psychosomatic disorders. *Activ Nerv Sup (Prague)* 1971;**13**:190–1.

48 de Craen AJ, Roos PJ, Leonard de Vries A, *et al.* Effect of colour of drugs: systematic review of perceived effect of drugs and of their effectiveness. *BMJ* 1996;**313**:1624–6.

49 Cattaneo AD, Lucchilli PE, Filippucci G. Sedative effects of placebo treatment. *Eur J Clin Pharmacol* 1970;**3**:43–5.

50 Rickels K, Hesbacher PT, Weise CC, *et al.* Pills and improvement: a study of placebo response in psychoneurotic outpatients. *Psychopharmacologia* 1970;**16**:318–28.

51 Rickels K, Baumm C, Fales K. Evaluation of placebo responses in psychiatric outpatients under two experimental conditions. In: Bradley PB, Flugel F, Hoch PH, eds. *Neuropsychopharmacology*. Berlin: Springer-Verlag, 1964:80–4.

52 Hollander D, Harlan J. Antacids vs. placebos in peptic ulcer therapy: a controlled double-blind investigation. *JAMA* 1973;**226**:1181–5.

53 de Craen AJ, Moerman DE, Heisterkamp SH, *et al.* Placebo effect in the treatment of duodenal ulcer. *Br J Clin Pharmacol* 1999;**48**:853–60.

54 Hussain MZ, Ahad A. Tablet colour in anxiety states. *BMJ* 1970;**3**:466.

55 Grenfell RF, Briggs AH, Holland WC. A double-blind study of the treatment of hypertension. *JAMA* 1961;**176**:124–8.
56 Traut EF, Passarelli EW. Placebos in the treatment of rheumatoid arthritis and other rheumatic conditions. *Ann Rheum Dis* 1957;**16**:18–21.
57 de Cracn AJ, Tijssen JG, de Gans J, *et al.* Placebo effect in the acute treatment of migraine: subcutaneous placebos are better than oral placebos. *J Neurol* 2000;**247**: 183–8.
58 Payer L. *Medicine and Culture.* New York, An Owl Book: Henry Holt and Company, 1996.
59 Gaines AD. Medical/Psychiatric Knowledge in France and the United States: Culture and Sickness in History and Biology. In: Gaines AD, ed. *Ethnopsychology: The Cultural Construction of Professional and Folk Psychiatries.* New York: State University of New York Press, 1992:171–201.
60 Lilienfeld SO, Lynn SJ, Kirsch I, *et al.* Dissociative identity disorder and the sociocognitive model: recalling the lessons of the past. *Psychol Bull* 1999;**125**:507–23.
61 Hahn RA. *Sickness and Healing: an Anthropological Perspective.* New Haven: Yale University Press, 1995:56.
62 Coronary Drug Project Research Group (CDPRG). Influence of adherence to treatment and response of cholesterol on mortality in the coronary drug project. *N Engl J Med* 1980;**303**:1038–41.
63 Irvine J, Baker B, Smith J, *et al.* Poor adherence to placebo or amiodarone therapy predicts mortality: results from the CAMIAT study. Canadian Amiodarone Myocardial Infarction Arrhythmia Trial. *Psychosom Med* 1999;**61**:566–75.
64 Pennebaker JW. *Opening Up: The Healing Power of Confiding in Others.* New York: W. Morrow, 1990.
65 Pennebaker JW. Putting stress into words: health, linguistic, and therapeutic implications. *Behav Res Ther* 1993;**31**:539–48.
66 Kaplan GA, Camacho T. Perceived health and mortality: a nine-year follow-up of the human population laboratory cohort. *Am J Epidemiol* 1983;**117**:292–304.
67 Kaplan GA, Seeman TE, Cohen RD, *et al.* Mortality among the elderly in the alameda county study: behavioral and demographic risk factors. *Am J Public Health* 1987;**77**:307–12.
68 Idler EL, Kasl S. Health perceptions and survival: do global evaluations of health status really predict mortality? *J Gerontol* 1991;**46**:S55–65.
69 Maruta T, Colligan RC, Malinchoc M, *et al.* Optimists vs pessimists: survival rate among medical patients over a 30-year period. *Mayo Clin Proc* 2000;**75**:140–3.
70 Sherbourne CD, Hays RD, Ordway L, *et al.* Antecedents of adherence to medical recommendations: results from the medical outcomes study. *J Behav Med* 1992;**15**:447–68.
71 Roberts A, Kewman DB, Mercier L, *et al.* The power of nonspecific effects in healing. implications for psychosocial and biological treatments. *Clin Psych Rev* 1993;**13**: 375–91.
72 Kirsch I, Rosadino MJ. Do double-blind studies with informed consent yield externally valid results? An empirical test. *Psychopharmacology* 1993;**110**:437–42.
73 Sprafkin J, Gadow KD. Double-blind versus open evaluations of stimulant drug response in children with attention-deficit hyperactivity disorder. *J Child Adolesc Psychopharmacol* 1996;**6**:215–28.
74 Kaptchuk TJ, Edwards RA, Eisenberg DM. Complementary medicine: efficacy beyond the placebo effect. In: Ernst E, ed. *Complementary medicine: an objective appraisal.* Oxford: Butterworth-Heinemann, 1996:42–70.
75 Assendelft WJ, Koes BW, van der Heijden GJ, *et al.* The effectiveness of chiropractic for treatment of low back pain: an update and attempt at statistical pooling. *J Manipulative Physiol Ther* 1996;**19**:499–507.
76 Cherkin DC, MacCornack FA. Patient evaluations of low back pain care from family physicians and chiropractors. *West J Med* 1989;**150**:351–5.
77 Koes BW, Bouter LM, van Mameren H, *et al.* The effectiveness of manual therapy, physiotherapy, and treatment by the general practitioner for nonspecific back and neck complaints. a randomized clinical trial. *Spine* 1992;**17**:28–35.
78 Oths KS. Unintended Therapy: Psychotherapeutic Aspects of Chiropractic. In: Gaines AD, ed. *Ethnopsychology: The Cultural Construction of Professional and Folk Psychiatries.* New York: State University of New York Press, 1992:85–123.

79 Berkow RMD. *The Merck Manual of Diagnosis and Therapy*. Rahway, NJ: Merok Sharp & Dohme, 1987.
80 Wyman LC. *Blessingway. With Three Versions of the Myth Recorded and Translated From the Navajo by Berard Haile*. Tucson: University of Arizona Press, 1970.
81 Sandner D. *Navaho Symbols of Healing*. New York: Harvest//HBJ Book//Harcourt Brace Jovanovich, 1979.
82 Silko LM. *Ceremony*. New York: Viking Penguin Inc., 1988.
83 Witherspoon G. *Language and Art in the Navajo Universe*. Ann Arbor, MI: University of Michigan Press, 1977.
84 Reichard G. *Navajo Religion*. New York: Bollingen Foundation, 1970:112.
85 Levine JD, Gordon NC, Fields HL. The mechanism of placebo analgesia. *Lancet* 1978;**2**:654–7.
86 Levine JD, Gordon NC, Bornstein JC, *et al*. Role of pain in placebo analgesia. *Proc Natl Acad Sci USA* 1979;**76**:3528–31.
87 Fields HL, Levine JD. Biology of placebo analgesia. *Am J Med* 1981;**70**:745–6.
88 Gracely RH, Dubner R, Wolskee PJ, *et al*. Placebo and naloxone can alter post-surgical pain by separate mechanisms. *Nature* 1983;**306**:264–5.
89 Benedetti F, Amanzio M. The neurobiology of placebo analgesia: from endogenous opioids to cholecystokinin. *Prog Neurobiol* 1997;**52**:109–25.
90 Amanzio M, Benedetti F. Neuropharmacological dissection of placebo analgesia: expectation-activated opioid systems versus conditioning-activated specific subsystems. *J Neurosci* 1999;**19**:484–94.
91 Amanzio M, Pollo A, Maggi G, *et al*. Response variability to analgesics: a role for non-specific activation of endogenous opioids. *Pain* 2001;**90**:205–15.
92 Price DD. Assessing placebo effects without placebo groups: an untapped possibility? *Pain* 2001;**90**:201–3.
93 Petrie KJ, Booth RJ, Pennebaker JW, *et al*. Disclosure of trauma and immune response to a hepatitis B vaccination program. *J Consult Clin Psychol* 1995;**63**:787–92.
94 Bartrop RW, Luckhurst E, Lazarus L, *et al*. Depressed lymphocyte function after bereavement. *Lancet* 1977;**1**:834–6.
95 Spratt ML, Denney DR. Immune variables, depression, and plasma cortisol over time in suddenly bereaved parents. *J Neuropsych Clin Neurosci* 1991;**3**:299–306.
96 Kirsch I, Sapirstein G. Listening to prozac but hearing placebo: a meta-analysis of antidepressant medication. *Prevention and Treatment* 1998; **1**. http://journals.apa.org/prevention/(Accessed 20 June 2000).
97 Ader R. The role of conditioning in pharmacotherapy. In: Harrington A, ed. *The Placebo Effect: An Interdisciplinary Exploration*. Cambridge, MA: Harvard University Press, 1977: 138–65.
98 Kleijnen J, de Craen AJ, van Everdingen J, *et al*. Placebo effect in double-blind clinical trials: a review of interactions with medications. *Lancet* 1994;**344**:1347–9.
99 Pizzo PA, Robichaud KJ, Edwards BK, *et al*. Oral antibiotic prophylaxis in patients with cancer: a double-blind randomized placebo-controlled trial. *J Pediatr* 1983;**102**:125–33.
100 Hogarty GE, Goldberg SC. Drug and sociotherapy in the aftercare of schizophrenic patients. One-year relapse rates. *Arch Gen Psychiatry* 1973;**28**:54–64.
101 Horwitz RI, Viscoli CM, Berkman L, *et al*. Treatment adherence and risk of death after myocardial infarction. *Lancet* 1990;**336**:542–5.
102 Gallagher EJ, Viscoli CM, Horwitz RI. The relationship of treatment adherence to the risk of death after myocardial infarction in women. *JAMA* 1993;**270**:742–4.

# 5: Explanatory mechanisms for placebo effects: cognition, personality and social learning

RICHARD R BOOTZIN, OPHER CASPI

*Cure sometimes; heal often; comfort always* – Hippocrates

## Summary

To understand placebo effects, it is necessary to review a large and complex literature involving cognitive and behavioral mechanisms. We examine definitions of placebo effects, discuss distinctions between specific and non-specific effects of therapies, and examine parallels with common factors from the psychotherapy literature. A number of methodological problems in examining placebo effects are briefly discussed including natural history of the disorder, regression to the mean, therapist biases, reactivity of measurement, and confounded treatment procedures.

The promise of research from specific personality and cognitive explanatory mechanisms of placebo effects is mixed. The literature on personality traits as a means of predicting who will respond to placebos has failed to identify reliable predictors. Interpersonal and contextual variables have shown more promise. The evidence regarding features of the therapeutic relationship suggests that relationship skills can enhance the effectiveness of treatment interventions. Research on expectancy and meaning has shown promising relationships with placebo effects.

We provide a conceptual model that integrates across multiple explanatory mechanisms. Important features of the model are that the causal effects are reciprocal, synergistic, and recursive and involve factors that are both internal and external to the individual. The concluding section provides our recommendations for a research agenda on tests of theory and new methodologies to advance knowledge about placebo effects.

## Introduction

Placebos work, yet we do not understand how they work (their mechanism of action), to what degree they work (how much of the outcome variance they account for), and under what circumstances they work (the ability to predict their effect and to use that prediction in research and therapy). In the introduction to her edited book on the placebo effect, Harrington[1] aptly describes placebos as "the ghosts that haunt our house of biomedical objectivity, the creatures that rise up from the dark and expose the paradoxes and fissures in our own self-created definitions of the real and active factors in treatment".

Placebo and placebo effects are difficult to define. Placebos are often narrowly defined as biologically inert substances (i.e. the placebo pill) given within a health care context. However, the term, placebo, has been generalized and applied to medical procedures (for example, sham surgery), to psychological interventions (for example, attention-placebo treatments), and to incidental components of treatments that may affect outcome (for example, the patient-therapist relationship). A thorough commentary that dealt with the multiple definitions of placebo and placebo effects in the literature led one author to declare his failure in defining the placebo effect in an unambiguous, logically consistent, and testable way.[2] Nonetheless, an examination of the various definitions of the placebo effect over the past three decades reveals an interesting process of evolution that is pertinent to the subject of this paper. This evolution can be best illustrated by the following definitions.

In the early 1960s, Shapiro[3] defined the placebo effect as "the psychological or psychophysiological effect produced by placebos". In 1980, Brody defined the placebo effect as "a change in a patient's illness attributable to the symbolic import of a treatment rather than a specific pharmacologic or physiologic property".[4] In a 1997 NIH publication, the placebo effect is defined as a "positive healing effect resulting from the use of any healing intervention, and that is presumed to be mediated by the symbolic effect of the intervention upon the patient".[5] Most recently, Brody[6] defined it as "a change in the body (or the body-mind unit) that occurs as a result of the symbolic significance which one attributes to an event or object in the healing environment". As one can note, the spirit and focus of these (and other) definitions have shifted from the effects of interventions that are presumed to have no active treatment properties to an inclusion of a plausible mechanism (i.e. symbolic effect or significance) and context (i.e. the healing environment). The later definitions are somewhat circular in that they presume a causal mechanism and context. As we will see, recent research points to symbolic effect and context as important aspects of placebo effects, but to include them as part of the definitions of placebo and placebo effects confuses cause with effect.

Research on placebo effects has followed the typical course of an artifact described by McGuire.[7] Placebo effects were first ignored, then treated as contaminants to be controlled, and finally investigated as variables of interest in their own right. While much research still focuses on controlling placebo effects as contaminants, there has been growing interest in recent years in studying and exploiting the placebo effect as a variable of interest in its own right.

Surprising as it may be, the definition and use of the placebo effect are different for clinical purposes than for outcome research purposes. This difference is rooted in the disparity between the focus of interest of each setting and results in two paradoxes. The first paradox is that there is a purposeful attempt to maximize the "placebo effect" in the clinic as a means of enhancing the effectiveness of treatments while controlling it in randomized clinical trials. In other words, whereas the placebo effect is a warmly welcomed ally in the clinical setting,[8] it is considered a nuisance to be controlled in most research settings. The second paradox is that maximizing the placebo effect in the clinic requires individualization of treatment that is the antithesis of the homogeneous, standardized intervention employed in clinical trials. A better understanding of the psychological explanatory mechanisms that underlie placebo effects requires a systematic approach that examines both domains, the clinic and research settings.

Unfortunately, there is still confusion between research methodologies that test efficacy versus ones that shed light on mechanisms of action. For some researchers, placebo control conditions are a means of setting a minimum standard of effectiveness for treatments. However, it is not the effectiveness of the treatment that is being evaluated but rather its mechanism of action. In the evaluation of medications, the assumption of the model being tested is that the effect of a medication consists of two components, a specific physiological and a non-specific psychological component, whereas the effect of a placebo consists of only one, the non-specific psychological component. Thus, it is not total effectiveness that is being evaluated, but the extent to which the physiological component adds significantly to the psychological component.[9]

In psychosocial intervention studies, placebo control groups are often called "attention placebo controls" to indicate that the attention received from the therapist is being controlled in addition to other non-specific or unspecified variables associated with treatment. As in pharmacology studies, the attention placebo control groups are used to identify why treatments are effective, not whether they are effective. Although a partition into physiological and psychological components is not relevant, an attempt to distinguish the specific effects derived from theory from the non-specific effects associated with all therapy is relevant.[9]

## Specific and non-specific treatments

"Placebo effect" and other "non-specific" effects of therapy are often used interchangeably, reflecting some confusion around cause and effect of therapy.[10] The popular definition of placebo as "non-specific" treatment is not entirely accurate. Although the placebo effect stems from the incidental elements of treatments,[11] the effects of the placebo can be highly specific. They include effects, such as pain reduction, healing of a peptic ulcer, bronchodilation in asthmatics and the like.

Specific elements of therapy (also called the defining or characteristic elements by Grünbaum[11]) are those therapeutic maneuvers derived from a particular theoretical orientation as being necessary for the amelioration of a symptom or disorder. By definition they are well-defined, theoretically derived, intentional actions or intervention strategies on the part of the therapist that are unique to a specific therapy. The application of these techniques is believed to be causally responsible for the outcome.

Non-specific elements, on the other hand, (called incidental elements by Grünbaum[11]) are those unspecified variables that accompany the characteristic elements, but which are not necessary for the therapy to be of the specified kind. They happen in conjunction with and after the therapy, and would not have happened, had the therapy not been given. Examples of these non-specific elements include the patient–therapist relationship, individual patient and therapist qualities during therapy, and elements of the treatment structure, change processes, and strategies.[12]

The medical encounter is one that is of particular importance as it often includes constituents, referred to as preliminary elements of treatment[13] that may affect patients' outcome even before treatment is eventually offered. The diagnostic process, for instance, may include elements that are perceived as meaningful to the patient and thus may trigger healing well before any medical advice is given.[14,15]

In psychotherapy research, non-specific factors have also been called common factors and refer to the common features of therapeutic interventions regardless of theoretical orientation.[16] Many of the common factors that are thought to produce positive benefit for patients involve the therapeutic relationship and the patient's expectations. We will discuss both of these aspects of the therapeutic encounter in more detail in later sections.

## Methodological issues

Before discussing the mechanisms that underlie the effectiveness of placebo effects, it is important to recognize that some effects attributed to placebos are methodological artifacts. This may seem contradictory in that we are advocating examining the placebo in its own right rather than as an artifact to be controlled. An evaluation of placebos and their mechanisms, however, requires attention to the research literature in which placebo effects have been found. That literature has variable quality and not all effects that are claimed to be placebo effects can in fact be attributed to placebos.

Among the alternative hypotheses to be considered are the natural history and course of the disorder, reliability of measurement and regression to the mean, reactivity of measurement, therapist and observer bias, and confounded therapeutic procedures. Since other papers in this workshop focus in more detail on some specific methodological issues, we will provide only an overview. Also see Kienle and Kiene[17] for a thorough discussion of methodological problems in identifying placebo effects.

*Natural history of the disorder*

Many disorders are cyclical or improve spontaneously. An important reason for including no treatment control groups in evaluating the effects of treatments has been to rule out the natural history of the disorder as an explanation for the observed improvement. The same difficulty occurs, of course, when attributing improvement to placebo interventions. Only when placebo interventions produce improvement in contrast to no treatment controls, can natural history be ruled out as an alternative explanation.

*Regression to the mean*

Regression to the mean refers to a statistical phenomenon that occurs when measures are subject to error or when there is within-patient random variability in measurements.[18] Individual scores that are high or low on one measurement occasion are likely to be closer to the mean of all scores on the second measurement occasion. The degree to which regression to the mean occurs in a study depends on the reliability of the measure and the extent to which patients are selected into a study on the basis of extreme measurements. Individuals generally seek treatment when symptoms are worse than usual and are recruited into research studies because they meet inclusion criteria such as having a sufficient number and intensity of symptoms. Individuals may show improvement, both in the clinic and in research studies, even in the absence of treatment effects because of the variability of the intensity of symptoms over time (a natural history effect) or because of the random error in the measures being used (regression to the mean). On subsequent occasions, then, there is likely to be demonstrated improvement even if the treatment or placebo had no effect. Here, too, having a no-treatment control is essential to rule out regression to the mean effects for the improvement of placebo interventions.

*Therapist and observer biases*

If raters evaluate improvement, but are not blind to whether the individual received a treatment or a placebo, it would not be surprising if the ratings were biased in favor of the intervention expected to be more effective. The same problem can occur when comparing placebo interventions, or minimal treatment, against no treatment. Blind assessment is essential. The need for blind assessment has led to the use of double blind designs in which neither the patient nor the physician know whether an active or placebo medication is being administered. Measurement biases and expectancies may still operate in double blind studies since patients and physicians can often guess accurately about whether the substance administered was the active medication or the placebo based on the strength of the reaction and side effects.[19]

*Reactivity of measurement and patient biases*

A parallel problem to observer bias is reactivity of measurement.[20] This refers to the extent to which patients are aware that they are being assessed. Measures vary in how reactive they are. Thus, measures that are archival (for example, number of sick days, data from patient charts, etc.) and were recorded for reasons other than the evaluation of the interventions at hand are less reactive than measures assessed directly as part of a study. In clinical trials, typically all measures are reactive. The patient is assessed before and after treatment and knows that the assessments are an evaluation of the effectiveness of the interventions. Since the patient is aware of the assessment, incentives for biasing the response may play a role. For example, at the beginning of treatment in a clinical setting or when being assessed against inclusion criteria in a clinical trial, patients may bias their responses to indicate increased severity so that they can qualify for treatment. At the end of treatment, patients may bias responses towards improvement as a means of being a good patient or subject and as a means to end therapy. This pattern is often referred to as a "hello-goodbye" effect and has the effect of demonstrating or exaggerating improvement even when little improvement has occurred.

*Confounded treatment procedures*

Identifying an intervention as a placebo does not necessarily make it so. Treatments that appear to be inert may include active elements. As others have mentioned, even sugar pills would have a physiological effect on someone with diabetes[11] and would not be considered a placebo in attempts to change blood sugar levels. It is worth re-emphasizing that placebos, by definition, do not contain the characteristic elements of treatment for a specific disorder. Consequently, substances which have active elements, whether physiological or psychological, are placebos only if and when those elements are incidental ingredients of the treatment being evaluated for a particular problem. This means that an intervention could be a placebo in one context, but a treatment in another.

In this paper, we place considerable emphasis on using explanatory mechanisms underlying placebo effects to enhance treatments. However, the "surprising" effectiveness of placebos is sometimes due to confounded treatment components. For example, in a study of the efficacy of bright light for sleep onset insomnia conducted by one of the authors of this paper,[21] subjects in all treatment groups, including a dim light placebo treatment, had to wake up earlier than usual in order to sit in front of a light box before starting their daily activities. Regularizing sleep/wake patterns is an effective way of improving sleep.[22] Consequently, improvements in the sleep of subjects of all groups, both treatment and placebo, may have been due in part to treatment elements that were part of the protocol. When identifying explanatory mechanisms underlying placebo effects, it is important to be aware of active treatment components that may have been incidental for the purpose of the study, but which could have contributed to the placebo's effectiveness.

## Explanatory mechanisms of placebo effects

How do placebos work? Among the mechanisms proposed that involve either direct or indirect effects on physiology and behavior are Pavlovian conditioning, cognitive and behavioral mechanisms, and sociocultural explanations. Other chapters focus on Pavlovian conditioning[23] and variations in what Moerman[24] calls the "meaning response" in different cultural contexts. We will focus on cognitive and behavioral explanatory mechanisms primarily from a social learning perspective. In a social learning perspective, learning is not simply a matter of reacting to stimuli. Individuals apply cognitive processes to the stimuli they encounter, selecting, organizing, and transforming them. It is the individual's interpretation of stimuli and not the stimuli themselves that influence behavior. In this section on explanatory mechanisms of placebo effects, we will examine cognitive and behavioral mechanisms including personality traits and characteristics of patients, the patient-therapist relationship, expectancy and meaning, and how these mechanisms produce change.

### Personality and placebo: correlation or causation?

Very few concepts appeal more to the logic of the human mind than the assumption that there must be an association between a placebo response and some underlying personality trait(s). The rationale is clear, i.e. personality traits account for a significant portion of human behavior and the placebo effect is just one more example of this repertoire of behavior. Researchers attempted to identify the psychological profile of placebo responders using primarily correlational studies.

That line of placebo research was the prevailing one during the sixties and the seventies. These efforts to identify a placebo responder personality type, and predict with any sort of confidence exactly who will respond to placebo and under what circumstances, have generally failed.[6,19,25]

Several recent published studies across different medical conditions and cultures re-examined the potential personality dimension of the placebo response. The following are a few examples. In contrast to studies indicating that increased anxiety is associated with placebo response in pain reduction,[26] a recent study on characteristics of placebo responses in medical treatment of premenstrual syndrome failed to find that anxiety or depression were associated with placebo response rate,[27] a study that used factor-analyzed symptom dimensions to predict outcome in patients with obsessive-compulsive disorder failed to show any predictors of placebo response,[28] and a study of panic disorder patients found that placebo responders reported less psychopathology.[29] Another study that looked at the placebo response in Parkinson's disease failed to find significant relationships with any proxy variables, such as demographics, education, and religion with placebo response rate.[30] Patients with type A pesonalities were shown in one study[31] to have a higher placebo response rate than those with type B. This, however, might be due to differences in the level of detection and report of symptoms.

In reviewing the research regarding placebo responders, Shapiro and Shapiro[19] conclude:

> ...personality traits found in one study differ from those reported in others. Contradictory findings can be the result of different clinical conditions, patient populations, research procedures, and settings. Some of the studies report, however, and it is commonly assumed, that (when compared with placebo nonreactors) placebo reactors are less intelligent; less educated; more frequently neurotic or psychotic; more frequently female; from lower social classes; more dependent, inadequate, immature, impulsive, atypical, depressed, religious, and stereotypic; and more likely to have symptoms of hypochondriasis, obsessive-compulsiveness, anger-hostility, bewilderment-confusion, and performance difficulties. In our studies and others there appear to be no consistent data relating either these variables or demographic variables such as age, sex, intelligence, race, social class, ethnicity, religiosity, or religious background to placebo reaction (pp. 39–40).

The capacity to elicit the placebo response is likely inherent in us all.[32] The placebo effect appears to be a contextual situational phenomenon more than an enduring personality trait. Two factors contributed to the shift in psychological inquiry in the science of placebo. They are (1) a failure of the placebo personality paradigm, and (2) a major revolution in the milieu of health care. Language such as the one used in an influential 1945 article,[33] advocating the use of placebo in "ignorant ... disappointed and displeased ... hopeless, [and] incurable case[s]" has been replaced by concepts such as patient empowerment that characterize modern therapeutic values. These two factors resulted in a shift in the focus of research from personality traits to a more detailed analysis of the interpersonal and situational context in which placebo effects occur.

### The therapeutic relationship and the placebo effect

The experience of the therapeutic relationship has been shown to facilitate change. It sometimes seems as if there is a set of desired qualities which may imbue the practitioner or the patient with some sort of special power. But it is the relationship, not the individual person, that provides the framework for change.[34] Does the placebo effect interaction explain the placebo effect? No, but we join many others in stressing the importance of that interplay. The placebo response depends on interactions between the clinician, the treatment process, and the patient.[35] The patient's perception of that interaction often ignites the healing/placebo process. The clinician is a therapeutic agent and the medical encounter is its playing field.[36] As Brody[37] points out, Houston's[38] article on the doctor as a therapeutic agent and Findley's[39] comment that "the physician is a vastly more important institution than the drug store" demonstrate how well this assertion is grounded.

Optimal care of patients requires that the placebo effect should be maximized.[40] Research suggests that the placebo response is more likely to occur in the clinic when the patient regards the clinician as experienced, competent, and optimistic[13,41] and when the clinician expects the treatment to help.[26,42] An attempt to formalize these qualities into a systematic clinical approach led recently to the development of the "sustained relationship" model between physicians and patients[43] as a way to enhance the effect of therapy, probably through maximizing the placebo effect.[44]

Benson and Epstein[45] suggested that placebo responses occur only when both patients and physicians are of like mind. According to that supposition, both need to share positive beliefs and expectations and have a good relationship. Thomas[36] conducted a study on the impact of a physician's positive attitude on patients' outcome and found that the physician's advice was a more effective placebo intervention than the administration of a placebo prescription medication. In a systematic analysis of all placebo controlled studies in ulcerative colitis,[46] only one variable, the number of study visits, was shown to predict increased placebo response. A plausible explanation might be that the more frequent the contacts with the health care provider in a supportive setting, the higher the chances that the patients will respond. One of the major elements in this perception of support relates to the physician's ability to attend to the needs of the patient.[13] And indeed, the derivation of the word, therapy, is from the Greek, to attend.[34]

Aspects of the patient-therapist relationship have also been a central focus of attempts to identify the common factors of psychotherapy. The search for common factors was stimulated by findings that therapies from different orientations had about equal effectiveness (for example, Smith, Glass, and Miller[47]). Some prominent recent examples include the National Institute of Health Treatment of Depression Collaborative Project[48] and the National Institute on Alcohol Abuse and Alcoholism evaluation of treatment of alcohol abuse.[49] Many concluded that it must be features that are common to all therapies that produce change. Among the features investigated in recent years have been the quality of the therapeutic relationship, emotional experiencing, patient expectations, the extent to which patients are given assignments outside of therapy to stimulate new learning, and focus on mastery and problem solving.[16]

Not everyone who has evaluated the therapy outcome literature has concluded that the commonalities are most important. For example, Andrews and Harvey[50] re-analyzed only the studies in which patients having clinical problems had sought or been referred for treatment from the larger Smith *et al.*[47] meta-analysis. They found that behavioral therapies had a significantly higher average effect size than verbal dynamic psychotherapies. More recently, in a large meta-analysis of treatments of alcoholism and alcohol abuse evaluated in clinical trials, Miller and his colleagues[51,52] ranked treatments by the extent to which they have consistently been found to produce significantly stronger or weaker effects than other treatments or control conditions. Contrary to the widely held belief that all treatments are equivalent, Miller and colleagues found that the treatments that were most consistently superior to alternative treatments were brief intervention, motivational enhancement, social skills training, and the community reinforcement approach. Treatments that were most consistently inferior to other treatments were educational lectures/films, general alcoholism counseling, psychotherapy, and confrontational counseling. Although not all techniques are equivalent, it is intriguing that motivational enhancement, which depends on therapist skills of empathy and providing feedback in a non-judgmental manner, is high on the list of effective treatments. It suggests that therapist skills may well interact with treatments to enhance their effectiveness.

Common factors, such as the therapeutic relationship, may be the necessary, but not sufficient, components of successful therapy without which a given technique would be devoid of meaning and therefore ineffective.[53] For example, Alexander, Barton, Schiavo, and Parsons,[54] in a study of the behavioral treatment of delinquents and their families, found that therapist relationship skills (affect-behavior integration, warmth and humor, directiveness, and self-confidence) accounted for 60% of the variance of outcome. However, an earlier study by these investigators of a Rogerian approach found therapist relationship skills alone were not effective in modifying the behavior of delinquent families.[55] Thus, relationship skills appear to enhance the effectiveness of interventions rather than substitute for them.

## Cognition

There are a variety of cognitive theories about how placebos produce change. These include changes in perception of symptoms, elicitation of hope, increases in outcome and efficacy expectations, changes in response expectancies, and changes in causal attributions and meaning networks. We provide an overview of this rich area of research. Cognitive theories show particular promise for helping to understand the mechanisms underlying placebo effects.

### *Signal detection theory*

A promising methodology for examining changes in the perception of symptoms produced by treatments and placebos is signal detection theory.[56] In signal detection theory, two independent indices are derived, the sensitivity in detecting differences between stimuli and the response bias of the judgments. For example, in evaluating pain judgments before and after treatment, it is possible to identify the extent to which changes in the judgments were due primarily to the extent to which the individual differentiated between stimuli more or less precisely (sensitivity) or shifted the overall criterion more conservatively or more liberally reflecting willingness or reluctance to report pain (response bias).

For example, in a study of acupuncture,[57] thermal sensitivity was measured on both treated and untreated arms before, during and after acupuncture. Results found that acupuncture increased the pain report criterion (response bias), but did not increase sensitivity. Because of the lack of change in sensitivity, the authors concluded that the improvement in acupuncture was likely due to suggestion rather than to analgesia.

In another example of the use of signal detection theory for understanding treatment and placebo effects, Losier, McGrath, and Klein[58] conducted a meta-analysis of 26 studies of the use of methylphenidate on continuous performance tests (CPT) in attention deficit hyperactivity disorder (ADHD) children and performed overall signal detection analyses. CPT is a form of a vigilance test in which children respond to targets and non-targets. Children with ADHD were found to be less sensitive to the difference between targets and non-targets than their normal counterparts, while showing a comparable response bias. Further, methylphenidate, when compared to placebo, improved sensitivity while not affecting response bias in both normal children and those with ADHD. Although the authors did not report analyses of the differences between methylphenidate and placebo compared to no treatment, an examination of the table of results indicates that both methylphenidate and placebo increased response bias slightly, but only methylphenidate increased sensitivity.

In both of the above examples, response bias, but not sensitivity, was found to be associated with placebo effects. Although promising, this methodology has been used infrequently in evaluating treatment and placebo effects. Additional research in these and other domains is needed to determine whether placebos can affect sensitivity as well as response bias.

*Hope*

In one of the early and influential cognitive theories, Jerome Frank[59,60,61] proposed that hope is the primary mechanism of change in folk traditions of healing, as well as in psychotherapy. He argued that psychotherapy patients suffer from a common disorder – demoralization, a chronic feeling of being overwhelmed and unable to cope effectively with problems. He proposed that all healing endeavors share:

- a patient in distress
- a clinician who is perceived as an expert in dealing with the patient's distress

- an acceptable explanation or "myth" provided by the clinician
- some sort of healing ritual conducted by the clinician that serves to instil hope and positive expectations in the patient.

For Frank, the specific ingredients of the clinician's technical interventions are important only because they provide a shared belief system between the patient and clinician and give form to prescribed rituals. The patient's expectancies are an important aspect of Frank's analysis, as they are for other theorists described below.

*Outcome and efficacy expectations*

Albert Bandura[62,63] has proposed that expectancies, particularly efficacy expectations, are critical in any analysis of therapeutic change. He distinguishes between outcome and efficacy expectations. Outcome expectations refer to consequences that follow actions while self-efficacy expectations are beliefs that one can successfully perform the actions required to achieve valued outcomes. Thus, for someone who is afraid of flying, an outcome expectancy would be the expectancy that if the individual takes a plane, the plane will crash, whereas an efficacy expectancy would be the expectancy that the individual will be able to cope with and manage his fear of flying.

Bandura's analysis of patients' expectancies has been the focus of considerable research dealing with health care outcomes. A recent review by Crow *et al.*[64] found that expectancy was related to a number of health care outcomes in three areas, preparation for medical procedures, management of chronic illness, and medical treatment. In studies evaluating preparation for medical procedures, skill training to reduce stress in complying with medical procedures (for example, relaxation training) that increased self-efficacy either alone or in combination with information about the medical procedures was more effective than information alone. The main health outcomes were less anxiety and reduced use of pain medication.

In the second research area, studies evaluating the management of chronic illness, training with regard to the management of the disorder which increased self-efficacy resulted in improvement in the patient's symptoms (for example, improved mood, less anxiety, reduced pain, and being less bothered by asthma) and improvement in the patient's disease status (for example, lowered blood pressure, immunological changes, and better metabolic control).

In the third research area, studies of medical treatment, when positive outcome expectancies were stated by the clinician as compared to cautious or skeptical expectancies, most studies provided evidence that positive outcome expectancies enhanced medical outcomes. The improvements, however, were primarily patient self-reports of reduced anxiety, pain, and distress, rather than objective physiological outcomes.

Three observations about the results of this review should be noted. First, it is impressive that self-management training programs increase self-efficacy and have positive health effects. But, it is unclear whether the improved health effects are due primarily to expectancies or to new skills that were learned. In the studies reviewed, the skills and expectancies change together. Bandura[63] has shown in previous research that efficacy expectations are better predictors of subsequent behavior than past performance or emotional responses. In the studies reviewed, however, it is not possible to separate the learning of new skills from increases in efficacy expectation. It may be that these studies provide examples of the use of characteristic, rather than incidental, treatment procedures to improve health outcomes. The implication for clinicians is still clear, however. Clinicians can increase the likelihood of positive outcomes by providing patients with information about medical procedures and teaching skills that increase self-efficacy.

Second, self-efficacy can be changed in many ways, including performance feedback, associative learning, observational learning, information, persuasion, feedback from autonomic responses, and other symbolic processes.[9] The more reliable the information upon which the expectancies are based, such as performance feedback[63] or associative learning over many trials,[65] the stronger the expectancy and the more likely that subsequent behavior will correspond to it. As mentioned above, Crow *et al.*[64] found improved functioning in response to medical treatment due to the expression of positive outcome expectancies by the clinician, i.e. the clinician predicted a likely positive outcome and expressed enthusiasm to the patient. The clinician's effort to "charge the intervention" through positive suggestion is an attempt to change the patient's outcome expectancies based on persuasion and the clinician's status. While such interventions may have immediate salutary effects, the danger would be that the patient's expectancies would be vulnerable to revision unless the clinician's information is confirmed. The vulnerability of such expectancies to revision may be one explanation for the finding that improvements in this area were limited to self-report assessments of distress.

Third, as the Crow *et al.*[64] results are examined, it appears that most of the positive results, whether on subjective or objective measures, are on measures that have broad impact in the individual such as anxiety and distress reduction, pain reduction, and changes in immunological functioning. This appears to be another version of the specific versus non-specific proposition of how active treatments versus placebos produce their effects. We will return to this issue in a later section.

*Response expectancies*

In a complementary view of Bandura's analysis of expectancy, Irving Kirsch[66,67] has proposed that response expectancies are the major determinant of placebo effects. Response expectancies are expectations held by the individual about one's own emotional and physiological responses such as anxiety, pain, sexual arousal, and mood. These responses are not considered by the individual to be volitional. The magnitude of placebo effects varies depending on the condition being treated and on various situational variables that affect response expectancies.[67] A wide range of conditions could affect response expectancies including the credibility of the rationale for the intervention, the likelihood of the response expected, the dose of the intervention, among others.

Expectations may be altered by even small variations in instructions and experimental designs in clinical research. For example, Kirsch and Weixel[68] found that differences between double blind and deceptive administration of placebos can produce different outcomes. In a study of response expectancies about coffee, subjects were administered decaffeinated coffee under two different instructional sets. In one, subjects were given the usual double blind administration as used in clinical trials, in which they were told that they might receive either caffeinated or decaffeinated coffee. Neither the subject nor the experimenter knew which beverage was being administered. In the other design, subjects were told that they would receive caffeinated coffee, when in fact they received decaffeinated coffee, a procedure more akin to what might happen in a clinical setting. The authors proposed that deceptive administration would have stronger effects on outcome than double blind administration because in double blind administration the subjects would be less certain about whether they actually were receiving caffeinated coffee.

The results were complex, but did confirm that the different protocols produced different effects. Subjects who received the deceptive administration had higher pulse rates 20 minutes after ingestion than those in the double blind condition and had significantly different patterns of responses across increased doses of the placebo on self-rated alertness and tension and systolic blood pressure. There were no differences between the experimental conditions on the behavioral outcome measures of digit-symbol, reaction time, and pursuit rotor task. However, expectancies about the effect of caffeine on these tasks were significantly correlated with performance across both experimental conditions.

In an article on expectations in clinical drug trials, Swartzman and Burkell[69] point out that even in double blind crossover designs, features of the design can influence the result. In a study comparing clonidine and placebo for postmenopausal hot flushes,[70] patients were informed that they would receive two courses of treatments (the active medication and placebo), although they were not informed about which intervention would be first. There was no statistically significant difference between clonidine and placebo before the crossover. Both treatments reduced hot flushes. After the crossover, however, patients who received the placebo as the first treatment continued to improve when they received clonidine. In contrast, patients who received clonidine as the first treatment, began to get worse after the crossover when they received the placebo. It appears that patients were able to infer which treatment they were receiving after the crossover since they could directly compare their reactions to the two interventions.

As illustrated by this study, response expectancies may play a role in all treatment effects, not just in placebo effects. Kirsch and Sapirstein[71] after conducting a meta-analysis of the effects of antidepressant medication, proposed that response expectancies are important not only in understanding the mechanisms that underlie placebo effects, but that they also account for a substantial degree of the effect produced by medications for psychiatric disorders such as depression. They speculate that medications for depression may be little more than active placebos that strengthen the patient's response expectancies by producing side effects. Thus, in their view, the difference between medication and placebo typically found in clinical trials for depression is equivalent to the difference between active and inert placebo.

In the absence of studies comparing antidepressants to active placebos, this is a difficult proposition to evaluate. Even so, it is a somewhat paradoxical argument for Kirsch. As described above, response expectancies, even for inert placebos, produce automatic emotional and physiological effects. Consequently, subjects given an inert placebo would be expected to experience targeted changes and side effects. Thus, even "inert" placebos would be active placebos. There may be differences in the number and intensity of side effects, but studies would be needed to demonstrate that the differences in perceived number and intensity of side effects affected the patient's response expectancies and therapeutic outcomes.

*Causal attributions and meaning*

Expectancy is only one of many cognitive constructs that have been investigated. An important line of research in social cognition has been focused on how individuals attach meaning and make causal inferences about their experiences. Attribution theorists have proposed that self-attributed behavior change has a greater probability of being maintained over time than does behavior change attributed to an external source such as a drug.[72] In a creative test of this hypothesis, Davison, Tsujimoto, and Glaros[73] administered a treatment package for insomnia that consisted of chloral hydrate (a hypnotic), a brief relaxation training procedure, and instructions to schedule and regularize bedtime behaviors. Subjects who demonstrated improvement in sleep onset latencies from this treatment regimen were told, after they improved, that they had received either an optimal dose of the drug or that they had received a dose that previous research indicated was ineffective. Subjects who were led to attribute their improvement to their own efforts, rather than to the drug, maintained their improvement after the drug was withdrawn. Subjects led to attribute their improvement to the drug returned to their baseline levels of sleep disturbance. Patients with many disorders may attribute their improvement to salient medical interventions. These attributions may make patients more vulnerable to relapses when the interventions are withdrawn.

Attribution theory is one way of understanding how individuals give meaning to their experiences. Meaning, as an explanatory concept, has received increased recent attention in the placebo literature.[24] In a book on the placebo response, Brody[6] proposes that "an encounter with a healer is most likely to produce a positive placebo response when it changes the meaning of the illness experience for that individual in a positive direction" (p. 84). According to Brody[6] three conditions are associated with this change in meaning:

1 the individual is listened to and receives an explanation for the illness that makes sense
2 the individual feels care and concern being expressed by the healer and others in the environment
3 the individual feels an enhanced sense of mastery or control over the illness or its symptoms.

In a recent hypothesized causal account of the placebo response, Brody[44] suggests that meaning precedes other causal mechanisms such as conditioning and expectancy.

Meaning is also used as a central explanatory construct in another, but related, literature. In an impressive set of studies, Pennebaker and other investigators have found that writing about one's deepest thoughts and feelings on a set number of 20 to 30 minute occasions has health consequences even months later (for a summary of this literature, see Pennebaker[74] and Moerman[24]). In examining changes in how individuals express their thoughts and feelings across the assigned occasions, Pennebaker[74] found that increases in causal and insight words are associated with improved health. He proposed that the construction of stories or narratives may be an important way that humans integrate emotional experiences into their lives. An alternative explanation of the beneficial effects of writing about emotional experiences is that the writing assignment may produce extinction of negative emotional associations through repetition and exposure.[75] If extinction of emotional reactivity associated with thoughts of events is an important part of the process, then the linguistic changes that Pennebaker observed may be consequences, rather than causes, of changes in emotional reactivity.

**How cognitive mechanisms produce change**

In a later section, we propose a conceptual causal model for placebo effects that differs significantly from both Brody's and Pennebaker's models. We believe that the patient's assignment of meaning to health problems and therapeutic rituals provides a summary context of the operation of a number of causal variables. We propose that causal effects are reciprocal, synergistic, and recursive and involve factors that are both internal and external to the individual.

One hypothesis that deserves separate attention is whether placebos produce their specific effects through mediation by broad, systemic biological and psychological effects. We, and other authors in this book, have noted that placebos have been shown to reduce stress, improve immunological functioning, and improve subjective wellbeing. There have been some contradictory results as well, but it appears that there have been enough studies that have similar findings to raise the question of whether placebo works primarily through mediation.

A recent meta-analysis of the psychotherapy literature has tried to answer that question. Stevens, Hynan, and Allen[76] conducted a meta-analysis of 80 studies to determine the relative magnitude of common factor and specific treatment effects as related to type of outcome measures, i.e. subjective wellbeing, symptoms, and life-functioning. If placebo and common factor effects are primarily mediated effects in which subjective wellbeing is affected first, the authors should have found that common factors were most strongly associated with changes in subjective wellbeing. The magnitude of common factor versus no treatment comparisons and common factor versus specific treatment comparisons did not differ across outcome domains. Thus, although there are likely many instances in which there are mediators of placebo effects, for example, concomitant changes in health behaviors and/or reductions in stress, placebos are as likely to directly affect symptoms and life-functioning as they are to affect subjective wellbeing.

Overall, in this meta-analysis, specific therapy was more effective than common factors and common factors were more effective than no treatment in each of three outcome domains.[76] The difference in effectiveness between specific therapy and common factors was particularly noteworthy for severe disorders in that in those comparisons, common factors did not produce significantly more improvement than no treatment. In the psychological literature, at least, placebo controls and common factors do not produce the same degree of change as does specific therapy (see also Lipsey and Wilson[77]). The importance of this finding is limited, however, since common factor control conditions are seldom as credible as specific treatments. Nevertheless, the finding from meta-analyses of a difference between common factors and specific therapy expands the point we made earlier about the therapeutic relationship that common factors, including the therapeutic relationship, can often enhance therapy, but do not substitute for it.

## Placebo and healing

The relationships between the placebo effect and healing deserve some discussion as these two terms mean different things to different people. We distinguish two forms of interplay between them: (1) the understandin biological events in which healing is used as a quasi synonymous terr cure, and (2) the therapeutic process in which healing is used to describe the process of enhancement of health and wellbeing. The former deals with the science of medicine; the latter with its art.

The power of placebo draws upon the innate ability of the body to heal itself spontaneously.[78] That innate capacity is best represented in the fundamental biological principle of homeostasis that is believed to exist in all living beings. Evidence exists that self-repair occurs at all levels of physiology and anatomy.[79] Nonetheless, like many other scientific concepts healing remains a theoretical construct that cannot be directly observed but only inferred. In other words, we observe certain manifestations that we hypothesize are related to healing (two examples for which are wound healing and DNA repair), but may also be manifestations of something else. That realization is extremely important to understand because the placebo effect, like healing, is an inferential construct, i.e. a label. Misattribution of cause and effect, especially when placebos are involved, poses an important methodological challenge that requires great attention and critical thinking. Thus, it is entirely possible that the same biological events are being labeled by different observers as spontaneous remission, spontaneous healing, or placebo effect depending on one's viewpoint, belief system and context.

In the second form of relationship between the two, the placebo effect is believed to promote health and healing. Healing refers to the process of restoring the patient's perception of connectedness, indestructibility, and control.[80] It is a journey rather than a destination.[81] Proponents of this viewpoint regard the activation of the placebo effect as a powerful method that should be exploited rather than discarded.[8,40,78] This assertion stems from the observation that mastery is an important element in the placebo effect[6,44] and that patient empowerment leads to better health outcomes.[82] Health here is regarded as that state of spiritual, emotional, cognitive, physical, social, and environmental functioning which facilitates the individual's development, i.e. the balanced, coherent and integrated adjustment of, and accommodation to, internal and external events.[34]

Recently the tension between the science of medicine and the art of its practice became even more relevant in light of the debate around the role of the placebo effect in the apparent success of some complementary and alternative medicine (CAM) modalities.[83–85] The nature of the debate is not without implications. If indeed the incidental elements of CAM are those that account for its effectiveness, then health care providers need not necessarily be skilled in any of the CAM techniques but rather should be trained to activate the placebo effect/healing system pathways.[86] However, if the therapeutic relationship enhances rather than substitutes for treatment, as we concluded earlier, then all practitioners need to be trained to activate healing pathways.

## A conceptual model for the placebo effect within the therapeutic process

A biomedical model that seeks to understand the mechanisms by which this intriguing phenomenon occurs has largely dominated placebo research in the last few decades. Whereas findings of that line of research can help understanding of the "mind-body connection"[87] another aspect still needs to be explored, i.e. how does the placebo effect fit into the therapeutic process?

Based on what we have discussed so far, we would like to propose a conceptual model for the placebo effect within the therapeutic process. Two theoretical assumptions underlie this model.

1 The placebo effect is not static. It constantly evolves and changes in response to other biological and psychological signals that play a role in the therapeutic process. In other words, the placebo effect is a dependent variable that covaries with various other independent variables, both internal and external to the individual.
2 The placebo effect always interacts (in a synergistic rather than in an additive way) to an unpredictable degree with other elements of the therapeutic intervention, such as biological and psychological treatments. Albeit methodologically very complex and difficult to test, that interaction implies that even in experimental arms of randomized controlled trials the placebo effect may account for some of the outcome we measure.

It should be emphasized that the assignment of meaning to health problems and therapeutic rituals by the patient provides a summary context of the operation of a number of causal variables. We believe these variables (such as conditioning, expectancy, information from the clinician, feedback through changes in the internal and external environment, etc.) affect each other reciprocally and recursively.

The core concept of the current model is the recognition that clinician–patient interaction results not only in the generation of a treatment plan by the clinician, but also influences the patient's formation of health status meaning, as explained above. A clinician's treatment plan can be in the form of a one-line prescription or a comprehensive multi-step multi-dimensional program. For example, a patient recovering from acute myocardial infarction could be advised to take several medications from now on or could be advised to take these medications as part of an entire rehabilitation program, which requires extensive lifestyle modifications.

The assignment of meaning by the patient, we argue, is at times equally important in determining the outcome as the recommended biological treatment itself. For example, that patient may be devastated by his recent heart attack if this was preceded by good health or he may be grateful for surviving it knowing that heart attacks carry an immediate mortality rate of about 30%. Reality perception is a complex phenomenon by itself that is highly influenced by sociocultural ecological factors, patient belief systems and the like. Yet, information and suggestions provided by a physician who is perceived as competent and confident may also play a role in the creation of meaning. Thus, the patient–doctor interaction provides an excellent opportunity to positively reframe the meaning of any medical condition. The patient's outlook has limited implications when it is considered in terms of a glass that is half empty or half full, but it has expanded implications when one considers the fact that cognitive reframing may lead to (1) the placebo effect through the creation of positive or negative expectations, and (2) the development of coping strategies that will determine the patient's future health-related behavior. That behavior not only manifests itself in adherence and compliance but also leads to other patient-initiated activities that join the physician-initiated recommended treatment to form the total package of care. Thus, for instance, the doctor may recommend antihypertensive medications to our heart attack survivor, but the patient may add to that any number of other self-initiated interventions, such as stress reduction, a healthier diet, physical activity and the like that may influence the clinical outcome.

According to the proposed conceptual model, the placebo effect can affect the medical outcome potentially in three different ways.

1 Directly – through the activation of innate homeostatic healing processes, often referred to as spontaneous healing regardless of what the biological treatment might be.

   For instance, the characteristic elements[11] of antibiotics in the case of viral pharyngitis may be ineffective, yet the incidental elements[11] may trigger the placebo effect. The healing effects of antibiotics on pharyngitis may depend more on the health care context (for example, the patient's faith in the physician who prescribes the treatment, the patient's belief in the potency and plausibility of the treatment, and the very act of taking action to treat an illness) than on the specific biological effectiveness of the antibiotic. Thomas[88] refers to our unwillingness to acknowledge the ineffectiveness of antibiotics as a therapeutic illusion produced by the effectiveness of the placebo effect. Thus, under some circumstances, the placebo effect can retard the advancement of knowledge by making it difficult to provide evidence that interventions are ineffective.

2 Indirectly – through patient behavior as a mediating variable.

   For instance, Horwitz and Horwitz[89] found that patients who adhered more to the placebo treatment, in clinical trials across conditions, had better outcomes than those who did not. One plausible explanation might be that those who adhered might also have engaged in other good health-related activities, and that the incidental element of adhering to the treatment protocol may have affected their outcome.

3 Interaction of active and indirect effects with the total package of care, as proposed by the second assumption that underlies this model.

That is, treatments may be more or less effective depending on the interaction of meaning with active change ingredients.

In summary, this conceptual model has two advantages over a framework that focuses on individual components.

- We hypothesize that the model better represents how individual components interact to produce change. Cause and effect are seldom linear and unifactorial. Our model emphasizes the multi-dimensional and interactive aspects of change.
- The model provides a framework in which to summarize the complex literature on placebo effects and to advance knowledge through future research.

In our view, increased focus on cognitive variables of expectancy and meaning provides a promising direction for future research. However, cognitive variables of the patient are only part of what produces change. As stressed throughout the chapter and emphasized by our integrative conceptual model, the interplay between the patient, the disorder, and the clinician is important.

## Future research goals

In reviewing the literature for this paper, it is clear to us that a thoughtful research agenda is required if we are to advance knowledge about placebo effects. More of the same is unlikely to do that. We have some suggestions for research at both the conceptual and methodological levels.

### Neuroimaging

To advance knowledge about placebo effects, we need studies that will test specific theories about biological and psychological mechanisms and how they are represented in the brain. This is a whole set of studies and could involve Pavlovian conditioning, changes in expectancy, or any of a number of hypothesized mechanisms of placebo effects. Advances in this area could help advance knowledge about brain–behavior interactions more generally and bring placebo research into the mainstream.

### Tests of theory

Neuroimaging is, of course, a method for testing some hypotheses about theory. Other theory testing research is also required. For example, the hypothesized effect of active versus inert placebos has been based primarily on speculation. What is needed is programmatic research that examines characteristics of placebos and elements in the therapeutic relationship and their effects. For example, if meaning is an important summary variable, then research that directly attempts to affect meaning within a therapeutic context and measure specific outcomes is required.

### Signal detection theory

As we noted, signal detection methodology is a promising way of attempting to learn about how placebos change perceptions and judgments. We expect that more precise information of the type provided by signal detection theory (i.e. sensitivity and response bias) would facilitate theory testing about placebo effects.

### Research on experimental designs

The clinical trial with random assignment to a placebo control is seen as the gold standard for clinical efficacy studies. Nevertheless, the use of placebo control groups is often difficult or even impossible to employ due to a variety of practical and ethical considerations. We know very little about the extent to which other experimental designs will provide the same information as clinical trials. There are many methodological issues in addition to the use of placebo control groups, such as strict versus loose inclusion criteria, how therapies for comorbid disorders should be treated, what are the consequences of attrition, and so forth, that also require investigation.

Finally, everyone recognizes that our knowledge about the magnitude and mechanisms of placebo effects rests on a relatively small set of studies in which there have been both placebo control groups and no-treatment groups. Although such studies are informative in separating placebo effects from measurement artifacts, we believe that it is important that we begin seriously to examine the extent to which other experimental designs and methodologies could help provide information about placebo effects.

In conclusion, as the papers for this book indicate, we have learned enough about placebo effects in the past decade to be intrigued by the possibilities and power associated with them. What is required now is programmatic research into the mechanisms by which placebos are believed to change health status and behavior and a thorough exploration of designs and methodologies that will help advance knowledge about placebo effects.

## References

1 Harrington A, ed. *The placebo effect: an interdisciplinary exploration*. Cambridge, MA: Harvard University Press, 1997:1.
2 Gøtzsche OC. Is there logic in the placebo? *Lancet* 1994;**344**:925–6.
3 Shapiro AK. Factors contributing to the placebo effect. Their implication for psychotherapy. *Am J Psychother* 1964;**18**:73–88.
4 Brody H. Placebos and the philosophy of medicine. *Clinical, conceptual and ethical issues*. Chicago: University of Chicago Press, 1980.
5 NIH. OAM sponsors placebo and nocebo conference. *CAM Newsletter*. 1997. MACROBUTTON HtmlResAnchor *http://altmed.od.nih.gov/nccam/cam/1997/jan/2.htm*

6 Brody H. *The placebo response*. New York: Harper Collins, 2000:9.
7 McGuire WJ. Suspiciousness of experimenter's intent. In: Rosenthal R, Rosnow RL, eds. *Artifact in behavioral research*. New York: Academic Press, 1969.
8 Ernst E, Herxheimer A. The power of placebo: let's use it to help as much as possible. *BMJ* 1996;**313**:1569–70.
9 Bootzin RR. The role of expectancy in behavior change. In: White L, Schwartz GE, Tursky B, eds. *Placebo: theory, research and mechanisms*. New York: Guilford Press, 1985.
10 Kaptchuk TJ. Powerful placebo: the dark side of the randomized controlled trial. *Lancet* 1998;**351**:1722–5.
11 Grünbaum A. Explication and implications of the placebo concept. In: White L, Schwartz GE, Tursky B, eds. *Placebo: theory, research and mechanisms*. New York: Guilford Press, 1985.
12 Grencavage LM, Norcross JC. Where are the commonalities among the therapeutic common factors? *Prof Psychol: Res Pract* 1990;**21**:372–8.
13 Barfod TS. Placebo therapy in dermatology. *Clin Dermatol* 1999;**17**:69–76.
14 Brody H. "My story is broken; can you help me fix it?" medical ethics and joint construction of narrative. *Lit Med* 1994;**13**:79–92.
15 Brody H, Waters DB. Diagnosis is treatment. *J Fam Pract* 1980;**10**:445–9.
16 Arkowitz H. Integrative theories of therapy. In: Wachtel PL, Messer SB, eds. *Theories of psychotherapy: origins and evolution*. Washington, DC: American Psychological Association, 1997.
17 Kienle GS, Kiene H. The powerful placebo effect: fact or fiction? *J Clin Epidemiol* 1997; **50**:1311–18.
18 Davis CE. Regression to the mean or placebo effect? This volume, chapter 7.
19 Shapiro AK, Shapiro E. *The powerful placebo: from ancient priest to modern physician*. Baltimore: The John Hopkins University Press, 1997.
20 Webb EJ, Campbell DT, Schwartz RD, Sechrest LB. *Unobtrusive measures: nonreactive research in social sciences*. Chicago: Rand McNally, 1966.
21 Bootzin RR, Lack L, Wright H. Efficacy of bright and dim light with and without stimulus control instructions for sleep onset insomnia. *Sleep Res Online* 1999;**2**(Supp. 1): 648.
22 Manber R, Bootzin RR, Acebo C, Carskadon MA. The effects of regularizing sleep-wake schedules on daytime sleepiness. *Sleep* 1996;**19**:432–41.
23 Siegel S. Explanatory mechanisms for placebo effects: Pavlovian conditioning. This volume, chapter 6.
24 Moerman DE. Explanatory mechanisms for placebo effects: cultural influences and the meaning response. This volume, chapter 4.
25 Doongaji DR, Vahia VN, Bharucha MP. On placebos, placebo responses and placebo responders. *J Postgrad Med* 1978;**24**:147–57.
26 Evans FJ. The placebo response in pain reduction. In: Bonica JJ, ed. *Advanced Neurology*: Vol. 4: *Pain*. New York: Raven Press, 1974:289–96.
27 Freeman EW, Rickels K. Characteristics of placebo responses in medical treatment of premenstrual syndrome. *Am J Psychiatry* 1999;**156**:1403–8.
28 Mataix-Cols D, Rauch SL, Manzo PA, Jenike MA, Baer L. Use of factor-analyzed symptom dimensions to predict outcome with serotonin reuptake inhibitors and placebo in the treatment of obsessive-compulsive disorder. *Am J Psychiatry* 1999;**156**: 1409–16.
29 Rosenberg NK, Mellegard M, Rosenberg R, Bech P, Ottosson J-O. Characteristics of panic disorder patients responding to placebo. *Acta Psychiatr Scand* 1991;**365**(Suppl):33–8.
30 Shetty N, Friedman JH, Keiburtz K, Marshall FJ, Oakes D. The placebo response in Parkinson's disease. *Clin Neuropharmacol* 1999;**22**:207–12.
31 Drici MD, Raybaud F, de Lunardo C, Iacono P, Gustovic P. Influence of the behavior pattern on the nocebo response of healthy volunteers. *Br J Clin Pharmacol* 1995;**39**: 204–6.
32 Spiro H. Clinical reflections on the placebo phenomenon. In: Harrington A, ed. *The placebo effect: an interdisciplinary exploration*. Cambridge, MA: Harvard University Press, 1997.
33 Pepper OHP. A note on the placebo. *Am J Pharmacol* 1945;**117**:409–12.
34 Mitchell A, Cormack M. *The therapeutic relationship in complementary health care*. Edinburgh: Churchill Livingstone, 1998.

35 Oh VM. The placebo effect: can we use it better? *BMJ* 1994;**309**:69–70.
36 Thomas KB. General practice consultations: is there any point in being positive? *BMJ* 1987;**294**:1200–2.
37 Brody H. The doctor as therapeutic agent: A placebo effect research agenda. In: Harrington A, ed. *The placebo effect: an interdisciplinary exploration*. Cambridge, MA: Harvard University Press, 1997.
38 Houston WR. The doctor himself as a therapeutic agent. *Ann Intern Med* 1938;**11**: 1416–25.
39 Findley T. The placebo and the physician. *Med Clin North Am* 1953;**37**:1821–6.
40 Benson H, Friedman R. Harnessing the power of the placebo effect and renaming it "remembered wellness." *Annu Rev Med* 1996;**47**:193–9.
41 Thomas KB. The placebo in general practice. *Lancet* 1994;**344**:1066–7.
42 Gracely RH, Dunbar R, Deeter WR, Wolskee PJ. Clinician's expectations influence placebo analgesia. [Letter] *Lancet* 1985;**1**(8419):43.
43 Leopold N, Cooper J, Clancy C. Sustained partnership in primary care. *J Fam Pract* 1996;**42**:129–37.
44 Brody H. The placebo response: recent research and implications for family medicine. *J Fam Pract* 2000;**49**:649–54.
45 Benson H, Epstein MD. The placebo effect: a neglected asset in the care of patients. JAMA 1975;**232**:1225–7.
46 Bernstein CN. Placebos in medicine. *Semin Gastrointest Dis* 1999;**10**:3–7.
47 Smith ML, Glass GV, Miller TJ. *The benefits of psychotherapy*. Baltimore: Johns Hopkins University Press, 1980.
48 Elkin I, Shea MT, Watkins JT, *et al.* National Institute of Mental Health Treatment of Depression Collaborative Research Program: general effectiveness of treatments. *Arch Gen Psychiatry* 1989;**46**:971–82.
49 Project MATCH Research Group. Matching alcoholism treatments to client heterogeneity: Project MATCH post-treatment drinking outcomes. *J Stud Alcohol* 1997; **58**:7–29.
50 Andrews G, Harvey R. Does psychotherapy benefit neurotic patients? A re-analysis of the Smith, Glass, and Miller data. *Arch Gen Psychiatry* 1981;**38**:1203–8.
51 Miller WR, Brown JM, Simpson TL, *et al.* What works? a methodological analysis of the alcohol treatment outcome literature. In: Hester RK, Miller WR, eds. *Handbook of alcoholism treatment approaches: effective alternatives*, 2nd ed. Boston: Allyn & Bacon, 1995.
52 Miller WR, Andrews NR, Wilbourne P, Bennett ME. A wealth of alternatives: Effective treatments for alcohol problems. In: Miller WR, Heather N, eds. *Treating addictive behaviors*, 2nd ed. New York: Plenum Press, 1998.
53 Grencavage L, Bootzin RR, Shoham Salomon V. Specific and nonspecific effects in psychological treatments. In: Costello CG, ed. *Basic issues in psychopathology*. New York: Guilford Press, 1993.
54 Alexander JF, Barton C, Schiavo RS, Parsons BV. Systems behavioral intervention with families of delinquents: therapists' characteristics, family behavior, and outcome. *J Consult Clin Psychol* 1976;**44**:656–64.
55 Parsons Jr BV, Alexander JF. Short-term family interventions: a therapy outcome study. *J Consult Clin Psychol* 1973;**41**:195–201.
56 Green DM, Swets JA. *Signal detection theory and psychophysics*. New York: Wiley, 1966.
57 Clark WC, Yang JC. Experimental pain following analgesic, placebo, and acupuncture: an introduction to signal detection theory. *Acupunct Electrother Res* 1976;**2**(1-sup-2): 87–103.
58 Losier BJ, McGrath PJ, Klein RM. Error patterns of the Continuous Performance Test in non-medicated and medicated samples of children with and without ADHD: a meta-analytic review. *J Child Psychol Psychiatry* 1996;**37**:971–87.
59 Frank JD. *Persuasion and healing*. Baltimore: Johns Hopkins University Press, 1961.
60 Frank JD. Therapeutic factors in psychotherapy. *Am J Psychother* 1971;**25**:350–61.
61 Frank JD. Therapeutic components shared by all psychotherapies. In: Hawey JH, Parks MM, eds. *Psychotherapy research and behavior change*. Washington, DC: American Psychological Association, 1981.
62 Bandura A. Self efficacy: toward a unifying theory of behavior change. *Psychol Rev* 1977; **84**:191–215.

63 Bandura A. *Self-efficacy: the exercise of control.* New York: Cambridge University Press, 1997.
64 Crow R, Gage H, Hampson S, Hart J, Kimber A, Thomas H. The role of expectancies in the placebo effect and their use in the delivery of health care: a systematic review. *Health Technol Assess* 1999;**3**:3.
65 Reiss S. Pavlovian conditioning and human fear: an expectancy model. *Behavior Therapy* 1980;**11**:380–96.
66 Kirsch I. Response expectancy as a determinant of experience and behavior. *Am Psychol* 1985;**40**:1189–202.
67 Kirsch I, Lynn SJ. Automaticity in clinical psychology. *Am Psychol* 1999;**54**:504–15.
68 Kirsch I, Weixel LJ. Double blind versus deceptive administration of a placebo. *Biomed Ther* 1988;**XVI**(3):242–6.
69 Swartzman LC, Burkell J. Expectations and the placebo effect in clinical drug trials: why we should not turn a blind eye to unblinding, and other cautionary notes. *Clin Pharmacol Ther* 1998;**64**(1):1–7.
70 Clayden JR, Bell JW, Pollar P. Menopausal flushing: double blind trial of a non-hormonal preparation. *BMJ* 1974;**1**:409–12.
71 Kirsch I, Sapirstein G. Listening to Prozac but hearing placebo: a meta-analysis of antidepressant medication. In: Kirsch I, ed. *How expectancies shape experience.* Washington, DC: American Psychological Association, 1999.
72 Valins S, Nisbett RE. *Attribution processes in the development and treatment of emotional disorders.* Morristown, NJ: General Learning Press, 1971.
73 Davison GC, Tsuimoto RN, Glaros AG. Attribution and the maintenance of behavior change in falling asleep. *J Abnorm Psychol* 1973;**82**:124–33.
74 Pennebaker JW. Writing about emotional experiences as a therapeutic process. *Psychol Sci* 1997;**8**:162–6.
75 Bootzin RR. Examining the theory and clinical utility of writing about emotional experiences. *Psychol Sci* 1997;**8**:167–9.
76 Stevens SE, Hynan MT, Allen M. A meta-analysis of common factor and specific treatment effects across the outcome domains of the phase model of psychotherapy. *Clin Psychol: Sci Pract* 2000;**7**:273–90.
77 Lipsey MW, Wilson DB. The efficacy of psychological, educational, and behavioral treatment. *Am Psychol* 1993;**48**:1181–209.
78 Bennet P. Placebo and healing. In: Pizzorno JE, Murray MT, eds. *Textbook of natural medicine.* Edinburgh, UK: Churchill Livingstone, 1999.
79 Weil A. *Spontaneous healing.* New York: Fawcett Columbine, 1995.
80 Cassell EJ *The healer's art.* Harmondsworth, UK: Penguin, 1978.
81 Maizes V, Caspi O. The principles and challenges of integrative medicine. *West J Med* 1999;**171**:148–9.
82 Greenfield S, Kaplan S, Ware JE. Expanding patient involvement in care: effects on patient outcomes. *Ann Intern Med* 1985;**102**:520–8.
83 Joyce CRB. Placebo and complementary medicine. *Lancet* 1994;**344**:1279–81.
84 Moerman DE. Placebo effects in medical care. In: Jonas W, Levin JS, eds. *Textbook of complementary and alternative medicine.* Baltimore: Williams and Wilkins, 1999.
85 Richardson P. The placebo effect in orthodox and complementary medicine. In: Vincent C, Furnham A, eds. *Complementary medicine.* West Sussex: Wiley, 1997.
86 Caspi O. On mainstreaming and integration of complementary and alternative medicine. *BMJ* 2000. *http://www.bmj.com/cgi/eletters/321/7262/683#EL6* (accessed August 21, 2001).
87 Dienstfrey H (ed.). Placebo and health. *Adv Mind Body Med* 2000;**16**:6–46.
88 Thomas KB. The placebo in general practice. *Lancet* 1994;**344**(8929):1066–7.
89 Horwitz RI, Horwitz SM. Adherence to treatment and health outcome. *Arch Intern Med* 1993;**153**:1863–8.

# 6: Explanatory mechanisms for placebo effects: Pavlovian conditioning*

SHEPARD SIEGEL

## Introduction

Sometimes innocuous treatments or inert substances have substantial physiological and behavioral effects. Depending upon one's definition of "placebo effect", these responses may be classified as instances of placebo effects. In a previous review of the contribution of Pavlovian conditioning to the placebo effect, Ader discussed the various definitions of the effect, and the theoretical biases that are incorporated in some definitions.[1] Some clinicians emphasize the fact that "placebo" is the first-person singular of the future tense of the Latin "placere" – to please – thus the placebo effect is a manifestation of the patient's attempt to please the clinician. Since the clinician's job is to make the patient better, the placebo effect is, according to this view, a therapeutic benefit resulting from (or attributed to) an inert substance or innocuous treatment – "A biomedically inert substance given in such a manner to produce *relief* is known as a placebo"[2] [emphasis added here, see also Shapiro, *et al.*[3]]. According to this view of the placebo as a therapeutic agent, if a pharmacologically ineffective potion attenuates depression, insomnia, or pain, the phenomenon is termed a placebo effect. For others, however, the placebo effect refers to *any* physiological response to an innocuous treatment that is not explained by the properties of the treatment (whether or not the response is salubrious). According to this second view, even if a patient claims that an innocuous substance makes

* Preparation of this article, and research from the author's laboratory summarized in the article, was supported by grants from the Natural Sciences and Engineering Research Council of Canada, the United States National Institute on Drug Abuse, and the Alcoholic Beverage Medical Research Foundation.

him or her ill, the patient is said to be experiencing a placebo effect. For example, some clinicians who are skeptical about the existence of "multiple chemical sensitivity" or environmental illness attribute these complaints to "placebo effects".[4,5] It is the latter sense of placebo effect that is relevant to this discussion of the contribution of Pavlovian conditioning to understanding the phenomenon: a response to a substance or treatment that is not explicable on the basis of the known properties of the substance or treatment (whether or not the response is therapeutic).

Most early observers of the placebo effect considered it a demonstration of human suggestibility: "It would seem to us inescapable that the placebo reaction must be a manifestation of suggestion, using the term in its broadest sense".[6] Others, however, emphasized the fact that phenomena resembling the placebo effects seen in medical practice could be reproduced in the laboratory with non-human animals (as well as humans). All that was necessary was to follow the procedures emphasized by Ivan Pavlov for developing new responses to previous neutral stimuli – a process called "Pavlovian conditioning":

> The placebo effect is usually attributed to some kind of 'suggestion' that operates, even if temporarily, to fulfill the patient's expectations about treatment ... The placebo effect can, however, be viewed in a different way. The elicitation of a specific reaction by arbitrary agents, such as the abatement of a symptom after the mere sight of a physician and his medicines, may be nothing more than simple conditioning of the sort originally demonstrated by Pavlov with animals.[7]

## What is Pavlovian conditioning?

Ivan Petrovich Pavlov won the Nobel Prize for physiology in 1904. He was awarded the prize for his studies of digestive reflexes, in dogs, using chronic observational methods (i.e. digestive reflexes were observed in intact, awake dogs). Because he used chronic preparations, Pavlov made some observations that, although not the basis for his Nobel Prize, would be the topic of his research for the remainder of his life.

In his Nobel Prize acceptance speech, Pavlov did not discuss the gastrointestinal work that formed the basis of the award. Rather, he presented an address entitled "The First Sure Steps along the Path of a New Investigation". The "new investigation" was the study of what we now call "conditional reflexes". Pavlov, then 55 years old, essentially abandoned his successful study of digestive physiology to devote his full energies to this new topic – one that he considered even more important.[8]

Pavlov observed that his dogs displayed digestive reflexes (such as gastric secretion), not only in response to stimuli that had reflexively elicited such responses (i.e. stimulation of receptors in the stomach), but also in response to stimuli that, in the past, had signaled such stimulation (for example, the presence of the person who fed the dog). Pavlov concluded that it would be impossible to understand digestive physiology without understanding the role of these "psychic" reflexes (as they were originally termed), as well as physiological reflexes. He developed procedures and terminology that are used today in the study of Pavlovian conditioning.

## The Pavlovian conditioning paradigm

Pavlovian conditioning (sometimes termed respondent, classical, or Type 1 conditioning) is defined by a set of operations in which a neutral conditional stimulus (CS) is paired with a biologically-significant unconditional stimulus (UCS). At the start of conditioning, the UCS reflexively (i.e. "unconditionally") elicits some response, termed the "unconditional response", or "unconditional reflex" (UCR). As a result of CS–UCS pairings, the CS becomes associated with the UCS. The acquisition of this association is revealed by the emergence of a new response to the previously neutral CS. Because this new response is conditional on CS–UCS pairings, it is termed the "conditional response", or "conditional reflex" (CR).* Pavlov realized that salivation was much easier to measure than gastric secretion, and the manipulation of cues such as tones and lights could be much more precise than manipulation of cues such as the sight of the person that normally fed the dogs. In Pavlov's well known work, the UCS was food or dilute acid injected into the mouth, the UCR salivation, and the CS some arbitrary cue (such as a tone of a certain pitch). After some pairings of CS and UCS, a new reflex develops. In this example, a tone elicits salivation.

The pairing responsible for Pavlovian conditioning may occur because an experimenter presents CSs and UCSs in the laboratory. Alternatively, such pairing may result adventitiously. The sight of an acidic food (for example, the sight of a lemon) normally is paired with this food in the mouth, thus the sight of a lemon typically serves as a CS. People salivate in response to the sight of a cut lemon, even before the salivation is unconditionally elicited by the citric acid stimulation of receptors in the mouth. The sight of the lemon is a "placebo treatment" that elicits the placebo response of salivation. Similarly, the sight of a drug and the preparations for drug administration typically precede the unconditional pharmacological effect, thus drug administration cues may serve as a CS. Nesse and colleagues[9] presented an example of such drug administration cues adventitiously becoming associated with a drug effect. They described the case of a woman who reported nausea (and sometimes vomited) when she encountered an odor that was present in a clinic. This woman was being treated for Hodgkin's disease with a regimen of MOPP

* Although Pavlov used the terms "unconditional" and "conditional" reflexes, the terms subsequently were unfortunately mistranslated from the original Russian as "unconditioned" and "conditioned" reflexes.[114]

chemotherapy (mechlorethamine, "Oncovin" (vincristine), procarbazine, and prednisone). Each MOPP injection induced nausea lasting for many hours. Nesse *et al.*[9] reported that about 44% of their patients being treated for lymphoma demonstrated such "pretreatment nausea", and suggested that "this syndrome of pretreatment nausea can be understood as a classically conditioned response"; certain odors have become aversive because of their association with chemotherapy-induced illness. Much subsequent research has attested to the value of Nesse *et al.*'s observations concerning the role of learning in aversions acquired by patients receiving chemotherapy.[10–12] On the basis of a conditioning analysis, the clinic odor is a "placebo treatment" that elicits a placebo response of nausea.

Several phenomena of Pavlovian conditioning are especially relevant to appreciating the potential contribution of conditioning to placebo effects.

### *Conditioning can occur with a long delay between the CS and UCS*

Typically, conditioning experiments involve presentation of the CS and UCS in close temporal contiguity, usually within seconds of each other. Such an arrangement of conditioning stimuli often is not necessary to establish an association. Rather, with some CSs and UCSs, the interval may be minutes or hours. For example, with a variety of chemical UCS (for example, emetics, immunomodulators), CS–UCS associations can form even with very long delays between the two conditioning stimuli.[5,13] Thus, even if there is a considerable delay between the time the drug is administered and the time some drug effect is noted, pharmacological conditioning is still possible.

### *Conditioning can occur rapidly*

Although conditioning experiments frequently involve many CS–UCS pairings, there are many conditioning preparations in which an association is well established in only a single trial. The most thoroughly studied instances of such one-trial learning involve associations formed with flavor (or odor) CSs and chemical UCSs, although there is evidence that such rapid learning is a general feature of Pavlovian conditioning.[5] It is not necessary, then, for a patient to have extensive experience with active medication for a conditioning mediated placebo effect to occur.

### *Conditional responses display stimulus generalization*

Conditional responses may be elicited by stimuli that have never been paired with the CS. Such conditional responding to novel stimuli is termed "generalization". Typically, the greater the similarity between the novel assessment stimulus and the CS, the greater the strength of the generalized CR. To use an example described by Pavlov, "if a tone of 1000 d.v. [Hz] is established as a conditioned stimulus, many other tones spontaneously acquire similar properties, such properties diminishing proportionally to the intervals of these tones from the one of 1000 d.v. [Hz]".[14] Thus, the CR may be displayed in response to cues that are not exactly like those used during the acquisition of the learned response. Because of stimulus generalization, the CS that elicits the placebo effect need not be identical to the cues that accompanied administration of the active medication.

*Conditional responses are well retained but can be extinguished*

Once CRs are established, they are very well retained. That is, following CR acquisition, if neither the CS nor UCS is presented for a considerable period of time, there is little decrement in CR strength.[15] Indeed, patients who have acquired the CR of illness as a result of chemotherapy for cancer sometimes display conditional illness in response to treatment related cues several years after they have completed treatment.[16] Although CRs are very resistant to decrement merely as a function of the passage of time, they can be weakened by repeated presentation of the CS in the absence of the UCS. Such repeated presentations of the CS alone to an organism that had acquired a CR as a result of prior CS–UCS pairings is termed "extinction". If the placebo effect is a CR, it should be well retained, but should be subject to extinction by repeated presentation of the administration cues in the absence of the active medication.

## Pavlovian conditioning of pharmacological responses

The idea that predrug cues are effective CSs in Pavlovian conditioning can be traced to the very earliest studies of Pavlovian conditioning. When Pavlov's salivary conditioning work was translated into English[17] it stimulated considerable interest among some Western investigators. One of the earliest observations of Pavlovian conditioning of a salivary response in an American laboratory is especially relevant to a conditioning analysis of the placebo effect. Collins and Tatum[18] were studying the effects of chronic morphine administration in dogs. They injected eight dogs with morphine daily for seven or eight days. Each injection elicited copious salivation. As an apparently serendipitous observation made in the course of these studies, they found every dog displayed salivation as a CR: "The entrance into the dog room of the person conducting the experiment was in most cases sufficient to precipitate this copious salivation. The sight of a hypodermic syringe never failed to produce a secretion of saliva ...".[18] Thus, it would appear that drugs, in common with food, could serve as UCSs. In a subsequent study of morphine conditioning, Kleitman and Crisler[19] similarly reported that dogs that had been injected with morphine after placement in a temporary restraint displayed profuse salivation (and occasionally anticipatory vomiting and sleep) when placed in the restraint, prior to any drug injection.

In fact, when the results of additional research from Pavlov's laboratory were finally translated and published in English two years after the Collins and Tatum report, it was apparent that the Soviet scientists had, independently, made similar observations. Pavlov[14] described the results of research by Krylov. In Krylov's experiments, a dog was repeatedly injected with morphine. After five or six such injections, it was observed that "the preliminaries of injection"[14] elicited many morphine-like responses, including salivation. Additional research, primarily by Soviet and Eastern European investigators (or Western scientists trained in Pavlov's laboratory), demonstrated that a wide variety of drugs are effective UCSs in the classical conditioning procedure, and that many visceral and behavioral responses can be affected by initially neutral cues that signal the effects of these drugs.[20–22] Some of the early findings are quite striking. For example, both Dolin[21] and Perez-Cruet and Gantt[23] demonstrated conditional catalepsy. They repeatedly induced a cataleptic state in dogs by widely-spaced injections of bulbocapnine. After about 10 drug administrations, catalepsy could be induced as a CR simply by presenting bulbocapnine-paired cues. More recently, similar findings of conditional catalepsy have been reported in mice repeatedly injected with SCH 23390, a selective antagonist of D(I)-like dopamine receptors.[24]

Reiss[25] suggested that insulin shocklike behaviors were subject to Pavlovian conditioning. He injected rats with a large dose of insulin on 10 occasions and observed the temporal characteristics of the "slight neuromuscular twitching, head stroking, retardation of normal movements, and semi-coma" elicited by the hormone. He noted that "a reaction not unlike that of the established insulin reaction" could be induced in these rats by injection of physiological saline. Similar findings have been reported in dogs[26] and in patients with a history of insulin shock therapy.[27]

Throughout the late 1920s and early 1930s, there were many reports of conditional modifications of defensive blood reactions related to immunity (Ader presented a review of early conditional immunomodulation studies[28]).

The early findings of conditional pharmacological responses (primarily by Russian investigators) certainly were dramatic, and there were many empirical demonstrations that a variety of effects of many drugs could be conditioned. However, the research typically was not described in great detail and there appeared to be methodological inadequacies. Gregory Razran, who translated much of the early research by Pavlov and his students (including pharmacological conditioning research), described the field as "literally clogged with unintegrated empirical findings".[29] However, the work was potentially so important that it nevertheless deserved serious consideration – "No one, it seems, suggests throwing out the modern Russian baby along with its indigenous methodological bath".[30] A considerable amount of subsequent, more methodologically adequate, research has confirmed the fact that drugs are effective UCSs in Pavlovian conditioning. There are many contemporary demonstrations of conditioning of behavioral, biochemical, and intracellular pharmacological responses.[1,31–33]

## Pavlovian conditioning as a mechanism of the placebo effect

Although there was a considerable amount of research on the conditioning of drug effects in the early part of the 20th century, there was not much recognition of the importance of the placebo effect until mid-century. In 1957, both Kurland[34] and Gliedman, Gantt, and Teitelbaum[35] independently suggested that the pharmacological conditioning research was relevant to the clinical phenomenon. Perhaps the best known of the early advocates for a conditioning interpretation of the placebo effect was Herrnstein, who published a paper in *Science* in 1962 titled "Placebo Effect in the Rat".[7] He demonstrated that scopolamine alters the pattern of operant responding for sweetened milk in rats in a particular manner, and, in rats with a history of scopolamine administration, injection of saline had a similar effect on milk motivated responding. Herrnstein concluded that the injection procedure acted as a CS, which was paired with unconditional effects of scopolamine. After 14 such pairings, merely presenting the CS (injection of an inert substance) caused scopolamine-like alteration of behavior.

According to Herrnstein's conditioning analysis of the placebo effect, the phenomenon does *not* result from any patient-healer dynamic, nor is it a phenomenon of human suggestibility ("... we are disposed to speak of nonverbal animals as conditionable rather than suggestible"[7]). Rather it is yet another instance of Pavlovian conditioning – a phenomenon seen in many species with many cues (not just predrug or pretreatment cues) and many responses (not just drug or treatment elicited therapeutic benefits): "Viewed as conditioning, the placebo effect is merely a particular instance of a phylogenetically widespread behavioral phenomenon, and not a manifestation of man's special symbolic capacities".[7]

There has been a considerable amount of research that has attempted to explain the placebo effect as a CR. Although there are many findings that support the conditioning analysis of the effect, there also are some contrary findings and contradictory data. The purpose of this chapter is to review the evidence that Pavlovian conditioning mediates the placebo effect, and then to indicate findings that are problematic for a simple conditioning interpretation of all placebo effects.

## Examples of placebo effects attributable to Pavlovian conditioning

It would not be possible to summarize the very extensive pharmacological conditioning/placebo effect literature in this paper (for prior reviews[36–40]). Rather, what follows are some illustrations of placebo phenomena that have been attributed to Pavlovian conditioning.

**Multiple chemical sensitivity**

Environmental illness, or multiple chemical sensitivity (MCS), is a controversial medical diagnosis. It may be applied to patients who complain of illness when exposed to various, commonly encountered (typically odiferous) stimuli that others do not find aversive. Some "clinical ecologists" have attributed MCS to pathology resulting from exposure (or accidental overexposure) to pollutants, insecticides, airborne irritants, or other toxic agents (i.e. MCS is a UCR). Others, as previously indicated, have attributed at least some cases of MCS to a placebo effect attributable to Pavlovian conditioning. According to this view, MCS is a CR.

As would be expected on the basis of a conditioning account of MCS, the respiratory effects of airborne irritants can be conditioned.[41,42] As summarized by Wood and Coleman:[42]

> If airborne concentrations of irritants are sufficiently aversive, they may act as unconditioned stimuli necessary for respondent conditioning to occur. Subsequent exposure to previously ineffective concentrations, or to other stimuli associated with chemical irritation, might result in the elicitation of conditioned responses that are unpleasant in and of themselves or have behavioral or other effects.

Case reports suggest that some individuals may have acquired their MCS in a manner consistent with an aversion-learning analysis. For example, Bolla-Wilson, Wilson, and Bleecker[43] describe cases in which individuals became ill after accidental exposure to high levels of odorous toxic agents (for example, insecticides or solvents) and thereafter reported various symptoms (headaches, nausea, pain in extremities) in response to a variety of odors. That is, the illness-associated odor (for example, odor of insecticide) as well as other odors (for example, cigarette smoke, car fumes) elicited uncomfortable somatic symptoms. In contrast, MCS patients rarely, if ever, develop their symptoms following exposure to odorless substances:

> We have never seen the development of these [MCS] episodic symptoms after significant exposures to odorless toxic substances such as lead or arsenic. Therefore, it appears that the person must be exposed to an odorous toxicant (solvents, chlordane) for conditioning to take place and for generalization to other substances to occur.[43]

As described by Bolla-Wilson *et al.*, MCS symptoms may be explained as aversions to the odor paired with illness upon the occasion of accidental exposure, and stimulus generalization from the illness-paired odor to other odors: "the causal mechanism for prolonged physical symptoms and sensitivity to common environmental substances can best be conceptualized in a classical conditioning model."[43]

The extensive literature concerning the contribution of Pavlovian conditioning to MCS has been reviewed elsewhere.[5,13] The MCS model is useful for illustrating the polarized views that result when symptoms are interpreted as CRs, rather than as UCRs. For example, there are those that assert that since MCS is a CR, it is not a "medical disorder", and those who think otherwise are "masquerading the placebo effect as science".[4]

## Non-medical drug use

Although placebo effects are seen as relevant in evaluating the effects of drugs in medical practice, most drugs are used non-medically. People ingest enormous amounts of licit psychoactive drugs (caffeine, nicotine, and alcohol). Because these drugs are typically administered orally, there are naturally-occurring cues that signal the imminent pharmacological stimulation, and thus that may serve as CSs – the flavor of the drug in the medium in which it is consumed. In addition to licit non-medical drug use, many drugs are used illicitly.

### *Caffeine*

Zwyghuizen-Doorenbos, Roehrs, Lipschutz, Timms, and Roth[44] conducted an experiment to determine if the effects of caffeine can be conditioned. Men received either caffeinated or decaffeinated ("placebo") coffee twice a day for two days. On the third ("conditioning test") day men in both groups received the placebo beverage. Alertness was measured using standardized tests of daytime sleepiness and auditory vigilance performance. On the conditioning test, those subjects that received caffeine on the two prior days were more alert than were those subjects that received the placebo.

Although the Zwyghuizen-Doorenbos *et al.*[44] results provide evidence that the effects of caffeine can be conditioned, it may not be necessary to administer conditioning sessions in the laboratory. Most adult drinkers of a caffeinated beverage have had many thousands of pairings of a distinctive gustatory cue (CS) with the systemic effects of caffeine (UCS). It might be expected, then, that (without any prior laboratory training) presentation of the CS alone (i.e. decaffeinated coffee) should elicit a placebo response.

Both Knowles[45] and Flaten and Blumenthal[46] provided evidence that some effects of coffee, attributable to caffeine, are mimicked by decaffeinated coffee, and suggested that their results were relevant to a Pavlovian conditioning interpretation of the placebo effect. For example, Flaten and Blumenthal reported that, in women who were experienced coffee drinkers, decaffeinated coffee increased some subjective (for example, rated alertness) and physiological (for example, startle reflex magnitude) arousal responses. They concluded that their results

> showed that presentation of caffeine-associated stimuli increased arousal as did caffeine itself. The behavior of this conditioned response is similar to the behavior of a placebo response. Thus, it is concluded that caffeine use is a model in which placebo responses and their effects on treatment may be studied.[46]

*Nicotine*

Robinson, Houtsmuller, Moolchan, and Pickworth[47] recently have summarized the results of many studies that have evaluated the effects of "placebo cigarettes" in cigarette smokers. Recently, tobacco-based denicotinized cigarettes have been developed for research purposes. Robinson *et al.* report findings indicating that these placebo cigarettes that closely duplicate the sensory aspects of smoking (in the absence of actual nicotine) reduce subjective measures of tobacco craving, desire to smoke, and tobacco withdrawal. Although it would appear that the placebo cigarettes elicited cigarette-like CRs, further research is needed. As indicated by the authors, it is possible that these apparent cigarette placebo responses are due to the unconditional effects of chemical constituents (other than nicotine) in the placebo cigarettes (for example, tar, carbon monoxide), rather than to the sensory aspects of the denicotinized cigarette (i.e. a CR).

*Alcohol*

Most college students have considerable experience in which the taste of beer is paired with the systemic effect of alcohol. Newlin[48] evaluated several responses elicited by a CS for beer (dealcoholized beer) in female college students. He found that the response to the "alcohol placebo" was, like the response to alcohol, an increase in heart rate and increase in reported intoxication.

Do alcoholics have a greater placebo response to alcohol-associated cues than do non-alcoholics? Meyer and Dolinsky[49] evaluated levels of plasma testosterone and leuteinizing hormone when men were presented with a frosted mug of beer which they could handle and smell, but not drink. Half the men were inpatient alcoholics, and half were non-alcoholic control subjects. Holding and sniffing the beer resulted in decreased plasma testosterone and leuteinizing hormone in alcoholic (but not control) subjects. As summarized by Meyer and Dolinsky, alcohol consumption unconditionally elicits a decrease in these hormones, thus the more experienced drinkers appeared to have a greater CR to naturally occurring alcohol associated cues.

*Illicit drug use*

Several clinicians have observed that drug addicts sometimes respond to drug-related stimuli with drug-like intoxication. For example, Levine[50] described the phenomenon of "needle freaks" – some intravenous narcotics users display compulsive injection without resulting drug effect (for example, injection of tap water). Siegel[51] described a study in which 20 users of cocaine (intranasal and smoked) were provided with a vial of oil containing the aroma of cocaine. He found that, for some subjects, the cocaine-odor elicited some aspects of the cocaine experience: "Thirteen users recognized the smell and reported mild, albeit transient (1 to 2 seconds), cocaine-like effects of heightened arousal and alertness". For some users, the cocaine-aroma reduced craving for cocaine.

## Medical drug use

Typically drugs administered for medical reasons are signaled by a variety of events that are uniquely present at the time of drug administration, for example, the sight of the medication, the flavor of an orally ingested drug, the piercing of the skin with a hypodermic needle, or the clinic environment. There have been many, many studies of the conditioning of the effects of such therapeutically-administered drugs, and the contribution of such conditioning to placebo effects. Only a few illustrative examples are summarized here.

### *Immunological placebo effects*

Over a century ago MacKenzie[52] reported that some people who are allergic to flowers display an allergic reaction when presented with something that superficially looks like a flower, but contains no pollen – an artificial flower. The association between the visual features of the flower (CS) and the pollen (UCS) results in the allergic reaction to the non-antigenic artificial flower. Extensive recent research, much of it by Ader and colleagues, has convincingly demonstrated that:

- immunological responses may be modified by Pavlovian conditioning
- these immunological CRs may contribute to placebo effects both in humans and in non-human animals
- conditional immunological responses may be profitably exploited in pharmacotherapy.[1,36]

A recent study with humans illustrates the phenomenon of conditional immunosuppression.[53] The subjects were patients receiving cyclophosphamide as a treatment for multiple sclerosis (MS). They ingested an anise-flavored syrup prior to intravenous administration of the immunosuppressive drug (at doses ranging from 1100 to 1826 mg, each drug administration inducing substantial leukopenia). On a test session, in a double blind manner, they ingested the syrup and were infused with a small, ineffective dose of cyclophosphamide (10 mg, less than 1% of the effective dose). Eight out of ten subjects displayed decreased peripheral leukocyte counts on this test session. As indicated by the authors, such a placebo elicited leukopenia has important clinical implications. For example, patients with prior experience with immunosuppressants may acquire an immunosuppressive CR to drug-associated stimuli. Such patients would be "placebo responders" in subsequent experiments: "It is possible that previously treated patients participating in a clinical trial and receiving a placebo in a double blind manner actually show a suppression of a clinically relevant immune response that modifies the disease course".

Moreover, the fact that such a clinically relevant immune response may be displayed as a CR suggests that it may be possible to reduce the dose of drug administered during treatment: "It is possible that conditioned responses could enable reduction of the cumulative doses, or extension of the duration of benefit, of conventional immunosuppressive treatments of immune-mediated diseases such as MS".

An earlier study by Ader and Cohen[54] supported Giang *et al.*'s[53] suggestion that placebo effects, established by conditioning, may be exploited for therapeutic benefit. Ader and Cohen used NZ/B mice, which are genetically disposed to develop a disease that is considered to be a model of systemic lupus erythematosus. Since these mice have autoimmune disease, cyclophosphamide is beneficial inasmuch as it retards onset of the disease and subsequent morbidity. Conditioned mice received CS cyclophosphamide paired presentations interspersed with CS alone exposures. Mice in this group had delays in the onset of disease that were statistically not different from animals which received twice as much cyclophosphamide, but no CS.

*Cardiac placebo effects*

Bykov[20] presented the results of many studies (likely conducted many years before the 1959 English translation of his book) in which previously neutral stimuli, after being paired with a drug that modifies electrocardiographic activity, become capable of similarly modifying the electrocardiogram. For example, after about 100 pairings of a "bicycle horn" with intravenous injection of nitroglycerin in a dog, the sound of the horn alone altered the electrocardiogram in the same manner as the drug – heart rate increased, and the S-T segment and T wave of the electrocardiogram displayed nitroglycerin-like alterations: "The similarity between the conditioned and the unconditioned response is astonishingly clear".[20] As is the case in many of the early Russian studies, important details of the experimental procedure were not provided, but Bykov's findings of cardiac conditioning in dogs repeatedly administered nitroglycerin were essentially replicated by Lang, Ross, and Glover.[55] Lang *et al.* recognized that their findings might be relevant to understanding placebo effects: "The fact that conditional responses can be induced by drugs and that physiological changes are elicited by stimuli associated with repeated drug administration has important clinical implications … Placebo reactions may be more explicable when considered in terms of learning concepts and conditional responses".

Subsequently, Lang and Rand[56] evaluated conditioning of the effects of sublingual nitroglycerin in three healthy women. Sessions were conducted three times per week. For each session, the subject was given a peppermint-flavored tablet of nitroglycerin sublingually. After varying numbers of such drug sessions (but at least eight), a peppermint-flavored placebo tablet was substituted for the nitroglycerin tablet. Every subject responded to the placebo tablet with tachycardia (but the conditional increase in heart rate was consistently less than that unconditionally induced by the drug). Following some of the administrations of nitroglycerin, the subjects reported palpitations and headache. They also reported these symptoms following some of the placebo administrations. Lang and Rand interpreted their findings as a demonstration of pharmacological conditioning: "These effects are interpreted as conditional responses established with the active tablet serving as the unconditional stimulus and the placebo as the conditional stimulus". Moreover, they noted that their findings were relevant to understanding the placebo effect, especially in subjects that had been repeatedly subject to clinical trials: "Despite the use of double blind and objective techniques, placebo reactions occur in anginal patients. In many instances, it seems probable that these reactions would be more properly described as conditional responses induced by active drugs used previously". That is, Lang and Rand suggested that prior drug experience might be an important factor in determining the magnitude of the placebo effect. More recently, this has been characterized as a sequence effects variable.

## Sequence effects and extinction

As discussed by Ader,[1] "if learning processes were not involved in placebo effects – that is, if the placebo effect were simply attributable to faith in the system or in one's physician, or perhaps a function of some personal characteristic – one would expect that one placebo would be as effective as another and that a placebo would be equally effective no matter when it was administered". In contrast, if the placebo effect is a CR it should be most effective following a period of active drug treatment (i.e. following the CS–UCS pairings necessary to establish a CR), rather than when it is given prior to such treatment. There is evidence that such sequence effects exist. For example, Sunshine, Laska, Meisner, and Morgan[57] found that there was a substantial placebo effect in patients receiving either an analgesic (aspirin or indomethacin) or placebo as a second or third medication (all subjects having received an analgesic previously). In these circumstances, the placebo was as effective as the drug in relieving pain. In contrast, in subjects with no prior experimental treatment histories who received either of the analgesic drugs or the placebo as a first medication, aspirin and indomethacin were more effective than the placebo. Subsequently, Kantor, Sunshine, Laska, Meisner, and Hopper[58] reached a similar conclusion in studies of analgesics in patients with postsurgical pain. Various analgesic drugs (aspirin, codeine, pentazocine) and placebo were compared. Two drug presentations were used, the second always being a placebo. The effectiveness of the placebo in attenuating pain depended on the preceding drug – the placebo elicited analgesia only when it followed an effective analgesic. When a placebo followed a placebo, the responses were identical. The existence of such sequence effects is consistent with the conditioning analysis of placebo effects.

As discussed by Ader[1] and Kantor *et al.*,[58] such sequence effects also have important implications for "crossover designs" widely used in drug trials. If a patient receives Drug 2 sometime after completion of a series of Drug 1 administrations, the response to Drug 2 will depend on both the unconditional effects of Drug 2 and a placebo effect – conditional responding acquired during Drug 1 administrations. The usual procedure of imposing a "wash out" period between Drug 1 and Drug 2 will not affect the CR, because, as indicated earlier, CRs do not diminish appreciably merely as a function of the passage of time: "Wash-out periods may eliminate the presence or effects of prior drug(s), but they cannot eliminate a learned response ... the effects of conditioning can be eliminated only by extinguishing the conditioned response, that is, by presenting the CS without the UCS".[1]

Indeed, if the placebo response is a CR, it should be subject to extinction; the effectiveness of the placebo should decrease over the course of repeated administrations. Several clinicians have noted that the effectiveness of a placebo appears to decrease over the course of successive administrations.[34,59]

## Pavlovian conditioning, placebos, and modulation of the effect of a drug

In most examples of pharmacological conditioning described thus far, the CR that constitutes the placebo effect is manifest as a response elicited by drug-associated cues in the absence of the drug. Such conditioning should also be manifest as an alteration in the response to the drug. For example, Tatarenko[60] reported that psychiatric patients who underwent a regimen of insulin shock therapy not only displayed insulinoid behaviors in anticipation of the central effects of the hormone, but also reported that these CRs summated with the unconditional effects of insulin. That is, it became possible to induce comas with a fraction of the insulin dose usually required.

Previously discussed findings indicated that the effects of caffeine were conditionable, i.e. decaffeinated coffee had caffeine-like effects in experienced coffee drinkers. Some time ago, Stanley and Schlosberg[61] presented evidence that the CR to caffeine may be manifest as an altered response to a caffeine-containing beverage. Stanley and Schlosberg reported that, in tea drinkers, the effects of tea on simple and complex reaction time were observable immediately after the tea was ingested – too soon for chemical stimulation of central receptors. They concluded that

> the rapid appearance of the tea effect cannot be ascribed to the pharmacological action of caffeine; some of the other ingredients or characteristics of a cup of tea may be important determinants of the effect ... i.e. the taste of tea has become

a conditioned stimulus for evoking a reaction produced originally by the diverse factors, including caffeine, and by the variety of conditions usually present during consumption of the tea.

These investigators went on to note that "although this learned effect would seem to be a most appropriate subject for psychological study, it appears to have been completely neglected".

The fact that a pharmacological CR may modulate a drug effect has important implications for pharmacology and for medicine. For example, CRs may progressively augment the effect of a drug over the course of repeated administrations. Recall that Pavlov[14] summarized research by Krylov indicating that dogs repeatedly injected with morphine display a morphine-like salivary CR in response to drug paired cues. In his own description of this morphine conditioning research, Krylov[62] noted not only a salivary CR, but also that the salivary effect of morphine increased over the course of successive administrations. Such an enhancement of the effects of a drug over the course of repeated administrations is termed "reverse tolerance", or "sensitization".

The enhancement of the behavioral activating effects of amphetamine over the course of repeated administrations provides another example of drug sensitization mediated by Pavlovian conditioning. Amphetamine unconditionally elicits an increase in locomotor activity, and such hyperactivity becomes conditioned to drug administration cues.[63] In rats repeatedly injected with amphetamine, the activity-inducing effect of the drug becomes progressively more pronounced, and this sensitization can be interpreted as a summation of the pharmacological CR with the unconditional effects of the stimulant.[64] More recently, Chinen and Frussa-Filho[24] provided evidence that sensitization to the cataleptic effect of a dopamine antagonist is attributable to a conditional cataleptic response summating with the unconditional cataleptic effect of the dopamine antagonist.

The fact that a drug effect may be enhanced by a pharmacological CR may be exploited in pharmacotherapeutic regimens. It may be possible to occasionally replace a drug with deleterious side effects with a lower dosage of the drug. This lower dose, although normally ineffective, would now be effective in this drug experienced patient because the unconditional drug effect would be augmented by a conditional drug effect.[1,65]

## Conditional compensatory responses

In the examples provided thus far, the CR mimics the drug effect. For example, nitroglycerin increases heart rate in dogs and people, and nitroglycerine associated CSs similarly increase heart rate. Such findings are consistent with Pavlov's[14] neurological theory of CR formation, which specifies that the CR is similar to the UCR. However, there are findings that, at least upon initial inspection, seem to be quite different, and these findings complicate the Pavlovian conditioning analysis of placebo effects.

Early in the study of the conditioning of drug responses it became apparent that some pharmacological CRs did not appear to look anything like the pharmacological UCR. In 1929 Mulinos and Lieb[66] noted that atropine causes a decrease in salivation, but the CR following training with atropine is an *increase* in salivation (a finding subsequently replicated).[67,68] In 1937, Subkov and Zilov provided additional evidence that the CR might actually compensate for the drug effect.[69] They injected dogs with epinephrine on a number of occasions (one injection every few days). Each injection caused a pronounced increase in heart rate. On a final test session they injected an inert substance (Ringer's solution). On this test, a *decrease* in heart rate was observed. Thus, again, the CR did not appear to be a replica of the UCR; rather, the CR appeared to be an adaptive preparation for the impending pharmacological perturbation. Subkov and Zilov cautioned against "the widely accepted view that the external modifications of the conditional reflex must always be identical with the response of the organism to the unconditional stimulus".

Additional research provided evidence of such compensatory CRs with a variety of effects of many different drugs. For example, chlorpromazine decreases activity, but the CR seen following training with this tranquilizer is an increase in activity.[70] Similar findings of a CR of hyperactivity have been reported with respect to conditioning of the activity suppressive effect of a $GABA_A$ agonist.[71] If hypoglycemia is repeatedly induced by insulin injections, injection of an inert substance leads to a hyperglycemic response.[72–74] Conversely, if hyperglycemia is repeatedly induced, either by intragastric or injected glucose, the preparations for administration lead to a hypoglycemic response.[75–77] Many other examples of such compensatory pharmacological CRs have been provided elsewhere.[33,78]

Sometimes, with the same pharmacological UCS, some components of the CR mimic the observed drug effect and some appear compensatory to the drug effect. For example, insulin (at a sufficiently high dose) has distinctive motor effects (decreased activity, convulsions, and non-responsiveness to peripherally applied stimulation), and decreases blood glucose concentration. The CR following training with insulin consists (as previously indicated) of an insulin-like pattern of motor behavior,[25] but, simultaneously, a compensatory hyperglycemic response.[73] Amphetamine increases activity and body temperature. Although the CR to amphetamine consists of an amphetamine-like increase in activity,[64] it also consists of an amphetamine-compensatory decrease in temperature.[79] Similarly, although the CR to caffeine consists of a caffeine-like increase in alertness,[44] it also consists of a caffeine-compensatory decrease in salivation.[80]

Much research on placebo effects concern placebo elicited analgesia. It is tempting to speculate that some instances of such placebo analgesia are due to a CR elicited by drug administration cues that have, in the past, been paired with active analgesic drugs. There are, in fact, many studies involving conditioning of the effects of morphine, and the results of these studies are problematic for a conditioning analysis of placebo elicited analgesia (at least when applied to opioid analgesics). When CRs are noted in these morphine conditioning experiments, they typically are not analgesia, but rather *hyper*aglesia – extraordinary sensitivity to painful stimuli.[81–84]

Indeed, about 25 years ago, in an evaluation of the literature on the conditioning of drug (including morphine) responses, Siegel concluded that "conditioned drug responses are commonly opposite in direction to the unconditioned effect of the drug".[84] We now know that this conclusion was somewhat superficial. Research in pharmacological conditioning has advanced in the last 25 years to the extent that we can make some sense out of the apparently conflicting findings concerning the topography of the pharmacological CR.

## Compensatory responding and the identification of stimuli and responses in Pavlovian conditioning

Recently there have been important analyses of pharmacological conditioning that have directly addressed the fact that CRs sometimes appear to mimic the UCR, and sometimes appear to mirror the UCR.[33,78,85–87] To a great extent, the apparent paradox is resolved if the UCR is defined correctly. The UCR is the response of the central nervous system (CNS) to the UCS. Chemical UCSs directly induce many responses which initiate CNS mediated homeostatic regulatory counter-responses. For example, an injection of glucose will, of course, elevate the glucose concentration in the blood. This hyperglycemia is *not* the UCR (i.e. it is not a response initiated by the CNS). Rather, the hyperglycemia that results from injected glucose is the UCS. The elevated glucose level is detected by receptors in the hypothalamus, and responses are initiated that decrease blood glucose concentration (for example, insulin secretion). The UCR is the response mediated by the central nervous system. In this example, the UCR to injected glucose is (in common with the CR) a hypoglycemic response. Most other examples of compensatory conditioning may be understood in this manner. As summarized by Dworkin,[78] "conditioned drug responses, when adequately isolated, dissected, and understood, exemplify in an uncomplicated way the phenomenon first described by Pavlov: the conditioned reflex resembles the unconditioned reflex".

## Compensatory CRs, drug tolerance, drug withdrawal, and the placebo effect

The existence of compensatory pharmacological CRs has implications for understanding the role of conditioning in phenomena of drug addiction – specifically, drug tolerance and withdrawal symptoms. In addition, such CRs have implications for a Pavlovian conditioning analysis of placebo effects.

## Compensatory CRs and tolerance

As indicated previously, drug-like CRs progressively augment the effect of a drug over repeated administrations, and contribute to drug sensitization, or reverse tolerance.[24,64] Similarly, drug-compensatory CRs progressively attenuate the effect of some drugs over the course of repeated administrations. Such a decreasing effect of a drug over the course of repeated administrations is termed *tolerance.*

There is now a very extensive literature[33,87] indicating that tolerance to a variety of effects of many drugs is, in part, mediated by compensatory CRs. That is, as the drug is consistently administered in the presence of the usual predrug cues, the association between these drug administration cues and the systemic effect of the drug grows stronger (i.e. drug compensatory CRs increase in magnitude). These drug anticipatory responses increasingly attenuate the effect of the drug over the course of repeated administrations. As expected on the basis of a conditioning interpretation of tolerance, tolerance is more pronounced when the drug is administered in the usual drug administration environment than when it is administered elsewhere: "Speaking casually, tolerance is more pronounced when a drug is expected than when it is unexpected".[88]

Such drug expectation even affects tolerance to the lethal effects of drugs. Many studies have evaluated overdose to a variety of drugs (heroin, ethanol, pentobarbital) and species (mice, rats, and humans). The results of these studies indicate that organisms with a history of drug administration are less likely to die following administration of a high dose of the drug if they received the drug in the context of the usual predrug cues than if they received the drug elsewhere – the drug compensatory CR can decrease drug lethality in non-human animals[89–91] and humans.[92–95] This compensatory CR type placebo effect promotes survival when it is displayed in the context of drug associated stimuli.

## Compensatory CRs and withdrawal symptoms

Drug tolerance is highly correlated with drug withdrawal symptoms. Moreover, withdrawal symptoms are compensatory responses: "As a general pharmacological principle, it can be asserted that withdrawal effects are usually opposite to acute drug effects".[86] According to the conditioning analysis, the relationship between tolerance and withdrawal, and the drug compensatory characteristics of withdrawal symptoms, are attributable to the fact they are both manifestations of the same drug compensatory CR.

When the drug is administered in the context of the usual drug administration cues, compensatory CRs attenuate the drug effect and contribute to tolerance. However, if there is no drug effect (i.e. the usual cues for drug administration are present, but the usual drug is not administered), these CRs achieve full expression because they do not interact with the drug effect. Such pharmacological CRs, displayed in such circumstances, are termed "withdrawal symptoms".

There is much experimental (both human and non-human animal) and epidemiological evidence that so-called "withdrawal symptoms", seen long after the last exposure to a drug, are especially pronounced in the presence of drug related cues[96,97] that is, "it is the anticipation of the drug, rather than the drug itself, that is responsible for these symptoms ... some drug 'withdrawal symptoms' are, more accurately, drug 'preparation symptoms'".[98]

On the basis of an analysis of the placebo effect that emphasizes Pavlovian conditioning, drug withdrawal symptoms (seen long after the last drug administrations) are placebo effects. They are manifestations of a pharmacological CR, albeit a drug compensatory CR.[99]

### Compensatory CRs and placebo effects

A placebo effect was defined at the beginning of this article as "a response to a substance or treatment that is not explicable on the basis of the known properties of the substance or treatment (whether or not the response is therapeutic)". Thus, drug compensatory CRs with no obvious beneficial significance (for example, hyperalgesia in response to morphine associated cues[82]), in common with drug-like CRs with palpable therapeutic value (for example, immunosuppression in response to cyclophosphamide associated cues in a patient suffering from an autoimmune disorder[53]), are placebo effects.*

Sometimes placebos have untoward effects. An individual expecting a sleeping pill may respond to an inert substance with increased sleeplessness,[100] or an individual expecting an analgesic may respond to an inert substance with increased pain sensitivity.[88] The status of such contratherapeutic placebo effects – sometimes termed "negative placebo effects"[101] or "nocebo reactions"[102] – is controversial. It is tempting to speculate, however, that some instances of the phenomenon may be due to drug compensatory CRs.

## Compensatory conditional responding – unresolved issues

Although the understanding that the compensatory CR is actually in the same direction as the pharmacological UCR (when the UCS and UCR have

* Whether or not a CR is "adaptive", in an evolutionary sense, cannot be determined simply by evaluation of the therapeutic efficacy of the CR. A compensatory CR of hyperalgesia in the patient with a history of morphine administration may exacerbate symptoms, but it also is a manifestation of one mechanism of drug tolerance, which decreases the likelihood of overdose.[33] (For a fuller discussion of Pavlovian conditioning and the evolution of behavioral mechanisms see Siegel and Allan[111]).

been appropriately delineated) has been fruitful, there are still some conflicting findings that have yet to be resolved. For example, there is extensive evidence that the CR following training with insulin (and its hypoglycemic effect) is a *hyper*glycemic response,[78] but some investigators have reported contrary findings.[103–105] Although, as summarized above, Newlin[48] reported that female college students respond to a CS for an alcoholic beverage with an alcohol-like CR, this same investigator also has reported that male college students respond with alcohol-compensatory CRs.[106] Although there are many findings that rats respond to a CS for the immunosuppressant, cyclophosphamide, with a CR of immunosuppression,[107] there also are findings where apparently similar conditioning procedures lead to the development of a CR of immunoenhancement.[108–110] Elucidation of the basis for such conflicting findings awaits the results of additional research.

A promising area for further investigation involves evaluation of the distinction, made by Ader,[1] between conditional *pharmacological* and conditional *pharmacotherapeutic* responses. Most experimental research on conditional drug responses involves the analysis of conditional pharmacological responses. That is, in a laboratory setting, healthy humans or non-human animals are exposed to neutral CSs and pharmacological UCSs, and the development of the CR is evaluated.

> In contrast, a conditioned pharmacotherapeutic response involves exposing 'patients', or, perhaps, a species of animal – animals that spontaneously develop a particular disease or in which a dysregulated physiological state has been induced experimentally – to one or more pairings of a neutral CS and pharmacologic agent that unconditionally elicits one or more physiological responses calculated to correct the naturally occurring or experimentally induced physiologic imbalance.[1]

Ader suggested that although conditional compensatory responses, in anticipation of a pharmacologically induced perturbation, act as a homeostatic mechanism in the normal, healthy organism (see also Siegel and Allan[111]), they may exacerbate the pathology in the organism in which the same drug has a therapeutic benefit. Thus, the direction of the pharmacological CR, and the nature of the placebo effect attributable to pharmacological conditioning, may be determined by whether or not the drug has a therapeutic effect in the subject.

## Conclusions

The major advantage of a conditioning interpretation of the placebo effect is that drug responses are readily conditionable, and such conditioning can be seen in non-human animals, as well as humans. Thus, not only does conditioning provide a simple, mechanistic interpretation of the phenomenon, but it also provides a model in which mediating biochemical or physiological processes may readily be investigated in non-human animals.

There are at least two major reasons why *all* placebo effects cannot readily be attributable to Pavlovian conditioning. The first reason is that, as indicated above, pharmacological CRs often do not mimic the drug effect. Thus, it would be difficult to explain placebo elicited analgesia as a CR in an organism with prior experience with opiates because the CR following training with morphine is hyperalgesia, rather than analgesia (although it is possible that further research will elaborate the conditions under which conditional analgesia and hyperalgesia may be seen). The second reason is that people can, apparently, have placebo responses without previous drug experience.[70,*] Kirsch and colleagues have suggested that "a contemporary informational view of classical conditioning"[112] – expectancy theory – can address a range of placebo phenomena not readily interpretable by a traditional Pavlovian conditioning analysis. Interestingly, almost 30 years ago Pihl and Altman noted, "the fact that the results of these studies support the notion that the placebo effect can be the result of simple conditioning does not derogate the expectancy hypothesis".[70]

As suggested by Ader,[1] it likely is simplistic to speak of a single placebo effect. Several different explanations for the placebo effect have been proposed.[113] Some placebo effects seem best explained by Pavlovian conditioning, and others by expectancy theory, spontaneous remission, regression to the mean, confounded treatment procedures, therapist biases, or altered patient symptom reporting criteria. It is likely that understanding of the various placebo effects (rather than attempting to understand *the* placebo effect) is necessary to fully appreciate the mechanisms whereby inert substances or treatments may sometimes have substantial medical consequences.

## References

1 Ader R. The role of conditioning in pharmacotherapy. In: Harrington A, ed. *The placebo effect: An interdisciplinary exploration.* Cambridge, MA: Harvard University Press, 1997.

2 Brody H. *Placebos and the philosophy of medicine.* Chicago: University of Chicago Press, 1980:1.

3 Shapiro AK, Shapiro E. *The powerful placebo: From ancient priest to modern medicine.* Baltimore: Johns Hopkins University Press, 1997.

4 Robb N. Some MDs displeased as MSNS board gives nod to complementary medicine section. *Can Med Assoc J* 1994;**150**:1462–5.

---

* Although a straightforward Pavlovian conditioning analysis would seem to require that the patient exhibiting a placebo effect has prior pairings of predrug cues with the systemic effect of the drug, such pairings may not actually be necessary for verbal organisms, i.e. humans. Later developments in conditioning theory, by Pavlov and his students, addressed the unique role of language. Pavlov suggested that language constitutes the "second signalling system": "Words have built up a second system of signalling reality, which is peculiar to us, being a signal of the primary signals".[115] Humans need not experience actual CS-UCS pairings to acquire a CR, since such information can be conveyed by the second signalling system. It is possible that a conditioning analysis of the placebo effect that acknowledges a role for the second signalling system may address the fact that some instances of the placebo effect may be seen in patients without a history of explicit pairings of a predrug CS and pharmacological UCS.

5 Siegel S. Multiple chemical sensitivity as a conditional response. *Toxicol Indus Health* 1999;**15**:323–30.
6 Tibbetts RW, Hawkings JR. The placebo response. *J Mental Sci* 1956;**102**:60–6.
7 Herrnstein RJ. Placebo effect in the rat. *Science* 1962;**138**:677–8.
8 Babkin BP. *Pavlov: A biography*. Chicago: University of Chicago Press, 1949.
9 Nesse RM, Carli T, Curtis GC, Kleinman PD. Pretreatment nausea in cancer chemotherapy: A conditioned response? *Psychosom Med* 1980;**42**:33–6.
10 Bernstein IL. Aversion conditioning in response to cancer and cancer treatment. *Clin Psychol Rev* 1991;**11**:185–91.
11 Jacobson PB, Bovbjerg DH, Schwartz MD, *et al*. Formation of food aversions in cancer patients receiving repeated infusions of chemotherapy. *Behav Res Ther* 1993;**31**:739–48.
12 Stockhorst U, Klosterhalfen S, Klosterhalfen W, Winkelmann M, Steingrueber HJ. Anticipatory nausea in cancer patients receiving chemotherapy: classical conditioning etiology and therapeutical implications. *Integrative Physiol Behav Sci* 1993;**23**:177–81.
13 Siegel S, Kreutzer R. Pavlovian conditioning and multiple chemical sensitivity. *Environ Health Perspectives* 1997;**105**:521–6.
14 Pavlov IP. *Conditioned reflexes*. London: Oxford University Press, 1927.
15 Kimble GA. *Hilgard and Marquis' conditioning and learning*. New York: Appleton-Century-Crofts, 1961:281.
16 Hursti T, Fredrickson M, Börjeson S, Füres CJ, Peterson C, Steinbeck G. Extinction of conditioned nausea after chemotherapy is associated with personality differences. *J Psychosocial Oncol* 1992;**10**:59–78.
17 Pavlov IP. *The work of the digestive glands*. London: Charles Griffin, 1910.
18 Collins KH, Tatum AL. A conditioned reflex established by chronic morphine poisoning. *Am J Physiol* 1925;**74**:14–15.
19 Kleitman N, Crisler G. A quantitative study of the salivary conditioned reflex. *Am J Physiol* 1927;**79**:571–614.
20 Bykov KM. *The cerebral cortex and the internal organs*. Moscow: Foreign Languages Publishing House, 1959.
21 Konradi G. Activity of the nervous system. In: Bykov KM, ed. *Text-book of physiology*. Moscow: Foreign Languages Publishing House, 1960.
22 Loucks RB. Humoral conditioning in mammals. *J Psychol* 1937;**4**:295–307.
23 Perez-Cruet J, Gantt WH. Conditional catalepsy to bulbocapnine: cardiac, respiratory, and motor components. *Fed Proc* 1959;**18**:118.
24 Chinen CC, Frussa-Filho R. Conditioning to injection procedures and repeated testing increase SCH 23390-induced catalepsy in mice. *Neuropsychopharmacol* 1999;**21**:670–8.
25 Reiss WJ. Conditioning of a hyperinsulin type of behavior in the white rat. *J Comp Physiol Psychol* 1950;**51**:301–3.
26 Hecht T, Baumann R, Hecht K. The somatic and vegetative-regulatory behavior of the healthy organism during conditioning of the insulin effect. *Life Sci* 1967;**2**:96–112.
27 Kantorovich NY, Rybking IV. On certain mechanisms in the development of insulin hypoglycemia. *Journal of Neuropathology and Psychiatry* (Nekotorik tesereralinik mekanismak v rasvitii gipoglikemii. *Zhurnal Neuropatologii i Psikhiatrii*) 1957;**57**:86.
28 Ader R. A historical account of conditioned immunobiologic responses. In: Ader R, ed. *Psychoneuroimmunology*. New York: Academic Press, 1981.
29 Razran G. The observable unconscious and the inferable conscious in current Soviet psychophysiology: interoceptive conditioning, semantic conditioning and the orienting reflex. *Psychol Rev* 1961;**68**:81–147.
30 Razran G. Russian Physiologists' psychology and American experimental psychology: A historical and a systematic collation and a look into the future. *Psychol Bull* 1965;**63**:42–64.
31 Baptista MAS, Siegel S, MacQueen G, Young LT. Pre-drug cues modulate morphine tolerance, striatal c-Fos, and AP-1 DNA binding. *NeuroReport* 1998;**9**:3387–90.
32 Siegel S. Learning and psychopharmacology. In: Jarvik ME, ed. *Psychopharmacology in the practice of medicine*. New York: Appleton-Century-Crofts, 1977.
33 Siegel S, Baptista MAS, Kim JA, McDonald RV, Weise-Kelly L. Pavlovian psychopharmacology: The associative basis of tolerance. *Exp Clin Psychopharmacol* 2000;**8**:276–93.
34 Kurland AA. The drug placebo: Its psychodynamic and conditional reflex action. *Behav Sci* 1957;**2**:101–10.

35 Gliedman LH, Gantt WH, Teitelbaum HA. Some implications of conditional reflex studies for placebo research. *Am J Psychiat* 1957;**113**:1103–7.

36 Ader R. The placebo effect as a conditioned response. In: Ader R, Weiner H, Baum A, eds. *Experimental foundations of behavioral medicine: Conditioning approaches*. Hillsdale, NJ: Lawrence Erlbaum Associates, 1988.

37 Archer T. The role of conditioning in the use of placebo. *Nordic J Psychiat* 1995;**49**: 43–53.

38 Siegel S. Drug anticipatory responses in animals. In: White L, Tursky B, Schwartz G, eds. *Placebo: Theory, research, and mechanisms*. New York: Guilford Press, 1985.

39 Wickramasekera I. A conditioned response model of the placebo effect. *Biofeedback and Self-Regulation* 1980;**5**:5–18.

40 Wickramasekera I. A conditioned response model of the placebo effect: Predictions from the model. In: White L, Tursky B, Schwartz G, eds. *Placebo: Theory, research, and mechanisms*. New York: Guilford Press, 1985.

41 Alarie Y. Irritating properties of airborne materials to the upper respiratory tract. *Arch Environ Health* 1966;**13**:433–49.

42 Wood RJ, Coleman JB. Behavioral evaluation of the irritant properties of formaldehyde. *Toxicol Appl Pharmacol* 1995;**130**:67–72.

43 Bolla-Wilson K, Wilson RJ, Bleecker ML. Conditioning of physical symptoms after neurotoxic exposure. *J Occup Med* 1988;**30**:684–6.

44 Zwyghuizen-Doorenbos A, Roehrs TA, Lipschutz L, Timms V, Roth T. Effects of caffeine on alertness. *Psychopharmacology* 1990;**100**:36–9.

45 Knowles JB. Conditioning and the placebo effect: The effects of decaffeinated coffee on simple reaction time in habitual coffee drinkers. *Behav Res Ther* 1993;**1**:151–7.

46 Flaten MA, Blumenthal TD. Caffeine-associated stimuli elicit conditioned responses: an experimental model of the placebo effect. *Psychopharmacology* 1999;**145**:105–12.

47 Robinson ML, Houtsmuller EJ, Moolchan ET, Pickworth WB. Placebo cigarettes in smoking research. *Exp Clin Psychopharmacol* 2000;**8**:326–32.

48 Newlin DB. Placebo responding in same direction as alcohol in women. *Alc: Clin Exp Res* 1989;**13**:36–9.

49 Meyer RE, Dolinsky ZS. Ethanol beverage anticipation: effects on plasma testosterone and luteinizing hormone levels – a pilot study. *J Stud Alcohol* 1990;**51**:350–5.

50 Levine DG. "Needle freaks": Compulsive self-injection by drug users. *Am J Psychiat* 1974;**131**:297–300.

51 Siegel RK. Cocaine aroma in the treatment of cocaine dependency. *J Clin Psychopharmacol* 1984;**4**:61–2.

52 MacKenzie JN. The production of the so-called 'rose cold' by means of an artificial rose. *Am J Med Sci* 1896;**91**:45–7.

53 Giang DW, Goodman AD, Schiffer RB, et al. Conditioning of cyclophosphamide-induced leukopenia in humans. *J Neuropsych Clin Neurosci* 1996;**8**:194–201.

54 Ader R, Cohen N. Behaviorally conditioned immunosuppression and murine systemic lupus erythematosus. *Science* 1982;**215**:1534–6.

55 Lang WJ, Ross P, Glover A. Conditional responses induced by hypotensive drugs. *Eur J Pharmacol* 1967;**2**:169–74.

56 Lang W, Rand MA. A placebo response as a conditional reflex to glyceryl trinitrate. *Med J Aust* 1969;**1**:912–14.

57 Sunshine AE, Laska E, Meisner M, Morgan S. Analgesic studies of indomethacin as analyzed by computer techniques. *Clin Pharmacol Ther* 1964;**5**:699–707.

58 Kantor TG, Sunshine A, Laska E, Meisner M, Hopper M. Oral analgesic studies: Pentazocine hydrochloride, codeine, aspirin, and placebo and their influence on response to placebo. *Clin Pharmacol Ther* 1966;**7**:447–54.

59 Lasagna L, Mosteller F, von Felsinger JM, Beecher HK. A study of the placebo response. *Am J Med* 1954;**16**:770–9.

60 Tatarenko NP. Pathophysiology of schizophrenia. *Journal of Neuropathology and Psychiatry* (K pätofiziolgii shizofrenii. *Zhurnal Neuropatologii i Psikhiatrii*) 1954;**54**:710–14 (Available as Technical Translation 1720 from the National Research Council of Canada).

61 Stanley WC, Schlosberg H. The psychophysiological effects of tea. *J Psychol* 1953;**36**:435–48.

62 Krylov V. Additional data on the study of conditioned reflexes on chemical stimuli. *Biol Abstr* 1933;7:871.

63 Pickens R, Dougherty J. Conditioning the activity effects of drugs. In: Thompson T, Schuster C, eds. *Stimulus properties of drugs*. New York: Appleton-Century-Crofts, 1971.
64 Tilson HA, Rech RH. Prior drug experience and effects of amphetamine on schedule controlled behavior. *Pharmacol Biochem Behav* 1973;**1**:129–132.
65 Ader R, Grota LJ, Moynihan JA, Grota LJ, Cohen N. Conditioned enhancement of antibody production using antigen as the unconditioned stimulus. *Brain Behav Immunol* 1973;7:334–42.
66 Mulinos MG, Lieb CC. Pharmacology of learning. *Am J Physiol* 1929;**90**:456–7.
67 Lang WJ, Brown ML, Gershon S, Korol B. Classical and physiologic adaptive conditioned responses to anticholinergic drugs in conscious dogs. *Int J Neuropharmacol* 1966;**5**:311–15.
68 Wikler A. Recent progress in research on the neurophysiologic basis of morphine addiction. *Am J Psychiat* 1948;**105**:329–38.
69 Subkov AA, Zilov GN. The role of conditioned reflex adaptation in the origin of hyperergic reactions. *Bulletin de Biologie et de Medecine Experimentale* 1937;**4**:294–6.
70 Pihl RO, Altman J. An experimental analysis of the placebo effect. *J Clin Pharmacol* 1971;**11**:91–5.
71 Jodogne C, Tirelli E. Modulation of tolerance to the $GABA_A$ agonist THIP by environmental cues. *Behav Brain Res* 1990;**36**:33–40.
72 Siegel S. Conditioning of insulin-induced glycemia. *J Comp Physiol Psychol* 1972;**78**: 233–41.
73 Siegel S. Conditioning insulin effects. *J Comp Physiol Psychol* 1975;**89**:189–99.
74 Woods SC, Shogren RE. Glycemic responses following conditioning with different doses of insulin in rats. *J Comp Physiol Psychol* 1972;**81**:220–5.
75 Deutsch R. Conditioned hypoglycemia: A mechanism for saccharin-induced sensitivity to insulin in the rat. *J Comp Physiol Psychol* 1974;**86**:350–8.
76 Matysiak J, Green L. On the directionality of classically-conditioned glycemic responses. *Physiol Behav* 1984;**32**:5–9.
77 Mityushov MI. Uslovnorleflektornaya inkretsiya insulina [The conditional-reflex incretion of insulin]. *Zhurnal Vysshei Nervnoi Deiatel* [*Journal of Higher Nervous Activity*] 1954;**4**:206–12. Translated by Overduin J, Dworkin BR, Jansen A. Introduction and commentary on MI Mityushov (1994) "Conditioned reflex incretion of insulin." *Integrative Physiol Behav Sci* 1997;**32**:228–46.
78 Dworkin BR. *Learning and physiological regulation*. Chicago: University of Chicago Press, 1993.
79 Obál F. The fundamentals of the central nervous control of vegetative homeostasis. *Acta Physiol Acad Sci Hung* 1966;**30**:15–29.
80 Rozin P, Reff D, Mark M, Schull J. Conditioned responses in human tolerance to caffeine. *Bull Psychon Soc* 1984;**22**:117–20.
81 Grisel JE, Wiertelak EP, Watkins LR, Maier SF. Route of morphine administration modulates conditioned analgesic tolerance and hyperalgesia. *Pharmacol Biochem Behav* 1994;**49**:1029–35.
82 Kim JA, Siegel S, Patenall VRA. Drug-onset cues as signals: intra-administration associations and tolerance. *J Exp Psychol: Anim Behav Proc* 1999;**25**:491–504.
83 Krank MD. Conditioned hyperalgesia depends on the pain sensitivity measure. *Behav Neurosci* 1987;**101**:854–7.
84 Siegel S. Evidence from rats that morphine tolerance is a learned response. *J Comp Physiol Psychol* 1975;**89**:498–506.
85 Eikelboom R, Stewart J. Conditioning of drug-induced physiological responses. *Psychol Rev* 1982;**89**:507–28.
86 Poulos CX, Cappell H. Homeostatic theory of drug tolerance: A general model of physiological adaptations. *Psychol Rev* 1991;**98**:390–408.
87 Ramsay DS, Woods SC. Biological consequences of drug administration: Implications for acute and chronic tolerance. *Psychol Rev* 1997;**104**:170–93.
88 Siegel S. Classical conditioning and opiate tolerance and withdrawal. In: Balfour DJK, ed. *Psychotropic drugs of abuse*. New York: Pergamon, 1990.
89 Melchior CL. Conditioned tolerance provides protection against ethanol lethality. *Pharmacol Biochem Behav* 1990;**37**:205–6.
90 Siegel S, Hinson RE, Krank MD, McCully J. Heroin "overdose" death: the contribution of drug-associated environmental cues. *Science* 1982;**216**:436–7.

91 Vila CJ. Death by pentobarbital overdose mediated by Pavlovian conditioning. *Pharmacol Biochem Behav* 1989;**32**:365–6.

92 Gutiérrez-Cebollada J, de la Torre R, Ortuño J, Garcés JM, Camí J. Psychotropic drug consumption and other factors associated with heroin overdose. *Drug Alc Dep* 1994;**35**:169–74.

93 Siegel S. Pavlovian conditioning and heroin overdose: Reports by overdose victims. *Bull Psychon Soc* 1984;**22**:428–430.

94 Siegel S, Ellsworth DW. Pavlovian conditioning and death from apparent overdose of medically prescribed morphine: a case report. *Bull Psychon Soc* 1986;**24**:278–80.

95 Siegel S, Kim JA. Absence of cross-tolerance and the situational-specificity of tolerance. *Palliat Med* 2000;**14**:75–7.

96 Deffner-Rappold C, Azorlosa JL, Baker JD. Acquisition and extinction of context-specific morphine withdrawal. *Psychobiol* 1996;**24**:219–26.

97 Kelsey JE, Aranow JS, Matthews RT. Context-specific morphine withdrawal in rats: duration and effects of clonidine. *Behav Neurosci* 1990;**104**:704–10.

98 Siegel S. Feedforward processes in drug tolerance. In: Lister RG, Weingartner HJ, eds. *Perspectives in cognitive neuroscience*. New York: Oxford University Press, 1991.

99 Siegel S. Drug anticipation and drug addiction. *Addiction* 1999;**94**:1113–24.

100 Storms MD, Nisbett RE. Insomnia and the attribution process. *J Personal Soc Psychol* 1970;**16**:319–28.

101 Kellogg R, Baron RS. Attribution theory, insomnia, and the reverse placebo effect: a reversal of Storms and Nisbett's findings. *J Personal Soc Psychol* 1975;**32**:231–6.

102 Kennedy WP. The nocebo reaction. *Medical World* 1961;**91**:203–5.

103 Alvarez-Buyalla R, Carrasco-Zanini J. A conditioned reflex which reproduces the hypoglycemic effect of insulin. *Acta Physiologica Latino Americana* 1960;**10**:153–8.

104 Alvarez-Buyalla R, Segura ET, Alvarez-Buyalla ER. Participation of the hypophysis in the conditioned reflex which reproduces the hypoglycemic effect of insulin. *Acta Physiologica Latino Americana* 1961;**11**:113–19.

105 Segura ET. Insulin like conditioned hypoglycemic response in dogs. *Acta Physiologica Latino Americana* 1962;**12**:342–5.

106 Newlin DB. Human conditioned compensatory response to alcohol cues: initial evidence. *Alcohol* 1985;**2**:507–9.

107 Ader R, Cohen N. CNS-Immune system interactions: conditioning phenomena. *Behav Brain Sci* 1985;**8**:379–94.

108 Krank MD, MacQueen GM. Conditioned compensatory responses elicited by environmental signals for cyclophosphamide-induced suppression of the immune system. *Psychobiol* 1988;**16**:229–35.

109 MacQueen GM, Siegel S. Conditional immunomodulation following training with cyclophosphamide. *Behav Neurosci* 1989;**103**:638–47.

110 MacQueen GM, Siegel S, Landry JO. Acquisition and extinction of conditional immunoenhancement following training with cyclophosphamide. *Psychobiol* 1990;**18**: 287–92.

111 Siegel S, Allan LG. Learning and homeostasis: drug addiction and the McCollough effect. *Psychol Bull* 1998;**124**:230–9.

112 Kirsch I. Specifying nonspecifics: Psychological mechanisms of the placebo effect. In: Harrington A, ed. *The placebo effect: An interdisciplinary exploration*. Cambridge, MA: Harvard University Press, 1997.

113 Bootzin RR, Caspi O. Explanatory mechanisms for placebo effects: cognition, personality and social learning. This volume, chapter 5.

114 Woodworth RS, Schlosberg H. *Experimental psychology*. New York: Henry Holt, 1958.

115 Pavlov IP. *Conditioned reflexes and psychiatry* (WH Gantt, trans.). New York: International Publishers, 1941.

# 7: Regression to the mean or placebo effect?

CLARENCE E DAVIS

## Summary

Regression to the mean refers to the tendency for the value of a variable that is far from its expected value on one measurement to be closer to the expected value on a subsequent measurement. This is a mathematical property of all measurements subject to random error. The entry requirements of many clinical studies often require that patients have one or more measurements above some minimum level. Subsequent measurements then tend to be lower, because of regression to the mean, even if no biologically or psychologically mediated placebo effects are present. In actual clinical studies regression to the mean and placebo effects often appear together as a composite. In this chapter I will first clarify the difference between placebo effects and regression to the mean. I will then review the mathematics of regression to the mean, illustrate the concepts using computer-simulated data, explain why regression to the mean is commonly present in clinical trial measurements, and clarify how regression to the mean can mistakenly be seen as apparent placebo effects or treatment effects. Studies to elucidate placebo effects need to be designed to separate such effects from regression to the mean and other measurement artifacts as outlined in this chapter and elsewhere in this book.

## Introduction

The placebo effect has been defined variously since the initial attempt of Beecher to quantify therapeutic effects of placebos.[1–5] However, common to these definitions is a focus on psychological or psychophysiological changes. These biological changes, described in animal as well as human subjects,[6] have been attributed to expectancy, cognition, personality, and social learning[5] alone or in combination with Pavlovian conditioning,[7] and are said to take on meaning within the subject's cultural context.[4] Importantly, most definitions specifically exclude investigator, observer, and subject biases; the Hawthorne effect;* specific biological effects attributable to physical or chemical properties of the placebo (for example, hypersensitivity reactions to a coloring agent in a placebo tablet); natural history of the disorder (for example, improvement in nasal congestion due to clearing of a viral upper respiratory infection by the patient's immune response); and regression to the mean.

Yet many investigators fail to account for these artifacts. For example, Kienle and Kiene[8] recently re-analyzed the 15 studies in Beecher's original analysis of placebo effects using three criteria for acknowledging that a placebo effect was present: "(1) A *placebo* had to be given. (2) The event had to be an *effect* of the placebo treatment, i.e. the event would not have happened without placebo administration. (3) The event had to be relevant for the disease or symptom, i.e. it had to be a *therapeutic* event". They determined that in none of the 15 studies previously analyzed by Beecher could a placebo effect be established by their criteria. Rather, they concluded that in several of the studies, what had been attributed by Beecher to an effect of placebo treatment itself could be explained as "spontaneous improvement" or "spontaneous fluctuation of symptoms", both of which they regarded as special forms of regression to the mean. An earlier publication in the statistical literature[10] also concluded that "most improvements attributed to the placebo effect are actually instances of statistical regression".

The reason to cite these works is not to suggest that the biologically based placebo effect never occurs, but rather to illustrate two key points. The first is the important conceptual distinction between an *effect of a placebo on a patient* and *regression to the mean*. The former is postulated to be mediated by psychology or psychophysiology, while the latter is an artifact, albeit seen within a biological context, that is a mathematical property of all measurements whose precision is less than perfect. The second is the importance of accounting properly for regression to the mean in any study designed to quantify the placebo effect.

In the remainder of this chapter, I present a brief review of the mathematics of regression to the mean, provide graphical illustrations, explain why it is commonly present in clinical measurements, and illustrate how regression to the mean can create apparent treatment responses.

## Regression to the mean – definition

Regression to the mean refers to the phenomenon that a variable extreme on its first measurement will tend to be closer to the center of the distribution for a later measurement. For example, a person selected to be in a study because she has high blood cholesterol, will tend to have slightly lower blood cholesterol at a second, later measurement. Regression to the mean often appears together with the placebo effect in clinical trials, since

* This refers to the effect of being under study on the persons being studied.[9]

the criteria for inclusion of a participant in a clinical trial often require selection for being extreme.

Sir Francis Galton[11] first described regression to the mean in 1886:

> It is some years since I made an extensive series of experiments on the produce of seeds of different size but of the same species ... It appeared from these experiments that the offspring did not tend to resemble their parent seeds in size, but to be always more mediocre than they were – to be smaller than the parents, if the parents were large; to be larger than the parents, if the parents were small; ...

The experiments showed further that "the filial regression towards mediocrity was directly proportional to the parent deviation from it". Galton later replaced "regression towards mediocrity" with regression toward the mean, the term that is widely used today.

To make mathematically explicit what regression to the mean is, consider the following. Let $Y_1$ be the first measure and $Y_2$ be the second measure in a pair. In the cholesterol example, $Y_1$ is the first cholesterol measure and $Y_2$ the second; in Galton's example, $Y_1$ is the size of the parent seed and $Y_2$ of the offspring. We assume that $Y_1$ and $Y_2$ are distributed as a bivariate normal random variable with

$$E(Y_1) = E(Y_2) = \mu$$
$$\text{var}(Y_1) = \text{var}(Y_2) = \sigma^2$$
$$\text{and corr}(Y_1, Y_2) = \rho.$$
$$E(Y_2 - Y_1 \mid Y_1 > k) = -c\sigma(1 - \rho) \neq 0, \text{ where}$$
$$c = \frac{\phi\{(k - \mu)/\sigma\}}{(1 - \Phi\{(k - \mu)/\sigma\})},$$

$\phi(\cdot)$ is the probability density function of the standard normal distribution and $\Phi(\cdot)$ is the corresponding cumulative distribution function. In words, this equation shows that the second measure will not have the same average as the first measure. Moreover, the second measure will tend to be closer to the mean of the overall distribution than the first. Thus the difference between the means of the two measures is due to inherent variation, which leads to a less than perfect correlation between the two measures. The key element is the correlation coefficient $\rho$. When $\rho$ is one, there is no regression to the mean.

While the above mathematical description is based on an assumption of bivariate normality, Das and Mulder[12] have derived a corresponding formula that holds much more generally.

In studies of biologic measures, perfect correlation is seldom observed. However, the correlation may be very close to one in some instances. For example, if the measurement is height in middle-aged adults, and if the measurement is made with care, it is likely that the correlation between two measures on the same individual at different times, will be very close to

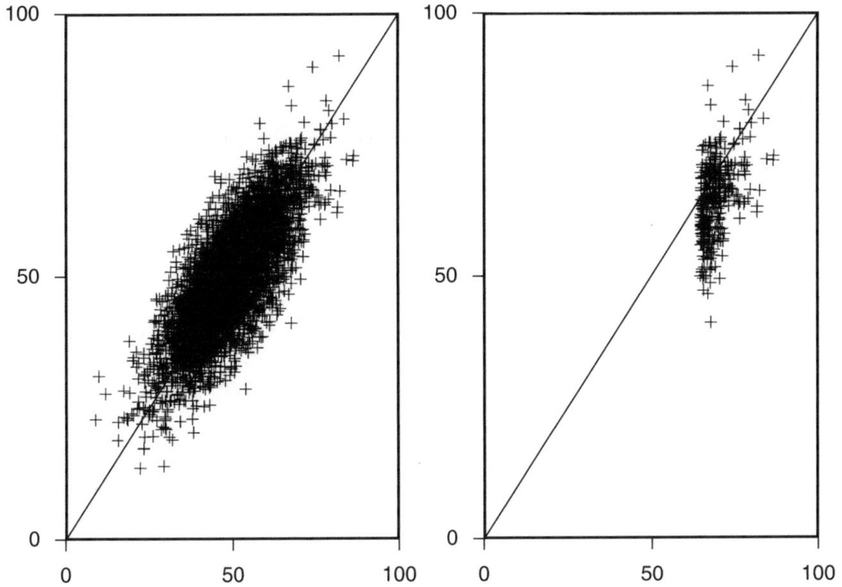


Figure 7.1A and 7.1B Computer simulated bivariate normal data (n = 5000) with mean 50, standard deviation 10, and correlation coefficient 0·75. The first measurement ($Y_1$) is shown on the horizontal axis and the second measurement ($Y_2$) is shown on the vertical axis. Figure 7.1A includes all data and it is easily seen that the data points are symmetrically distributed about the diagonal line $Y_1 = Y_2$. Figure 7.1B includes only those data points (n = 341) with $Y_1 > 65$. The tendency for $Y_2$ to be less than $Y_1$ in Figure 7.1B is apparent.

one. For most other biologic measures the correlation is not close to one. For example, in studies of blood cholesterol, the correlation has been found[13] to be approximately 0·8. A minimum standard of 0·75 has been proposed for the correlation in health measurement scales used in clinical research.[14] To illustrate how regression to the mean affects data on two successive measurements on the same subject, I have presented the results of several computer simulations of bivariate normal data ($Y_1$, $Y_2$) where the means and standard deviations of the first ($Y_1$) and second ($Y_2$) measurements on each subject are 50 and 10. Figures 7.1A and 7.1B are scatter plots of the first and second measurements ($Y_1$, $Y_2$) in a population with a correlation coefficient 0·75. In each graph the first measurement ($Y_1$) is plotted on the horizontal axis and the second measurement ($Y_2$) is plotted on the vertical axis. In Figure 7.1A the entire distribution is shown and it is easily seen that the data points are symmetrically distributed around the line $Y_1 = Y_2$. In Figure 7.1B only those pairs of data points with $Y_1 > 65$ are included. The tendency for the second measurement to be less than the first is visually apparent from the graph.

Figure 7.2 contains three box and whisker plots of the difference ($Y_2 - Y_1$) between the second and first measurements in three populations,

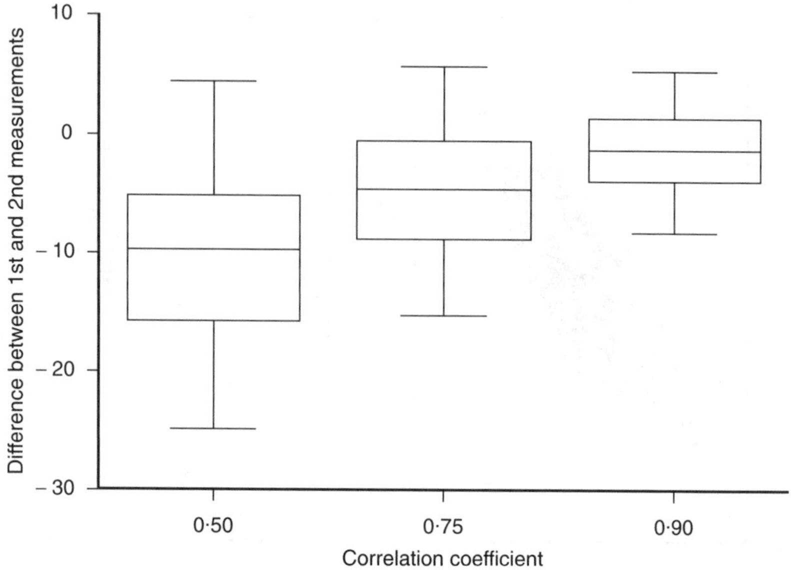


Figure 7.2 Computer simulated bivariate normal data with mean 50, standard deviation 10, and correlation coefficients 0·50, 0·75, and 0·90. The box and whisker plots show the distributions of $Y_2 - Y_1$, where $Y_1$ and $Y_2$ are the first and second measurements, respectively, in a population selected for $Y_1 > 65$. On each graph the horizontal line within the box represents the median, the upper and lower boundaries of the box represent the 75th and 25th percentiles, respectively, and the upper and lower capped bars represent the 95th and 5th percentiles, respectively. The smaller the measurement error, the closer the correlation between the first and second measurements is to 1, and the less pronounced is the regression to the mean.

with correlation coefficients of 0·50, 0·75, and 0·90 respectively, where in each case only those pairs of data points with $Y_1 > 65$ are included. The median difference is less than 0 in each case, illustrating the tendency for $Y_2$ to be less than $Y_1$. The lower the correlation, the more the distribution of the differences is shifted to values less than 0. Differences in the extent of measurement error (represented by differences in the correlation coefficient) and differences in the selection criteria for the study can produce varying magnitudes of regression to the mean. The smaller the measurement error, the closer the correlation between measurements is to 1 and the smaller is the regression to the mean. If measurement error were absent the correlation coefficient would be 1 and there would be no regression to the mean.

All of these effects are purely mathematical properties of the correlated data. They have nothing to do with psychology or physiology. In actual studies, these effects will typically be superimposed upon placebo effects that are mediated through psychological or psychophysiological pathways.

Figures 7.3A–C illustrate why regression to the mean occurs. Figure 7.3A shows the population distribution of a variable $X_1$. From this population individuals are selected for whom $X_1 > k$. In Figure 7.3B, the resulting

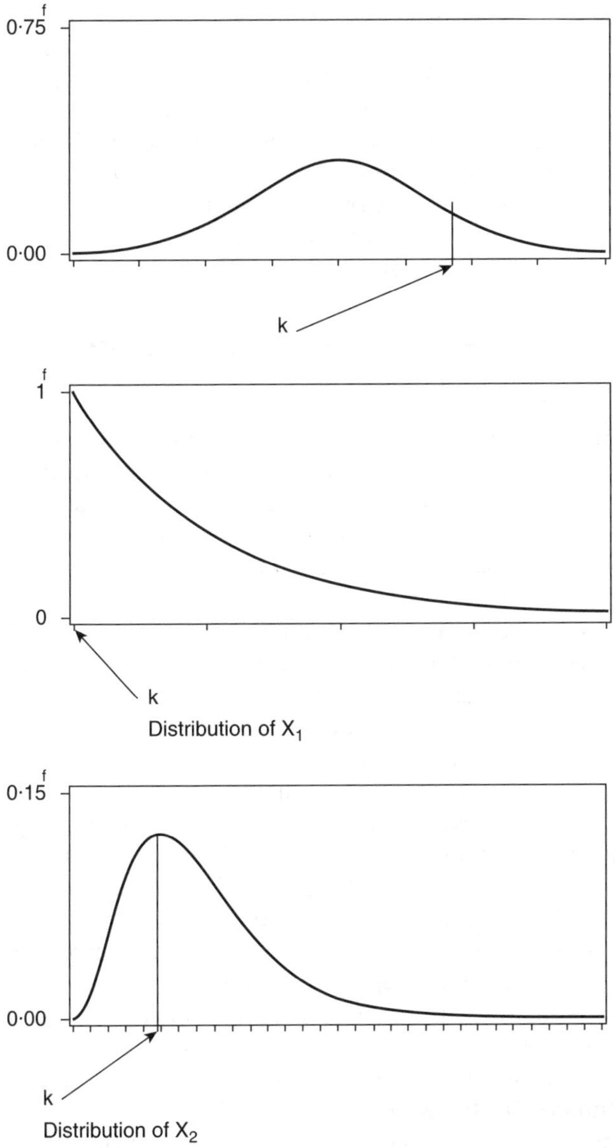


Figure 7.3A–C Graphical depiction of regression to the mean. Figure 7.3A shows the population distribution of a variable X. Individuals are selected whose first measurement of this variable is above some level, $X_1 > k$. Figure 7.3B shows the resulting distribution of $X_1$ for the selected individuals. This is necessarily a truncated distribution since the selected individuals were required to have $X_1 > k$. Figure 7.3C shows the distribution of the second measurement $X_2$ for this population. For at least some of the individuals $X_2 < k$ and it is clear that the mean of this distribution will be slightly smaller than that of the distribution in Figure 7.3B. The amount of regression to the mean will depend on the magnitude of k and on the correlation ρ between the first and second measurements.

distribution of $X_1$ for those persons selected because the first measure is extreme is a truncated distribution, since necessarily all such individuals have $X_1 > k$. However, when the second measurement $X_2$ is made some of the individuals in the study will have values less than k either because of biologic variability or because of random variation in the measurement. This results in the distribution shown in Figure 7.3C; a distribution which will clearly have a slightly smaller mean than that in Figure 7.3B. The amount of regression to the mean will depend on how close $\rho$ is to one and on the extremity of the cut point k through the formula discussed above.

## Regression to the mean and placebo effects: a composite

The implication of regression to the mean is that in uncontrolled studies where participants are selected because of extreme measurements, the intervention effect and the regression to the mean effect will be confounded. However, in controlled experiments, such as randomized controlled clinical trials, one can estimate the intervention effect by subtracting the mean effect in the control group from that in the intervention group. If the control group is given a placebo, it will not be possible to estimate the effect of the placebo due to the confounding with regression to the mean. For example, suppose we are conducting a trial of a medication to prevent migraine headaches and we select for study, persons who have had at least six attacks in the last six months. Participants are randomly assigned to receive the new medication or a suitable placebo. We will obtain an unbiased estimate of the medication effect on the frequency of migraines by comparing the mean number of attacks in the treated group with the mean in the placebo group. The theory of regression to the mean predicts that the mean number of attacks in the placebo group during the study will be less than that prior to the study. Thus, if we observe a decrease in the mean attack rate in the placebo group, we cannot attribute it to a placebo effect.

If precise estimates of $\mu$, $\sigma$, and $\rho$ were available, we could estimate the effects of regression to the mean using the formulation given earlier and thus by subtraction obtain an estimate of the placebo effect. However, precise estimates are rarely (if ever) available. The other obvious way to estimate the placebo effect is to randomly assign participants to placebo or no intervention. In this case the placebo effect can be estimated in the same way we estimate the intervention effects as described above.

Given the above description of regression to the mean, the question remains: does regression to the mean explain the placebo effect in all instances? Certainly, in situations where participants in a clinical trial are selected for having extreme values (for example, high blood pressure or many migraine headaches), regression to the mean will explain much of what has been described as placebo effect. Even in situations where we do not select patients on extreme values, for example in a cancer clinical trial, we may be selecting the patients when they are at a peak or nadir of their illness experience, even though we do not explicitly make this an inclusion criterion. Thus the vagaries of selection may lead to an apparent placebo effect through regression to the mean.

On the other hand, there are situations when it is difficult to explain away changes in the placebo group by selection processes alone. In the Lipid Research Clinics Coronary Primary Prevention Trial,[15] middle-aged men with high cholesterol were randomly assigned to receive the cholesterol lowering drug cholestyramine or placebo. One of the known side effects of cholestyramine is constipation. At baseline, 3% of the men in each group reported constipation in the past month. One year into the study, 39% of the cholestyramine treated men reported constipation, while 10% of the placebo treated men reported constipation. The men were selected for the trial based on elevated cholesterol and being free of coronary heart disease, but not on the basis of the presence or absence of constipation. It is difficult to imagine that regression to the mean led to the increase in reported constipation, unless one hypothesizes a strong association between high cholesterol, lack of heart disease, and constipation. These data seem then to be consistent with a placebo effect. I would be remiss if I did not point out another alternative to the placebo effect in this example. The informed consent given to each man before randomization, informed him that one of the potential side effects of cholestyramine was constipation. I would ask the behavioral scientists if it is possible that the mention of constipation in the informed consent could lead to an increase in the proportion reporting symptoms after receiving the masked medication.

I conclude that regression to the mean is a possible explanation for many reported instances of a placebo effect. However, I do not believe that regression to the mean could explain all reported placebo effects. Nevertheless, any research designed to measure a placebo effect must carefully consider how regression to the mean might influence the results. Statistical methods to account for regression to the mean in clinical trials and observational studies have been published by a number of authors.[16–18]

Future studies to quantify the magnitude of the placebo effect in various settings can benefit from study designs and data-analytic methods commonly used to estimate treatment effect in randomized, double blind, controlled clinical trials in the presence of regression. In trials to specifically quantify the effect of a placebo intervention, it can be useful to include a "no-treatment" arm for comparison.[5,10] In such a trial the placebo arm would be the intervention arm and the "no-treatment" arm would be the control group.

## References


1 Beecher HK. The powerful placebo. *JAMA* 1955;**159**:1602–6.
2 Shapiro AK. Factors contributing to the placebo effect. Their implication for psychotherapy. *Am J Psychother* 1964;**18**:73–88.
3 Brody H. *Placebos and the Philosophy of Medicine. Clinical, Conceptual, and Ethical Issues*. Chicago: University of Chicago Press, 1980.

4 Moerman DE. Explanatory mechanisms for placebo effects: cultural influences and the meaning response. This volume, chapter 4.
5 Bootzin RR, Caspi O. Explanatory mechanisms for placebo effects: cognition, personality and social learning. This volume, chapter 5.
6 Price DD, Soerensen LV. Endogenous opioid and non-opioid pathways as mediators of placebo analgesia. This volume, chapter 9.
7 Siegel S. Explanatory mechanisms for placebo effects: Pavlovian conditioning. This volume, chapter 6.
8 Kienle GS, Kiene H. The powerful placebo effect: Fact or fiction? *J Clin Epidemiol* 1997; **50**:1311–18.
9 Last JM. *A Dictionary of Epidemiology*. New York: Oxford University Press, 1983:43.
10 McDonald CJ, Mazzuca SA, McCabe GP. How much of the placebo 'effect' is really statistical regression? *Stat Med* 1983;**2**:417–27.
11 Galton F. Regression towards mediocrity in hereditary stature. *J Anthrop Inst* 1886; **15**:246–63.
12 Das P, Mulder PCH. Regression to the mode. *Statis Neerl* 1983;**37**:15–20.
13 Davis CE. The effect of regression to the mean in epidemiologic and clinical studies. *Am J Epidemiol* 1976;**5**:493–8.
14 Streiner DL, Norman GR. Health measurement scales: a practical guide to their development and use. New York: Oxford University Press, 1989:89–90.
15 Lipid Research Clinics Program. The Lipid Research Clinics Coronary Primary Prevention Trial Results. *JAMA* 1984;**25**:351–64.
16 Chambless LE, Roeback JR. Methods for assessing difference between groups in change when initial measurement is subject to intra-individual variation. *Stat Med* 1993; **12**:1213–37.
17 Whittemore AS. Errors-in-variables regression using Stein estimates. *The American Statistician* 1989;**43**:226–8.
18 Lin HM, Hughes MD. Use of historical marker data for assessing treatment effects in phase I/II trials when subject selection is determined by baseline marker level. *Biometrics* 1995;**51**:1053–63.

# *Section 3:* Elucidating placebo effects: intervening psychophysiology

# 8: Neuroendocrine mediators of placebo effects on immunity

FARIDEH ESKANDARI, ESTHER M STERNBERG

## Summary

Many lines of research have recently established the numerous routes by which the immune and central nervous systems communicate. These suggest mechanisms by which factors such as the social world, beliefs and expectations might influence neuroendocrine and neural responses which could in turn affect immune responses and therefore disease expression. The placebo effect represents one phenomenon linking belief to wellbeing that can be analyzed systematically to provide insights into how beliefs might affect immune responses and disease expression or severity. Placebo effects have been explained by Pavlovian conditioning, cognition (for example, expectancy), personality, and social learning, alone or in combination, and these factors transduce meaning from the individual's cultural context. These psychosocial mechanisms evoke intervening psychophysiological events that involve multiple systems, including the autonomic nervous, endocrine, and immune systems, endorphin and motor pathways, and cardiovascular and gastrointestinal processes. The transducing mechanism by which placebo interventions convert meaning into the modification of physiologic responses is not known. Indeed, no studies fully trace the pathways of cognition/expectancy, personality, social learning, and social psychological interactions to regulation of psychophysiological responses. Some brain centers appear to be specifically involved depending on the environmental stimulus, such as insular cortex in taste aversion studies. Once the information is processed, several common central pathways are activated, including the hypothalamic-pituitary-adrenal axis, peripheral nervous system and autonomic nervous system. Neurohormones and neurotransmitters released into the peripheral blood or through nerve pathways that innervate immune organs then affect immune responses and disease expression.

## Introduction

The belief that mind plays an important role in physical illness goes back to the earliest days of medicine. From the time of the ancient Greeks to the beginning of the 20th century it was generally accepted by both physician and the patient that the mind can affect the course of illness and it seemed natural to apply this concept in medical treatments of disease. Until recently, however, this concept was dismissed by the scientific and medical community as unfounded.

However, many lines of research have recently established the numerous routes by which the immune, endocrine and central nervous systems communicate and interruptions or perturbations of each can alter the severity, course and susceptibility and resistance to diseases.[1–5] These suggest mechanisms by which factors such as the social world, beliefs and expectations might influence neuroendocrine and neural responses which could in turn affect immune responses and therefore disease expression. The placebo effect represents one phenomenon linking belief to wellbeing that can be analyzed systematically to provide insights into how beliefs might affect immune responses and disease expression or severity.

Placebo effects have been explained by Pavlovian conditioning, cognition (for example, expectancy), personality, and social learning, alone or in combination, and these factors transduce meaning from the individual's cultural context. These psychosocial mechanisms evoke intervening psychophysiological events that involve multiple systems, including the autonomic nervous, endocrine, and immune systems, endorphin and motor pathways, and cardiovascular and gastrointestinal processes.

The transducing mechanism by which placebo interventions convert meaning into the modification of physiologic responses is not known. Indeed, no studies fully trace the pathways of cognition/expectancy, personality, social learning, and social psychological interactions to regulation of psychophysiological responses. Two mediating physiological processes that have been studied extensively are the immune system and the opioid and non-opioid mechanisms involved in placebo analgesia.[6–17] This chapter focuses on psychoneuroendocrine immunology.

In addition to sending regulatory signals to the immune system, the central nervous system (CNS) receives and produces cytokine signals.[18] This afferent arm of CNS-immune communication will not be discussed in this chapter because the mechanisms relevant to the placebo effect more likely occur through efferent mechanisms.

Evidence that many environmental factors may modify expression of complex diseases such as autoimmune or inflammatory disease comes from genetic studies. Such studies indicate that expression of complex traits and illnesses, such as inflammatory or autoimmune disease, are multigenic and polygenic. That is, these traits are determined by many genes, each with small effect. In complex illnesses such as inflammatory disease and arthritis, any one genetic locus generally contributes only 35–40% of the variance of expression of a quantitative trait, with the remainder determined by so-called environmental factors.[19–21] Amongst the many environmental factors that could potentially influence expression of such complex diseases are developmental and social conditions, cultural beliefs and expectations, stressful situations and the placebo effect.

Cultural, social and emotional factors have profound effects on placebo responses, however these are discussed elsewhere in this volume. Conditioned learning experiments provide important insights into the physiological, neural and molecular mechanisms of placebo effect. Studies of cultural influences on psychological aspects such as expectancy also provide insights into mechanisms of placebo on health. The biology of how a symbolic meaning (placebo) can elicit biological changes is much more complicated than that of simple forms of conditioned learning. However, such studies shed light on how symbolic meanings could affect neuronal and neuroendocrine responses that in turn regulate immune responses. They can thus serve as a foundation to further build on the understanding of the biology of placebo effects on immunity. Conditioning has been discussed in detail in another chapter in this book.[22] In this chapter we will focus mainly on the underlying biology of conditioned learning and mechanisms by which such higher brain processes might alter immune responses through effects on neuroendocrine and neuronal systems.

Studies of mechanisms of placebo analgesic effects could also shed light on mechanisms of placebo effects on immunity. These have been well studied and are discussed elsewhere in this volume (see Chapter 9). While many of the pathways of placebo analgesia may be specific to placebo effects on pain, some are more general and thus will inform further analysis of placebo effects on immunity. Briefly, it is known that many ascending pain-related pathways terminate within cortical and subcortical structures such as hypothalamic nuclei, amygdala and midbrain periacqueductal grey that represent origins of pain modulatory pathways.[23] These same brain structures are related to learning and memory, threat-elicited defensive behavior and pain modulation and could also play a role in conditioning of the immune response in certain circumstances.

A full understanding of the biological mechanisms of placebo effects on immunity requires an analysis of the mechanisms by which beliefs and values, through psychological processes such as expectations and learning, could affect the brain and related physiologic structures, to ultimately alter immune responses.

## Overview of neural pathways mediating placebo effects on immunity

There is little doubt that learning processes contribute to the development and expression of immunoregulatory function. Brain centers involved in conditioning affect neuroendocrine, sympathetic and opioid

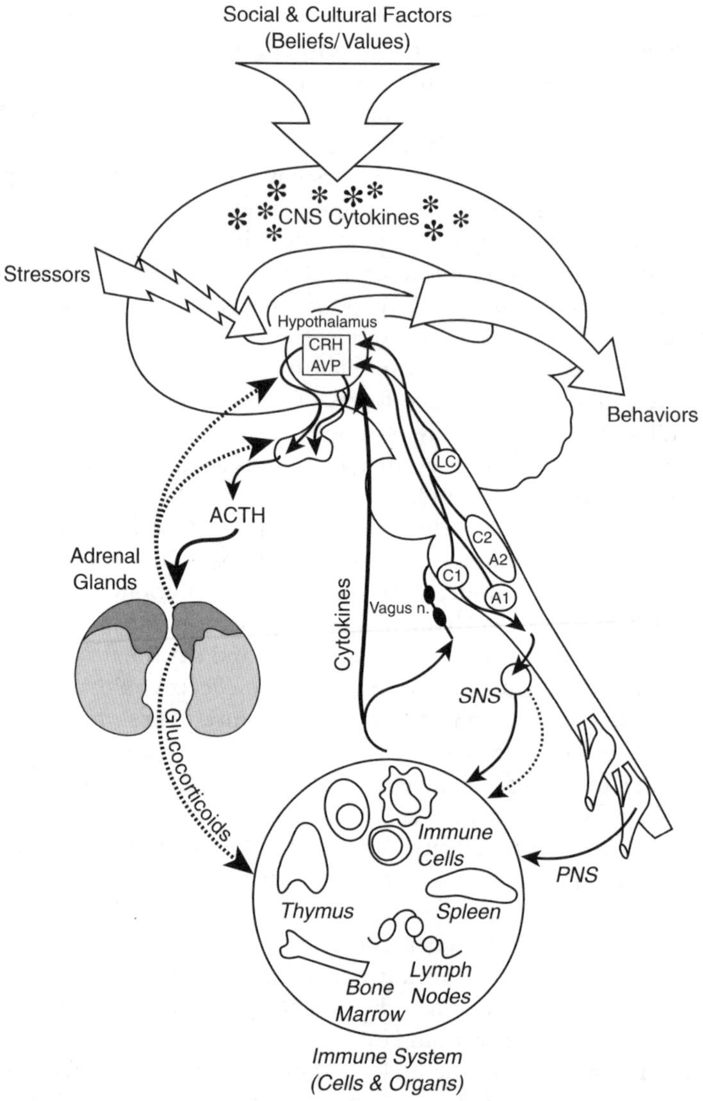


Figure 8.1 Interaction of the brain and immune system. Immune cells produce cytokines that stimulate the central nervous system through the blood stream or via nerves such as the vagus nerve. Stimulation of the hypothalamus results in the release of corticotropin releasing hormone (CRH) and arginine vasopressin (AVP). AVP acts as a co-stimulator with CRH resulting in release of adrenocorticotropin hormone (ACTH) from the anterior pituitary gland. ACTH causes the adrenal glands to release glucocorticoids, which modulate the immune system generally suppressing inflammation. Glucocorticoids also feedback and suppress hypothalamic CRH and pituitary ACTH release. CRH also acts on the brain stem to stimulate the sympathetic nervous system, which innervates immune organs and regulates inflammatory responses via noradrenergic mechanisms. Broken arrows (⋯→) indicate suppression and solid arrows (→) indicate stimulation.

pathways, whose released mediators may then alter immune responses. Placebo effects on immunity could occur through reduction of stress responses and/or stimulation of other neuropeptide pathways such as endogenous opiates.

The neuroendocrine stress response consists of hypothalamic–pituitary–adrenal (HPA) axis and autonomic nervous system responses (Figure 8.1). The HPA axis modulates immune responses systemically through the potent anti-inflammatory effects of the glucocorticoids.[24] The autonomic nervous system regulates the immune system regionally through innervation of immune organs such as the spleen, thymus and lymph nodes.[1] Glucocorticoids also regulate immunity regionally through their local production in immune organs such as thymus.[2,3] Peripheral nerves also regulate immune responses locally through innervation at sites of inflammation and release of neuropeptides.[4] Morphine decreases mitogen responsiveness and natural killer cell activity and could also affect immune responses indirectly through adrenergic effects.[5] At a cellular level, lymphocytes are also capable of receiving and generating neuroendocrine signals. By tapping into such pathways, signals from higher emotional or cognitive centers could affect release of neurohormones, neuropeptides and neurotransmitters that could then alter immune responses.

## Expectancy and conditioning

Expectancy and conditioning[25] have been proposed to mediate the placebo effect and themselves are modified by social and cultural factors. The complex interactions between conditioning and culturally and socially ingrained expectancies are discussed by Moerman.[26] In this chapter we will focus on neural mechanisms by which conditioning could modulate immune responses. An explanation of classical (Pavlovian) conditioning, is given earlier in this work.[22]

Conditioned alterations of immune responses have been clearly demonstrated in multiple studies. Immunogenic stimuli are capable of serving as unconditioned stimuli for the conditioning of other psychophysiological responses. In the seminal study by Ader and Cohen the effects of conditioning on immune response, saccharin-flavored water (the conditioned stimulus) was paired with an intraperitoneal injection of cyclophosphamide, an immunosuppressive (the unconditioned stimulus). Hemagglutinating antibody titers measured six days after antigen administration were not detectable in conditioned animals though they were in a randomized control group.[6] In 1982, the same scientists published a study, showing an improvement of autoimmune disease via classical conditioning of immunosuppression. In this study the groups of animals that received a solution of sodium saccharin paired with cyclophosphamide had a significantly lower proteinuria and mortality compared to a randomized group of non-conditioned animals.[7] These findings have been repeatedly reproduced in other studies in animals and more recently in some human studies.[8,10]

Other animal taste aversion conditioning studies with cyclosporine A causing immunosuppression have revealed significant reduction in granulocyte and lymphocyte number and function, reduced interleukin-2 and interferon γ synthesis by splenocytes, suppressed mitogen-induced lymphocyte proliferation in spleen and prolonged survival time of heterotopic heart allografts.[8,9]

In a human study cyclophosphamide was paired with a distinctively flavored drink in women with multiple sclerosis who were receiving monthly immunosuppressive therapy. After five or six sessions, the majority of patients exhibited leukopenia in response to the conditioned stimulus administered with a dose of cyclophosphamide (10mg) judged normally too small to produce leukopenia.[10] In another study on healthy tuberculin positive hospital employees, the delayed hypersensitivity reaction to tuberculin was diminished significantly by behavioral conditioning, which altered expectancy.[11]

Illnesses such as bronchial asthma have in the past been suggested to have some benefit from biofeedback and counter-conditioning. In one study 68% of children in the experimental biofeedback groups were able to decrease their airway resistance by 10–15%. The author postulated that the subjects' hypersensitivity to a large number of environmental irritants could be exacerbated through the process of classical conditioning. This author also suggested that the association of asthma with certain emotions could be established through the process of operant conditioning.[27] In a follow up study, the same author demonstrated deconditioning of exercise-induced asthma through the extinction procedure.[28] In a study of patients with moderate to severe psoriasis, mindfulness meditation-based stress reduction during phototherapy and photochemotherapy was associated with some improvement in disease.[29]

However, many of these studies employ subjective outcome measures and show wide variability in effects, probably partially accounted for by the small numbers of subjects studied. A more recent study, using objective outcome measures, has provided clear evidence that non-pharmacologic behavioral interventions such as writing about a stressful event, can positively affect autoimmune, inflammatory or allergic disease outcome in patients with rheumatoid arthritis and mild to moderately severe asthma.[30]

While the early studies are intriguing and more recent studies do provide some support for a role for conditioning behavioral and non-pharmacological interventions in treatment of some immune mediated diseases, further work must be performed to assess to what degree and at what point in the course of chronic immune, inflammatory or allergic illnesses, placebo, conditioning or behavioral interventions may alter disease course or severity. Full understanding of the neurobiological and neuroendocrine mechanisms of placebo will be crucial to identify intervention points in such illnesses, which may be responsive to placebo effects, as well as for identifying interventions that may be useful in specific cases.

## Neuronal and neuroendocrine mechanisms underlying conditioning of immune responses

Most of the literature relating to neuronal mechanisms of conditioning of the immune response do not fully trace the pathways of conditioning, learning and memory all the way through to regulation of immune diseases. Much work has been done to elucidate the neuronal pathways of conditioning, i.e. learning.[12–14,31–33] Some studies indicate brain centers important in regulating conditioning of immunity.[12–14] Many studies describe neuroendocrine and sympathetic regulation of immunity.[34–52] But few connect all these processes. This section will describe some of the recent findings relating conditioning pathways to immune responses.

### CNS centers involved in conditioning

Several CNS centers have been suggested to play a role in conditioning of different responses, such as pain and immunity. Some brain regions appear to be specifically involved depending on the response that is studied. These include the insular cortex in taste aversion,[12,13] the periaqueductal grey in analgesia.[53] Other regions appear to play a more general role in transducing the effects of placebo manipulations on a variety of responses. Thus, the hypothalamus, amygdala and various components of the autonomic nervous system may play a more general role in analgesic and immune effects of conditioning interventions.

Some evidence for brain regions that are involved in placebo effects comes from lesioning studies. Lesioning studies in rats in which the insular cortex region of the neocortex is ablated have been shown to disrupt the acquisition of conditioned immunosupression by taste aversions.[12] Similarly, lesioning studies of the amygdala interfered with acquisition of conditioned immunosuppressive responses but had no effect on the performance of pre-existing conditioned responses, when saccharin taste was paired with cyclophosphamide.[13] Other taste aversion studies have shown that the insular cortex and amygdala are involved in conditioned enhancement of antibody production, when gustative or odor stimuli were paired with antigenic stimulation. Lesioning of memory centers, such as the hippocampus, have not been shown to play a role in mediating taste aversion conditioning of the immune response.[14]

Thus, some of the effects of conditioning on immune responses, when the unconditioned stimulus involves taste, could be mediated through the insular cortex and through its connections with the hypothalamus and/or the autonomic nervous system. The amygdala could play a more general role in conditioned immune responses, when fear is involved, because of its clear role in fear responses and emotional enhancement of learning and memory.[31–33]

## Hypothalamic-pituitary-adrenal (HPA) axis

Once higher brain centers have been activated during a conditioned response, they can signal neuroendocrine responses in the hypothalamus and autonomic centers in the brain stem. Once activated, these centers release neurohormones and neurotransmitters that can influence immune responses.

Within several brain centers involved in both the hormonal stress response and fear conditioning, particularly the hypothalamus and amygdala, corticotropin releasing hormone (CRH) is a principal neuropeptide signal.[34] CRH is the main neuropeptide released from the hypothalamus, controlling the neuroendocrine stress response. CRH neurons also project extensively throughout the brain and mediate stress related patterns of behavior that fall under the category of fight or flight. CRH containing neurons and receptors present in amygdala, hypothalamus and locus coeruleus play a role in these behavior patterns.[34–36] CRH neurons, particularly in the amygdala, also interact with other neurotransmitter systems including dopaminergic, noradrenergic and serotoneric neurons.[34] The extent to which these neurotransmitter systems are involved in conditioning of the immune response has not been systematically investigated, although the effects of CRH on immune responses have been studied extensively.

Once released from the hypothalamus into the median eminence, CRH stimulates adrenocorticotropin hormone (ACTH) release from the pituitary, which in turn triggers glucocorticoid release from the adrenal glands. Through this route the central nervous system affects the immune system mainly through the largely immunosuppressive effects of the glucocorticoids. At physiologic concentrations, glucocorticoids are not totally immunosuppressive but specifically regulate the immune response. Thus, at lower concentrations, glucocorticoids cause a shift in immune responses from a proinflammatory cytokine pattern, of increased tumor necrosis factor $\alpha$, interleukin-1 to an anti-inflammatory cytokine pattern of increased interleukin-10 and endogenous IL-1 receptor antagonist.[37,38] In general, underactivity of the neuroendocrine stress response predisposes to enhanced susceptibility to inflammatory disease due to lack of suppression by glucocorticoids, while overactivity and excess glucocorticoid responses, as occur during stress, tend to suppress immune responses and predispose to infection.[39–41]

Thus, one mechanism by which conditioning could alter immune responses may be through modulation of the neuroendocrine stress response.[42,43] The relative contribution of this pathway to conditioning effects on immunity requires further evaluation.

## Autonomic nervous system

Other neural pathways through which conditioning might affect immune responses, include the autonomic and peripheral nervous systems. Immune organs, including thymus, spleen and lymph nodes, are innervated by sympathetic nerves.[44] Immune cells express neurotransmitter receptors, for example, adrenergic receptors on lymphocytes, which allow them to respond to neurotransmitters released from these nerves. Different lymphocyte populations have been shown to be differentially sensitive to β-adrenergic stimulation.[45] Systemic norepinephrine and epinephrine inhibit the production of type 1/proinflammatory cytokines, such as interleukin-12, tumor necrosis factor α and interferon γ and stimulate the production of type 2/anti-inflammatory cytokines such as interleukin-10 and transforming growth factor β. Through this mechanism, systemic catecholamines may cause a selective suppression of Th1 responses and cellular immunity and enhance Th2 response and humoral immunity. However, in certain local responses and under certain conditions, catecholamines may enhance regional immune responses, through induction of interleukin-1, tumor necrosis factor α and interleukin-8 production.[46]

Interruption of sympathetic innervation of immune organs has been shown to modulate inflammatory and infectious disease outcome and susceptibility.[50] Denervation of lymph node noradrenergic fibers is associated with exacerbation of inflammation, while systemic sympathectomy or denervation of joints is associated with decreased severity of inflammation. Dual activation of the sympathetic nervous system and HPA axis modulates host defenses to infection.[48] β-adrenergic activity has been shown to be involved in the expression of conditioned morphine induced immunomodulatory effects (see below) but is not required for acquisition of conditioned immune effects.

### Peripheral nervous system

The peripheral nervous system affects inflammation through neuropeptides, such as substance P, peripherally released CRH and vasoactive intestinal polypeptide. These molecules are released from nerve endings or synapses or may be synthesized and released by immune cells and tend to have proinflammatory effects.[4,49–52] Since substance P neurons are involved in ascending pain pathways, it is possible that these neurons could mediate conditioning effects on inflammatory responses, through pathways similar to those involved in placebo analgesia. This hypothesis however, has not been investigated.

### Opioid system

Opiate mediated mechanisms also have been shown to directly affect immune responses.[5,54,55] Pharmacologic intervention studies using opioid antagonists also indicate that opioid pathways play a role in conditioning of immune responses.[56]

Morphine decreases mitogen responsiveness and natural killer cell activity.[5,57,58] Opioids suppress many aspects of immune responses, including antimicrobial resistance, antibody production and delayed type hypersensitivity. This occurs in part through desensitization of chemokine receptors on neutrophils, monocytes and lymphocytes.[54,55]

Pharmacologic studies indicate that opioid receptor activity is involved in the acquisition of conditioned morphine induced immune alterations, as well as in the expression of a subset of these conditioned responses. The opioid antagonist, naltrexone when injected before conditioning, has been shown to prevent acquisition of the conditioned suppression of splenic lymphoproliferation, NK-cell activity and IL-2 production. Naltrexone injected before testing also blocked the expression of conditioned alterations in lymphoproliferative responses, attenuated the suppression of NK-cell activity at the highest dose and had no effect on IL-2 production.[56]

In addition to these direct effects, morphine could also affect immune responses indirectly through adrenergic effects, since it increases plasma levels of catecholamines.

## Placebo analgesia

Extensive research has been done to elucidate underlying mechanisms of placebo analgesia. These are reviewed in detail elsewhere in this volume.[59] A full understanding of these mechanisms will shed light on placebo effects on immune response modulation.

Some brain regions that have been shown to be involved in placebo analgesia include the central nucleus of amygdala, the periaqueductal-periventricular grey matter, the ventromedial medulla and the spinal cord dorsal horn. These are involved in opioid analgesia and presumably also play a role in placebo analgesia. Molecular mechanisms of placebo analgesia include opioid and non-opioid mechanisms including cholecystokinin, which appears to modulate endogenous opioid systems.[60] The opiate antagonist, naloxone, blocks some but not other forms of externally induced analgesia suggesting that both endogenous opiate and non-opiate systems must play a role in placebo analgesia. In one study placebo analgesia obtained by verbally induced expectancy was completely reversed by naloxone, whereas placebo analgesia obtained by conditioning was reversed by naloxone, only if the conditioning had been carried out with morphine. Conditioning with the non-opioid drug, ketorolac, produced an analgesic effect that was not naloxone reversible.[15]

## Complementary and alternative medicine (CAM)

Understanding the underlying neurobiology of the placebo effect and the mechanism of how placebos affect immunity might help to explain a portion of the health benefits of some psychosocial and mind-body CAM interventions. Some studies indicate that CAM practices such as meditation may alter autonomic function. For instance, autonomic nervous system activity has been shown to be heightened during meditation, as indicated by exaggerated heart beat variability.[16] This is contrary to the notion of autonomic quiescence during meditation. Such autonomic changes could potentially affect immune responses and thus alterations in autonomic function associated with these CAM therapies could potentially modify the course of immune disease.

Other studies, including pharmacological interventions using opioid antagonists such as naloxone, indicate that opioid mechanisms may contribute to the effectiveness of some other CAM therapies, such as acupuncture. Thus, the large majority of studies that have attempted to reverse acupuncture analgesia by naloxone have shown partial to complete reversal, consistent with an endogenous opioid component to this intervention. Similar reversals have been obtained in high intensity low frequency (acupuncture-like) transcutaneous electrical nerve stimulation (TENS) but not high frequency, low intensity TENS. Overall, these studies show that acupuncture and TENS activate both opiate and non-opiate systems depending on different parameters of stimulation.[17,61,62] Further studies of this nature will be required to fully elucidate underlying neurobiological and neurochemical mechanisms of these and other CAM interventions on immunity.

## Future approaches to further elucidation of placebo and conditioning effects on immunity

Neuroimaging studies have provided new insights to mapping of pain centers and thus hold promise for elucidating underlying neurobiology of some CAM practices.[63] It also has provided a new tool for understanding the pathophysiology of delirium.[64] In humans, neuroimaging techniques, such as positron emission tomography or functional magnetic resonance imaging, should in future be used to identify brain regions involved in placebo effects on immunity. Neuropharmacological studies should be applied to further identify molecular neurotransmitter and neuropeptide systems that are activated in response to placebo.

Animal studies employing systematic analysis of conditioning effects in inbred strains of animals with a well defined genetic background, lesioning studies or studies in gene knockout or transgenic animals, should also help to elucidate neuroanatomical and molecular pathways underlying the effects of conditioning on immune responses. Such approaches combined with other molecular technologies such as gene and protein expression arrays, may provide further insights into the patterns of genes that are altered by interventions, such as conditioning, that shed light on placebo effects.

## Conclusions

The mechanism by which conditioning, expectancy or placebo lead to modifications of physiologic responses, including immune responses is not known. No studies fully trace the pathways of conditioned learning and memory through transducing neuroendocrine and autonomic and opioid systems, to regulation of immune or other responses. Many studies address parts of this chain, particularly the effector endpoints of effects of adrenocortical steroids, endogenous opioids and catecholamines, acting singly or in concert, as mediators of conditioned alterations of immunity. Further studies are required to elucidate and connect neural pathways involved in perception of cultural and social factors, stress, beliefs and expectancy on these intervening neuroendocrine and neuronal transducing pathways on immune function and disease expression.

## References


1 Felten Y, Felten DL. Parallel development of noradrenergic innervation and cellular compartmentation in the rat spleen. *Exp Neurol* 1989;**103**:239–55.
2 Vacchio MS, Ashwell JD. Thymus-derived glucocorticoids regulate antigen-specific selection. *J Exp Med* 1997;**185**:2033–8.
3 Vacchio MS, Ashwell JD, King LB. A positive role for thymus-derived steroids in formation of the T-cell repertoire. *Ann NY Acad Sci* 1998;**840**:317–27.
4 Payan DG, Goetzl EJ. Dual roles of substance P: modulator of immune and neuroendocrine functions. *Ann NY Acad Sci* 1987;**512**:465–75.
5 Gomez-Flores R, Weber RJ. Inhibition of interleukin-2 production and downregulation of IL-2 and transferring receptors on rat splenic lymphocytes following PAG morphine administration: a role in natural killer and T-cell suppression. *J Interferon Cytokine Res* 1999;**19**:625–30.
6 Ader R, Cohen N. Behaviorally conditioned immunosuppression. *Psychosom Med* 1975;**37**:333–40.
7 Ader R. Behaviorally conditioned immunosuppression and murine systemic lupus erythematosus. *Science* 1982;**215**:1534–6.
8 Von Horsten S, Exton MS, Schult M, *et al.* Behaviorally conditioned effects of cyclosporine A on the immune system of rats: specific alterations of blood leukocyte numbers and decrease of granulocyte function. *J Neuroimmunol* 1998;**85**:193–201.
9 Exton MS, Horsten S, Schult M, *et al.* Behaviorally conditioned immunosuppression using cyclosporine A: central nervous system reduces IL-2 production via splenic innervation. *J Neuroimmunol* 1998;**88**:182–91.
10 Giang DW, Goodman AD, Schiffer RB, *et al.* Conditioning of cyclophosphamide-induced leukopenia in humans. *J Neuropsych Clin Neurosci* 1996;**8**:194–201.
11 Smith RG, McDaniel SM. Psychologically mediated effect on the delayed hypersensitivity reaction to tuberculin in humans. *Psychosom Med* 1983;**45**:65–70.
12 Ramirez-Amaya V, Alvarez-Borda B, Ormsby CE, Martinez RD, Perez-Montfort R, Bermudez-Rattoni F. Insular cortex lesions impair the acquisition of conditioned immunosuppression. *Brain Behav Immunol* 1996;**10**:103–14.
13 Ramirez-Amaya V, Alvarez-Borda B, Bermudez-Rattoni F. Differential effects of NMDA-induced lesions into the insular cortex and amygdala on the acquisition and evocation of conditioned immunosuppression. *Brain Behav Immunol* 1998;**12**:149–60.
14 Ramirez-Amaya V, Bermudez-Rattoni F. Conditioned enhancement of antibody production is disrupted by insular cortex and amygdala but not hippocampal lesions. *Brain Behav Immunol* 1999;**13**:46–60.
15 Amanzio M, Benedetti F. Neuropharmacological dissection of placebo analgesia: expectation-activated opioid systems versus conditioning-activated specific subsystems. *J Neurosci* 1999;**19**:484–94.
16 Peng CK, Mietus JE, Liu Y, *et al.* Exaggerated heart rate oscillations during two meditation techniques. *Int J Cardiol* 1999;**70**:101–7.
17 Price DD, Barrell JJ. Mechanisms of analgesia produced by hypnosis and placebo suggestions. In: Mayer EA, Saper CB, eds. *Progress in Brain Research 122. The Biological Basis for Third Body Interactions.* New York: Elsevier Science BV, 2000.
18 Dantzer R, Konsman JP, Bluthe RM, Kelley KW. Neural and humoral pathways of communication from the immune system to the brain: parallel or convergent? *Auton Neurosci* 2000;**85**:60–5.

19 Listwak S, Barrientos RM, Koike G, *et al.* Identification of a novel inflammation-protective locus in the Fischer rat. *Mamm Genome* 1999;**10**:362–5.

20 Joe B, Remmers EF, Dobbins DE, *et al.* Genetic dissection of collagen-induced arthritis in Chromosome 10 quantitative trait locus speed congenic rats: evidence for more than one regulatory locus and sex influences. *Immunogenetics* 2000;**51**:930–44.

21 Jafarian-Tehrani M, Sternberg EM. Animal models of neuroimmune interactions in inflammatory diseases. *J Neuroimmunol* 1999;**100**:13–20.

22 Siegel S. Explanatory mechanisms for placebo effects: Pavlovian conditioning. This volume, chapter 6.

23 Price DD. Psychological and neural mechanisms of the affective dimension of pain. *Science* 2000;**288**:1769–72.

24 Sternberg EM, Chrousos GP, Wilder RL, Gold PW. The stress response and the regulation of inflammatory disease. *Ann Intern Med* 1992;**117**:854–66.

25 Brody HB, Brody D. Placebo and health–II. Three perspectives on the placebo response: expectancy, conditioning and meaning. *Adv Mind Body Med* 2000;**16**:216–32.

26 Moerman DE. Explanatory mechanisms for placebo effects: cultural influences and the meaning response. This volume, chapter 4.

27 Khan AU. Effectiveness of biofeedback and counter-conditioning in the treatment of bronchial asthma. *J Psychosom Res* 1976;**21**:97–104.

28 Khan AU, Olson DL. Deconditioning of exercise-induced asthma. *Psychosom Med* 1977;**39**:382–92.

29 Kabat-Zinn J, Wheeler E, Light T, *et al.* Influence of a mindfulness meditation–based stress reduction intervention on rates of skin clearing in patients with moderate to severe psoriasis undergoing phototherapy (UVB) and photochemotherapy (PUVA). *Psychosom Med* 1998,**60**:625–32.

30 Smyth JM, Stone AA, Hurewitz A, Kaell A. Effects of writing about stressful experiences on symptom reduction in patients with asthma or rheumatoid arthritis: a randomized trial. *JAMA* 1999;**28**:1304–9.

31 Roozendaal B, Nguyen BT, Power AE, McGaugh JL. Basolateral amygdala noradrenergic influence enables enhancement of memory consolidation induced by hippocampal glucocorticoid receptor activation. *Proc Natl Acad Sci USA* 1999;**96**:11642–7.

32 Ferry B, Roozendaal B, McGaugh JL. Role of norepinephrine in mediating stress hormone regulation of long-term memory storage: a critical involvement of the amygdala. *Biol Psychiatry* 1999;**46**:1140–52.

33 Setlow B, Roozendaal B, McGaugh JL. Involvement of a basolateral amygdala complex-nucleus accumbens pathway in glucocorticoid-induced modulation of memory consolidation. *Eur J Neurosci* 2000;**12**:367–75.

34 Gray TS. Amygdaloid CRF pathways: Role in autonomic, neuroendocrine and behavioral responses to stress. *Ann NY Acad Sci* 1993;**697**:53–60.

35 Van Bockstaele EJ, Colago EE, Valentino RJ. Amygdaloid corticotropin-releasing factor targets locus coeruleus dendrites: substrate for the co-ordination of emotional and cognitive limbs of the stress response. *J Neuroendocrinol* 1998;**10**:743–57.

36 Lechner SM, Valentino RJ. Glucocorticoid receptor-immunoreactivity in corticotrophin-releasing factor afferents to the locus coeruleus. *Brain Res* 1999;**816**:17–28.

37 DeRijk R, Michelson D, Karp B, *et al.* Exercise and circadian rhythm-induced variation in plasma cortisol differentially regulate interleukin-1 beta (IL-1 beta), IL-6, and tumor necrosis factor-alpha production in humans: high sensitivity of TNF alpha and resistance of IL-6. *J Clin Endocrinol Metab* 1997;**82**:2182–91.

38 Elenkov IJ, Chrousos GP. Stress hormones, Th1/Th2 patterns, pro/anti-inflammatory cytokines and susceptibility to disease. *Trends Endocrinol Metab* 1999;**10**:359–68.

39 Sternberg EM. Emotions and disease: from balance of humors to balance of molecules. *Nature Med* 1997;**3**:264–7.

40 Sternberg EM. Neural-immune interactions in health and disease. *J Clin Invest* 1997; **100**:2641–7.

41 Sheridan JF, Feng NG, Bonneau RH, Allen CM, Huneycutt BS, Glaser R. Restraint stress differentially affects anti-viral cellular and humoral immune responses in mice. *J Neuroimmunol* 1991;**31**:245–55.

42 Moynihan JA, Kaip JD, Cohen N, Ader R. Immune deviation following stress odor exposure: role of endogenous opioids. *J Neuroimmunol* 2000;**102**:145–53.

43 Buske-Kirschbaum A, Grota L, Kirschbaum C, *et al.* Conditioned increase in peripheral blood mononuclear cell (PBMC) number and corticosterone secretion in the rat. *Pharmacol Biochem Behav* 1996;**55**:27–32.
44 Felten DL. Neural influence on immune responses: underlying suppositions and basic principles of neural-immune signaling. *Prog Brain Res* 2000;**122**:381–9.
45 Coussons-Read ME, Dykstra LA, Lysle DT. Pavlovian conditioning of morphine-induced alterations of immune status: evidence for peripheral beta-adrenergic receptor involvement. *Brain Behav Immun* 1994;**8**:204–17.
46 Elenkov IJ, Wilder RL, Chrousos GP, Vizi ES. The sympathetic nerve – an integrative interface between two supersystems: the brain and the immune system. *Pharmacol Rev* 2000;**52**:595–638.
47 ThyagaRajan S, Madden KS, Stevens SY, Felten DL. Effects of L-deprenyl treatment on noradrenergic innervation and immune reactivity in lymphoid organs of young F344 rats. *J Neuroimmunol* 1999;**96**:57–65.
48 Hermann G, Beck FM, Tovar CA, Malarkey WB, Allen C, Sheridan JF. Stress-induced changes attributable to the sympathetic nervous system during experimental influenza viral infection in DBA/2 inbred mouse strain. *J Neuroimmunol* 1994;**53**:173–80.
49 Crofford LJ, Sano H, Karalis K, *et al.* Local expression of corticotropin-releasing hormone in inflammatory arthritis. *Ann NY Acad Sci* 1995;**771**:459–71.
50 Takeba Y, Suzuki N, Kaneko A, Asai T, Sakane T. Evidence for neural regulation of inflammatory synovial cell functions by secreting calcitonin gene-related peptide and vasoactive intestinal peptide in patients with rheumatoid arthritis. *Arthritis Rheum* 1999;**42**:2418–29.
51 Hood VC, Cruwys SC, Urban L, Kidd BL. Differential role of neurokinin receptors in human lymphocyte and monocyte chemotaxis. *Regul Pept* 2000;**96**:17–21.
52 Dorsam G, Voice J, Kong Y, Goetzl EJ. Vasoactive intestinal peptide mediation of development and functions of T lymphocytes. *Ann NY Acad Sci* 2000;**921**:79–91.
53 Mayer DJ, Wolfle TL, Akil H, Carder B, Liebeskind JV. Analgesia from electrical stimulation in the brain stem of the rat. *Science* 1971;**174**:1351–4.
54 Grimm MC, Ben-Baruch A, Taub DD, *et al.* Opiates transdeactivate chemokine receptors: delta and mu opiate receptor-mediated heterologous desensitization. *J Exp Med* 1998;**188**:317–25.
55 Rogers TJ, Steele AD, Howard OMZ, Oppenheim JJ. Bidirectional heterologous desensitization of opioid and chemokine receptors. In: Conti A, Maestroni GJM, McCann SM, Sternberg EM, Lipton JM, Smith C, eds. *Neuroimmunomodulation Perspectives at the New Millennium*. New York: The New York Academy of Sciences, 2000.
56 Coussons-Reed ME, Dykstra LA, Lysle DT. Pavlovian conditioning of morphine-induced alterations of immune status: evidence for opioid receptor involvement. *J Neuroimmunol* 1994;**55**:135–42.
57 Mellon RD, Bayer BM. Role of central opioid receptor subtypes in morphine-induced alterations in peripheral lymphocyte activity. *Brain Res* 1998;**789**:56–67.
58 Mellon RD, Bayer BM. The effects of morphine, nicotine and epibatidine on lymphocyte activity and hypothalamic-pituitary-adrenal axis responses. *J Pharmacol Exp Ther* 1999; **288**:635–42.
59 Price DD, Soerensen LV. Endogenous opioid and non-opioid pathways as mediators of placebo analgesia. This volume, chapter 9.
60 Benedetti F, Amanzio M. The neurobiology of placebo analgesia: from endogenous opioid to cholecystokinin. *Prog Neurobiol* 1997;**52**:109–25.
61 Ulett GA, Han S, Han JS. Electroacupuncture: mechanisms and clinical application. *Biol Psychiatry* 1998;**44**:129–38.
62 Sluka KA, Deacon M, Stibal A, Strissel S, Terpstra A. Spinal blockade of opioid receptors prevents the analgesia produced by TENS in arthritic rats. *J Pharmacol Exp* 1999;**289**:840–6.
63 Iadarola MJ, Berman KF, Zeffiro TA, *et al.* Neural activation during acute capsaicin-evoked pain and allodynia assessed with PET. *Brain* 1998;**121**:931–47.
64 Lerner DM, Rosenstein DL. Neuroimaging in delirium and related conditions. *Semin Clin Neuropsychiatry* 2000;**5**:98–112.

# 9: Endogenous opioid and non-opioid pathways as mediators of placebo analgesia

DONALD D PRICE, LENE VASE SOERENSEN

## Introduction

Placebo effects have been explained by Pavlovian conditioning, cognition (for example, expectancy), personality, and social learning, alone or in combination, and these factors transduce meaning from the individual's cultural context. These psychosocial mechanisms evoke intervening psychophysiological events that involve multiple systems, including the autonomic nervous, endocrine, and immune systems, endorphin and motor pathways, and cardiovascular and gastrointestinal processes.

The transducing mechanism by which placebo interventions convert meaning into the modification of physiologic responses is not known. Indeed, no studies fully trace the pathways of cognition/expectancy, personality, social learning, and social psychological interactions to regulation of psychophysiological responses. Two mediating physiological processes that have been studied extensively are the immune system and the opioid and non-opioid mechanisms involved in placebo analgesia.

The purpose of this chapter is to provide a mechanistic foundation for explaining placebo analgesia. It is organized into two sections. The first section will briefly review the biological foundations of endogenous pain-inhibitory systems and the second section will provide some explanations of how endogenous pain-inhibitory circuitry is related to the psychological mechanisms of placebo analgesia. The interface between biological and psychological mechanisms will be a major focus of this chapter. The schematic of Figure 9.1 serves as a general guide.

An overarching theme of this chapter is that placebo analgesia involves multiple psychological factors and associated neural mechanisms, as implied by the number of points of synaptic interaction shown in Figure 9.1. Some of the same psychological factors, including conditioning, expectancy, meaning, and other cognitive factors are related to other types of placebo responses, including psychoactive, immunological, and cardiac responses. These factors are discussed within different contexts by other authors of this volume (Chapters 4, 5, 6 and 8).

## Biological foundations of endogenous pain-inhibitory systems

Considerable progress has been made in the past 35 years in identifying and characterizing neural circuitry that underlies the inhibition of pain. Many ascending pain related pathways terminate within cortical and subcortical structures that represent origins of pain modulatory pathways, structures such as hypothalamic nuclei, amygdala, and midbrain periaqueductal grey. Interestingly, these same brain structures are related to three currently active areas of psychology and neuroscience relevant to pain inhibition. These include learning and memory, threat-elicited defensive behavior, and pain modulation. For example, threat and modulation of pain are interrelated during the production of conditioned fear.[1–3] Furthermore, there is growing knowledge of the circuitry underlying each of these general phenomena. These three research areas relate in turn to questions about general neural mechanisms of pain inhibition. First, under what psychological and environmental circumstances do analgesic systems operate, that is, what triggers analgesic systems? Second, once triggered, what are the mechanisms by which the analgesic effect is produced? Third, what is the evidence that these psychological and physiological mechanisms of pain inhibition exist in humans?

### Animal studies of learning analgesia

Activation of analgesic mechanisms requires an extrinsic environmental cue or condition. For example, cues associated with past relief of pain may be visual (the pill or syringe), auditory (the nurse's voice), or pain itself (the prick of the needle associated with intravenous morphine). These cues may be effective for evoking endogenous analgesic mechanisms because they were present during previous effective treatments for pain or because they have symbolic meaning. For example, if the phrase "this is a powerful painkiller" accompanies an intravenous injection, analgesia may occur or be enhanced as a result of the meaning inherent in this phrase. The potential neurobiology of how symbolic meaning can elicit analgesia is much more problematical than that of simple forms of learning, such as classical conditioning. Nevertheless, animal models of learning analgesia are useful and have some applicability even to analgesia evoked by complex meanings (Animal models of conditioned responses have been explicated in Chapter 6).

Conditioned analgesic responses in animals can be robust and can be elicited in ways that have relevance to analgesia in humans, particularly placebo analgesia. The most extensively studied form of conditioned analgesia is that of fear-evoked defense responses. In studies of this phenomenon, rats are subjected to an inescapable noxious footshock leading to stress and analgesia.[1–5] The stress analgesia subsides, but when the rats are later returned to the apparatus in which the noxious stimulus was administered, the environmental context is sufficient to produce an analgesic effect. The inescapable footshock serves as the unconditioned stimulus and the environmental cues associated with the footshock serve as conditioned stimuli. Several trials of inescapable footshock result in a classically conditioned analgesia that can be evoked when rats are placed within the footshock apparatus. The analgesia associated with this kind of conditioning can be blocked by the opioid antagonist naloxone or by lesions of a specific neural circuit implicated in the production of defense behaviors in response to threat.[1] Watkins and Mayer[4] proposed this type of conditioned analgesia as a general model for placebo analgesia.

Specific central nervous system circuitry has been implicated in these forms of conditioned analgesia in animals. Hence, the extent to which these animal models of learned analgesia are applicable to psychologically mediated analgesia in humans is of theoretical importance in elucidating mechanisms of these forms of analgesia. The extent to which conditioning and fear/anxiety contribute to analgesia in humans is of particular interest because these factors are likely to contribute to placebo analgesia and analgesia due to threatening circumstances. This raises the question as to how such circuitry has a role in psychologically mediated analgesia.

## Endogenous pain-inhibitory systems: general considerations

It has become clear that information about tissue damage is not passively received by the nervous system. Rather, it is modulated even within the dorsal horn by complex inhibitory and facilitatory control systems. The discovery of these systems has fostered, and has in turn been fostered by, the notion that the central nervous system contains endogenous substances, endorphins, that possess analgesic properties. These concepts can be briefly examined by a consideration of opiate and non-opiate central nervous system pain modulatory mechanisms activated by environmental and psychological circumstances.

The first impetus for the detailed study of pain modulatory circuitry resulted from the observation that electrical stimulation of the periaqueductal grey region of the brain could powerfully suppress the perception of pain.[6,7] Further investigation of brain stimulation produced analgesia (SPA) provided considerable detail about the neural circuitry involved.[8] Significantly, at that time, several similarities were recognized between these observations and information emerging from a concomitant resurgence of interest in the mechanisms of opioid analgesia.[7] Two

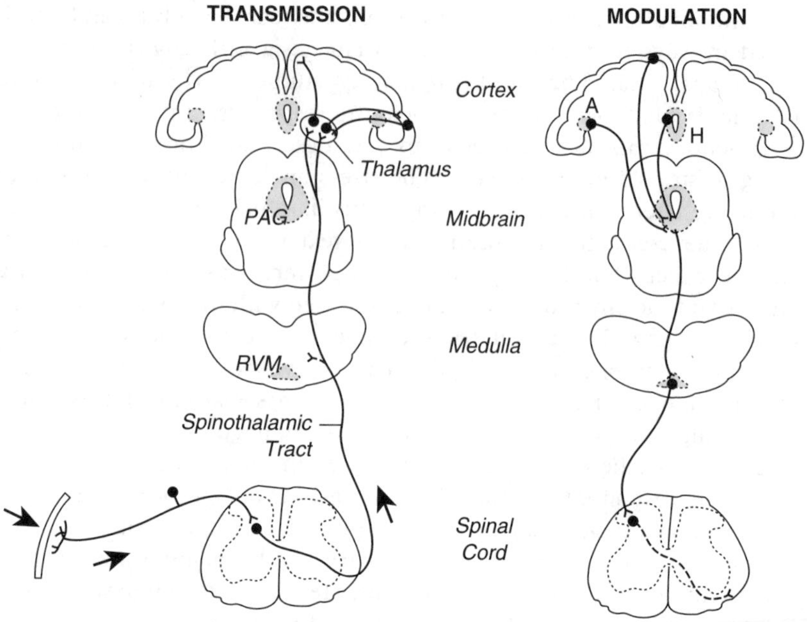


(From Fields and Price, 1997, Harvard University Press, with permission).

Figure 9.1 Transmission and modulation of pain transmission pathways. Note that the origin of pain modulatory pathways include the cerebral cortex, hypothalamus, amygdala, periaqueductal grey, and rostroventral medulla. Many of these structures are also central targets of ascending nociceptive pathways discussed in Chapter 5.

important parallel facts have resulted from these studies. First, effective loci for both opioid microinjection analgesia[9] and brain stimulation produced analgesia[7] reside within the periaqueductal and periventricular grey matter of the brain stem (Figure 9.1). Second, opioid analgesia and brain stimulation produced analgesia are both mediated in part by the activation of a centrifugal control system that descends from the brain and modulates pain transmission at the level of the dorsal horn (Figure 9.1).[7] Thus, the ultimate inhibition of the transmission of nociceptive information occurs, at least in part, at the initial processing stages in the dorsal horn by selective inhibition of nociceptive neurons.[10]

In addition, studies of brain stimulation produced analgesia provided direct evidence indicating that there are mechanisms extant in the central nervous system that depend upon endogenous opioids. Subanalgesic doses of morphine were shown to synergistically interact with subanalgesic levels of brain stimulation to produce behavioral analgesia.[11] Tolerance, a phenomenon invariably associated with repeated administration of opioids, was observed in response to the analgesic effects of brain stimulation and cross-tolerance was demonstrated between the analgesic effects of brain stimulation and systemic opioids.[12] Finally, brain stimulation produced analgesia could be at least partially antagonized by naloxone, a specific narcotic antagonist.[13,14] This last observation, in particular, could be most parsimoniously explained if electrical stimulation of the periaqueductal grey matter resulted in the release of an endogenous opioid-like factor. Indeed, naloxone antagonism of brain stimulation produced analgesia was a critical impetus leading to the eventual discovery of such a factor.[15] The identification of endogenous opioid mechanisms by naloxone antagonism has since been used in characterization of several types of analgesia, such as acupuncture analgesia, placebo analgesia, and stress analgesia.

Coincidental with work on brain stimulation analgesia, other discoveries of critical importance for our current concepts of endogenous analgesia systems were made. Several laboratories, almost simultaneously, reported the existence of stereospecific binding sites for opioids within the central nervous system.[16–18] Opiate receptor sites were subsequently shown to be localized to neuronal synaptic regions[19] and to overlap anatomically with loci involved in the neural processing of pain.[20] The existence of an opiate receptor again suggested the likelihood of an endogenous compound with opioid properties to occupy it. In 1975, Hughes[15] reported the isolation from neural tissue of a factor (enkephalin) with such properties. As with the opiate receptor, the anatomical distribution of endogenous opiate ligands shows overlap with sites involved in pain processing.[14]

Considerable data exist concerning the sites and mechanisms involved in the modulation of pain by the administration of exogenous opiates. Primarily, two lines of experimentation have been conducted. First, several areas in the central nervous system have been mapped and specific sites have been identified at which administration of opiates results in analgesia and the administration of opiate antagonists block analgesia. Second, brain locations wherein lesions block analgesic effects of exogenously administered opiates have been determined. Overall, these and other studies confirmed the importance of the periaqueductal region in opiate analgesia and provided an impetus for analysis of other brain areas (for example, amygdala[21]).

A brain area that has proved to be of considerable importance for opiate action is the anatomically complex region of the ventromedial medulla (Figure 9.1). This region consists of at least three distinct nuclei: the medially located nucleus raphe magnus (NRM), the more laterally situated nucleus reticularis paragigantocellularis (NRP), and the dorsolaterally located nucleus reticularis gigantocellularis (NRG). Microinjection of morphine into these brain areas results in analgesia, though some differences in sensitivity were found.[22–25]

A final region of critical importance is spinal cord dorsal horn (Figure 9.1). Relatively potent effects of intrathecal morphine microinjection have been consistently demonstrated.[26,27] This observation has had important clinical application since direct spinal cord application of opiates has been shown to have analgesic effects without the concomitant psychoactive effects observed with systemic administration.

Therefore, several general areas of the central nervous system are involved in opioid analgesia: the central nucleus of the amygdala, the periaqueductal-periventricular grey matter, the ventromedial medulla, and the spinal cord dorsal horn (Figure 9.1). The analgesic effects of a systemically administered opiate may produce analgesia by acting at any, all, or some combination of these distinct regions. The utilization of the microinjection of narcotic antagonists has provided at least partial answers to questions as to whether activation of each of these structures are necessary or sufficient for opioid analgesia.

This endogenous opioid analgesic system appears strategically organized in such a manner as to be activated by several types of external conditions, including both intense somatosensory stimulation and situations related to perceived threat or fear. Thus, the connections of this system, shown in Figure 9.1, demonstrate that the cerebral structures, the amygdala, the PAG and the hypothalamus all project to the RVM, which in turn projects to the spinal cord dorsal horn. The latter is an ultimate site of action of descending modulation of nociceptive transmission. At least some of these structures, including the amygdala, hypothalamus, and PAG, receive direct input from ascending pain related pathways. Thus, the circuitry for pain modulation is to some extent a feedback loop, in which stimuli that are likely to induce perceived fear or threat, such as painful stimuli, activate limbic, cortical, and subcortical structures involved in fear related defensive behaviors. The outputs of these structures converge on a common output region of the rostroventral medulla, that in turn projects to and modulates neurons of origin of central pain pathways.

## Output neurons of opiate descending modulatory systems

There now exists detailed knowledge of the neural mechanisms by which opioids act at the sites within the pain modulatory circuitry just described. Neurons at all of these levels are densely innervated by other neurons containing endogenous opioid peptides.[28,29] Furthermore, detailed knowledge exists of the neural mechanisms by which opioids act at some of these sites to produce analgesia.[30] To take just one of these sites, there are two distinct classes of pain modulating neurons in the RVM. One class is the *on cell* and it increases its impulse frequency just before withdrawal from a nociceptive stimulus. *On cells* are directly inhibited by endogenous opioids and they have a facilitatory influence on pain and withdrawal reflexes. The second class is the *off cell* and it decreases its impulse frequency just before withdrawal from a nociceptive stimulus. Although *off cells* are not directly affected by opioids, they are inhibited by *on cells*. Since opioids inhibit *on cells, off cells* increase their activity as a consequence of

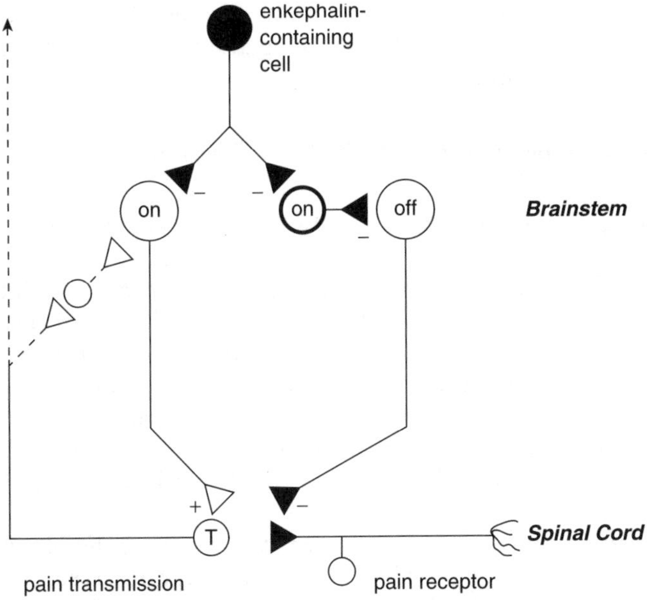


(From Fields and Price, 1997, Harvard University Press, with permission).

Figure 9.2 Opioid mediated pain modulating circuit.

opioid inhibition of *on cells*. In other words, *off cells* become disinhibited. Figure 9.2 illustrates this interaction.

The existence of *on cells* and *off cells* within the rostroventral medulla and elsewhere within the pain modulating system (for example, PAG) has important implications for how pain is modulated by various psychological conditions.[31] In the first place, the modulation of pain and pain behavior is bidirectional; pain can be enhanced or inhibited by these descending controls. Just as there exist local mechanisms within the dorsal horn that serve to produce hyperalgesia and allodynia as well as anti-nociception, so also there exist descending controls that serve to produce and enhance or inhibit these same phenomena. Pain sensitivity can be enhanced under certain psychological conditions and there even exists the possibility that pain can be generated in the complete absence of a peripheral nociceptive signal – a "virtual" pain. In the second place, the somewhat phasic nature of *on cell* and *off cell* responses suggests that the descending control of ascending nociceptive information may be more dynamic and dependent on moment-by-moment contingencies than previously acknowledged. For example, as will be discussed, placebo responses can be specifically located to one area of the body and can be quickly initiated and terminated, features that would be consistent with a phasic control system. Other types of descending controls may be more tonically active, such as when analgesia is produced by environmental stress or by prolonged somatosensory stimulation. It is possible that more tonic forms of analgesia may be activated by central modulatory neurons other than *off cells*, such as serotonergic "neutral" cells of the ventral medulla or by a combination of "neutral" and "off cells".

## Endogenous analgesia systems: evidence from animal research

The demonstration that opiates activate well-defined neural systems capable of potently blocking pain transmission suggests, but by no means proves, that the function of this system is to dynamically modulate the perceived intensity of noxious stimuli. If, in fact, this system has such a physiological role, then one might expect that the level of activity within the system would increase during various psychological circumstances. If such circumstances could be identified that produce analgesia, it would give credibility to the idea that invasive procedures, such as brain stimulation or narcotic drugs, inhibit pain by mimicking the natural activity within these pathways.

Hayes *et al.*[32,33] initiated the first systematic search for the physiological conditions that activate pain inhibitory systems. They observed that potent analgesia could be produced by such diverse stimuli as brief footshock, centrifugal rotation, and injection of intraperitoneal saline. Subsequent research from several laboratories has catalogued numerous types of external conditions that evoke analgesia in animals.[8] An important concept has emerged from these experiments. The opiate antagonist, naloxone, blocks some but not other forms of externally induced analgesia.[33] Therefore, it appears that non-opiate systems must exist in addition to the system activated by opiates described earlier.

Of interest is that some forms of analgesia produced by aversive conditions can be classically conditioned. For example, repeated pairings of cues associated with footshock, such as placement of the rat in the chamber where shocks have been applied, result in a condition wherein the cues alone are sufficient to evoke analgesia.[4] This conditioning activates an opioid analgesia system since conditioned analgesia is eliminated by systemic and intrathecal naloxone, morphine tolerance, and lesions of descending pathways of the endogenous pain modulatory circuit.[34] In addition, as would be expected, higher structures are involved in the conditioned analgesia since it is eliminated by decerebration and reduced by lesions of the (PAG).[4]

At the level of the spinal cord dorsal horn, complex neurotransmitter or neuromodulator mechanisms are also involved in these forms of learned analgesia. For example, cholecystokinin (CCK) appears to modulate endogenous opioid systems. Intrathecal application of CCK antagonizes analgesia from application of exogenous opiates as well as analgesia elicited by activation of endogenous opiates.[35,36] Also, CCK antagonists applied intrathecally potentiate pain relief as well as reverse opiate tolerance.[36] These findings suggest that other transmitters and/or modulators may interact with opiates to form complex circuits. These complex circuits relate, in turn, to the complexity of psychological factors that regulate pain and analgesia. For example, stimuli that signal safety to rats reduce the analgesic effects of morphine.[37] Furthermore, this anti-opiate effect occurs because the safety signal leads to the release of CCK in the spinal cord. As will be discussed, a similar CCK neuromodulatory mechanism may be involved in placebo analgesia in humans.

In sum, a review of the animal data provides strong evidence for the existence of endogenous pain modulatory circuitry and for at least some of the circumstances under which this circuitry is activated. These circumstances are largely those involving environmental threats or aversive stimulation, including pain itself. Knowledge of this circuitry and the conditions under which it is activated has clear and important implications for understanding general principles of pain inhibition in humans.

## Evidence for endogenous analgesia mechanisms in humans

It is very difficult to directly determine whether pain modulatory circuitry similar to that characterized in animal experiments exists in humans. Nevertheless, there are several independent, albeit indirect, lines of evidence supporting the likelihood that a similar pain modulatory system exists in humans. First, the brainstem-to-spinal-cord circuitry implicated in endogenous opioid analgesia is highly conserved in a variety of mammalian species, including marsupials, rodents, carnivores, and primates.[31] Importantly, the locations and extent of neurotransmitters, including opioid peptides, in this circuitry appears to be similar in a number of species, including humans.[38,39] The homogeneity of pain modulatory circuitry across this diversity of species leaves little doubt that such circuitry is present in humans. Second, opioid drugs that significantly reduce clinical pain are effective in inhibiting a variety of measures of nociceptive processing in other animal species, including nociceptive reflexes, more integrated escape behaviors, and nociceptive afferent neuron responses to painful stimuli.[30] In these animal species, analgesic effects of opioids are exerted in part through actions upon the neural circuitry that mediates learned analgesia.

In addition to these indirect lines of evidence, there exists a body of literature that relates to more direct determinations of endogenous opioid pain modulatory circuitry in humans. At this point, parallels can be drawn between the work described above and experimental and clinical studies in humans. These parallels are important because they highlight the potential relevance of this work to the very difficult problem of treating human pain syndromes. Throughout this discussion, it will be important to bear in mind that a number of distinct modulatory systems have been identified under controlled laboratory conditions. In the more naturalistic circumstances of clinical research, it is likely that more than one of these systems may be active at any given time, which may account for the variability and controversy in the clinical literature.

There are at least two situations available for study in which endogenous pain modulatory systems may be active in humans. The first involves the basal, tonic activity within these systems and allows the experimenter to assess whether pain inhibition occurs continuously, at least to some degree. The second involves clinical manipulations that attempt to activate pain inhibitory systems.

*Evidence for tonic pain modulatory mechanisms*

Attempts have been made to determine whether pain modulatory systems are tonically active. Studies of experimental pain that have used naloxone to infer the existence of a tonically active pain inhibitory system have found little support that it is tonically active.[40–42] On the other hand, naloxone appears to be more consistently effective in humans who are experiencing some level of clinical pain. In this regard, such results are consistent with the animal studies described above in which pain was observed to be an activator of endogenous analgesia systems. Thus, Levine *et al.*[43] and Gracely *et al.*[44] report that naloxone can increase the reported intensity of postoperative pain. In conclusion, endogenous opiate pain inhibitory systems seem to have little spontaneous activity under normal circumstances. However, when some level of pain is present for a critical amount of time, these systems seem to be activated.

*Conditions that may trigger endogenous analgesia mechanisms in humans*

Research on the involvement of endogenous opioids in pain modulation also has examined a number of environmental manipulations known to reduce clinical or experimental pain. This research has utilized two primary experimental strategies. The first is that of antagonizing or reversing the analgesia by a narcotic antagonist, usually naloxone. The rationale for this strategy is the same as that described above for animal experiments. The second strategy reasons that if endogenous opioids are involved in these forms of analgesia, then changes should be observed in the levels of these compounds in plasma or the central nervous system. The rationale for both types of tests is that if there exists physiological and psychological conditions under which endogenous opioids reduce pain, the resultant analgesia should be antagonized by naloxone and accompanied by measurable increases in levels of released endogenous opioids. In particular, the release of endogenous opioid peptides should be detectable during those conditions that activate endogenous pain inhibitory circuitry.

*Brain stimulation produced analgesia in humans*

As early as 1973, Richardson and Akil[45] reported the use of periventricular grey (PVG) stimulation to treat pain syndromes. Over 20 reports in the literature describe various studies of this technique that were published between 1973 and 1983[46] and the number of studies has greatly diminished since then. Evidence for analgesic effects was obtained in most studies, thereby corroborating animal studies of stimulation produced analgesia (SPA).[47] However, the numerous published studies indicate that the efficacy of this procedure is highly variable and the vast majority of clinical studies have poor outcome measures. Nevertheless, the studies are useful in providing some evidence that a central neural substrate of endogenous pain inhibitory mechanisms exists in humans and that it is generally similar to that of other mammalian species.

Several lines of evidence indicate a likely but not unequivocal role for endogenous opiates in SPA in humans. Opiate antagonists are reported to reduce SPA,[48,49] tolerance develops to SPA,[50] and dependence upon SPA has been reported.[49] Although somewhat controversial, there is evidence that endogenous opioids, primarily β endorphin, are released by electrical stimulation of the periaqueductal grey matter in pain patients.[45] At this point, it seems likely that endogenous opioids mediate, at least in part, the analgesia elicited by periaqueductal or periventricular grey stimulation in humans. The particular endogenous opioid and its site and mechanism of action have not been established.

*Counterirritation analgesia in man*

The observation that an acute painful stimulus can be used to alleviate ongoing pain has been known since antiquity and is known as counterirritation. Counterirritation has characteristics in common with acupuncture and some forms of transcutaneous electrical nerve stimulation or TENS. All use the application of somatic stimuli, either noxious or innocuous, to obtain relief from pain and pain relief often persists beyond the period of treatment when the treatment itself is intense or painful.

The large majority of studies that have attempted to reverse acupuncture analgesia by naloxone have shown partial to complete reversal, consistent with an endogenous opioid mechanism.[51] Similar reversals have been obtained for high intensity low frequency (acupuncture-like) transcutaneous electrical nerve stimulation (TENS) but not high frequency, low intensity TENS.[51] These results are strikingly consistent with reports in the animal literature. Overall, these studies show that acupuncture and TENS activate both opiate and non-opiate systems depending on different parameters of stimulation. The variable clinical outcomes observed following these treatments probably result from differential recruitment of segmental, extrasegmental, opiate, and non-opiate pain inhibitory systems, all of which are now known to be activated by these types of stimulation in animals.

Considering the diversity of stimulation conditions that result in the modulation of pain in humans, a generally convincing picture of mechanisms of pain modulation in humans emerges. The same types of somatosensory stimuli that result in analgesia in several mammalian species also reduce pain in humans and many of these stimuli activate endogenous opioid systems. Many important questions about the nature of this involvement remain unanswered. The most important of these are the particular endogenous opiate involved and its site of action. Answers to such questions are unlikely to come from human studies alone since invasive procedures are probably necessary to acquire such information. The consistency of the animal and human studies, however, suggests that such questions may be studied with animal models and verified in humans.

This section has presented a brief overview of the evidence for endogenous pain inhibitory circuitry that is activated in all mammals under a variety of physiological and psychological circumstances. This endogenous pain modulatory system utilizes opioid peptides at several levels of the neuraxis. There are good reasons to conclude that exogenous opioids activate this system at all of these levels to result in the inhibition of pain. However, for present purposes, the most important aspect of research on endogenous pain inhibitory systems is that pertaining to the demonstration of such a system in human beings and the development of strategies for identifying the psychological and physiological conditions under which this system operates. In the next section, several types of experiments will be discussed whereby the general psychological and neural mechanisms of placebo analgesia can be characterized to some degree. An important consequence of this approach is that it can be shown that placebo analgesia must depend on different general neural mechanisms. This is appropriate because they likely depend on different psychological mechanisms as well.

## Factors that co-determine the magnitude of placebo analgesic effects

In this section, we briefly consider the potential roles of classical conditioning, expectancy, desire for relief, anxiety, and distortions in memory as factors that may mediate placebo analgesia. Extensive explanations of these same factors are provided in Chapters 5 and 6 of this book.

### Classical conditioning

In accordance with animal research, modern studies of human placebo analgesia takes its point of departure within a classical conditioning paradigm. A landmark study of patients clearly showed that prior treatments with effective analgesic drugs enhance the analgesic effectiveness of a subsequent placebo.[52] In this study, a second medication, always placebo, followed graded doses of propoxyphene HCL (three dose levels), propoxyphene napsylate (three doses), or placebo. Thus, there were seven groups of patients with fourteen to twenty patients in each group. Their results showed convincing evidence of a "dose-response relationship" between the dose of the first medication and the analgesic response to the subsequent placebo, though the magnitudes of placebo effects were lower than their corresponding doses of the active drug. Placebo given as a second treatment was more effective as an analgesic when it followed a more potent analgesic, whereas placebo following a placebo continued to have the same slight analgesic effect as the first placebo administration. Their results support learning as a major factor in placebo analgesia. However, their results do not distinguish the contributions of conditioning versus expectation in producing placebo analgesia.

Voudouris *et al.*[53,54] provided the first experimental laboratory paradigm of human conditioned analgesia and showed that it is possible to condition placebo analgesia. They used the following subtle experimental design. Subjects were exposed to electric shock, with and without a placebo cream that was introduced as an effective analgesic. The shocks were given under three sessions: pretest, manipulation-test, and post-test. During the manipulation-test, the painful stimulus was decreased in intensity while the placebo cream was on but without the subject's knowledge. The result was that the placebo cream was connected with significant pain relief during the third as compared to the first session, although the painful stimulus intensities during the two sessions were exactly the same. The fact that the subjects obtained an experience of pain relieving effects of the cream disposed them to have a placebo response. According to Voudouris *et al.*[53,54] such a placebo effect is the result of conditioning. However, since there is no discrimination between conditioning and expectancy in the study it is not possible to deduce whether it is the conditioning or the resultant expectancy of pain relief that mediates the placebo effect.

Using a similar but better controlled experimental design, Voudouris *et al.*[55] studied the relative contribution of conditioning and verbally induced expectancy within placebo analgesia. Conditioning and expectancy were induced as follows. The conditioning group received neutral information about the placebo cream and obtained a positive experience of the placebo cream, as in their previous study. The expectancy group received only positive verbal information about the placebo cream. A placebo analgesic effect was obtained in the conditioning group but not in the expectancy group. At first glance, these results seem to support the conditioning hypothesis as opposed to the expectancy hypothesis. However, the subjects were only questioned about their expectancies *before* the conditioning manipulation, so there is no information of how the conditioning manipulation influenced their level of expectancy. Therefore, expectancy may still be the actual mediator of the observed placebo effect. Furthermore, the measurement of expectancy was overly simplistic. Voudouris *et al.*[55] did not measure expectancy in a detailed way since it was only one item on a questionnaire. Hence, it could not be compared directly with the actual pain ratings. Acknowledging some of these flaws, Voudouris *et al.*[55] conclude that the possibility that expectancy contributes to placebo analgesia cannot be excluded. However, they suggest that the concrete experience of reduced pain during conditioning trials may be more effective than verbal attempts to induce expectation of pain reduction, at least under their conditions. In the studies of Voudouris *et al.*[53–55] only pain intensity and not pain unpleasantness was measured even though the experience of pain consists of both dimensions. Therefore their studies do not address the question of whether placebo administration differentially influences the two dimensions of pain.

## Expectancy

Classical conditioning and expectancy do not have to be mutually exclusive. The stimulus substitution model can be extended to include cognitive elements[56] whereby the two approaches become complementary. According to this interpretation, what is obtained during conditioning is not an automatic association between the cream and the pain relief; it is an expectation that the cream will be followed by analgesia. Adopting this approach, Kirsch[57,58] introduced the concept of "response expectancies", denoting the circumstance that specific expectations cause specific responses. Response expectancies do not only emerge from conditioning, they may emerge from any sources of information such as observations of others and reading.

Montgomery and Kirsch[59] tested this interpretation of expectancy and conditioning by means of an experimental design that matched that of Voudouris and his colleagues[53–55] yet separately evaluated the relative contribution of conditioning and expectancy to placebo analgesia. The experimental design was improved by measuring expectancy both before and after the conditioning manipulation. Furthermore, expectancy was measured on a visual analogue scale from 0–10 by asking the subjects to estimate how much pain they expected to experience with or without the placebo cream. Conditioning and expectancy were induced as follows. The subjects in both groups obtained positive information about the placebo cream and both groups experienced reduction of pain stimuli during conditioning trials in which stimulus strength was reduced without the subjects' knowledge. The reduced stimulus intensities were given after application of placebo cream. However, the subjects in the expectancy group were told that the stimulus intensity was being reduced just prior to the conditioning trials, whereas subjects in the conditioning group were not told about the reduction (similar to the Voudouris *et al.* study[55]). A placebo analgesic effect occurred only in the latter group. The experiment showed that conditioning may cause a placebo effect only as long as the subjects do not know about the pain manipulation. Classical conditioning is not influenced by cognitive activity according to the stimulus substitution model and hence Montgomery and Kirsch[59] conclude that results of their study support the theory of response expectancies. As expectancy was measured both before and after the expectancy manipulation, it was possible to control for expectancy. Thus, it appeared that conditioning did not result in a placebo effect if expectancy was controlled for. Therefore, Montgomery and Kirsch[59] further conclude that even if conditioning may result in a placebo effect, it is mediated only by expectancy.

## Desire for pain relief

Desire for pain relief is an obvious possible mediator of placebo analgesia because of the well known influence of motivation on perception.[60] Placebo effects occur in clinical contexts wherein patients not only expect pain reduction but also have a strong need or desire for relief. Unfortunately, there have been very few explicit attempts to assess this factor in studies of placebo effects. A role of desire for relief is indirectly supported by the fact that placebo effects are larger in those experimental pain studies wherein threatening circumstances are present.[61]

Since this factor is not sufficiently addressed in studies of placebo, Price *et al.*[62] evaluated the potential influence of desire for pain relief in an experiment designed in a manner similar to that of Voudouris *et al.*[53–55] and Montgomery and Kirsch.[59] The experimental design was improved by measurement of both pain intensity and pain unpleasantness. The desire for the treatment to have a pain relieving effect was successfully increased in one group by giving them the prospects of receiving a large number of painful stimuli and decreased in a second group by telling them that only a few stimuli would be presented. Contrary to what was hypothesized, however, ratings of desire for pain relief were not significantly associated with the magnitudes of placebo analgesia.

Although this result casts some doubt on the possible contribution of desire for pain relief on placebo analgesia, there are reasons that the hypothesis should not be completely dismissed at this point. First, nearly all participants of the study had some degree of desire for pain relief as determined by their ratings of this factor. Second, desire for pain relief may be much more of a critical factor in placebo effects during clinical pain. Therefore, this factor needs to be assessed in clinical pain studies. Third, a study by Jensen and Karoly[63] showed that desire and motivation contribute to the placebo effect. Although the study was not about pain relief, they explicitly assessed the contribution of a desire for symptom change in a study of placebo manipulations suggesting possible sedative or stimulant effects. Jensen and Karoly[63] assessed separate contributions of *motivation* and *expectancy* to placebo responses. According to them, *motivation* referred to "the degree to which subjects desire to experience a symptom change" and *expectancy* was considered the subjects' expectation of symptom change. They manipulated both of these factors by separate instructions and then later checked (by subject self-ratings) to determine whether either or both factors had been influenced. They found that motivation accounted for a significant amount of variance in placebo responses that included perceived sedation in the case of placebo tranquilizers or perceived arousal in the case of placebo stimulants.

## Anxiety

Expectancy and desire are likely to interact in different ways under different circumstances whereby they give rise to a range of emotional states such as anxiety. Anxiety reflects a desire to avoid negative consequences coupled with an uncertain expectation of avoiding those consequences.[60,64,65] None of the studies discussed thus far have included explicit measures of anxiety, and therefore the possibility that anxiety partly mediates placebo analgesia cannot be ruled out. Unfortunately only a few studies have examined the contribution of anxiety to placebo analgesia and they present conflicting results. Some studies have found that levels of anxiety were related to the placebo effect[66,67] while other studies have not been able to prove such a relation.[68] Only one study has shown that placebo analgesia is primarily associated with a selective reduction in pain unpleasantness as opposed to pain intensity.[69]

It seems possible that anxiety may influence analgesia by two very different mechanisms whereby either reduced or enhanced levels of anxiety may be mediators of placebo analgesia. A reduction in anxiety may result from the very framing of the situation. If the patient is led to expect that the placebo will make the pain less distressing but not less intense, it is likely to result in an anti-anxiety effect in the form of a reduction in pain unpleasantness as opposed to pain intensity.[70] Alternatively, since high levels of anxiety may be accompanied by stress, it is also possible that highly enhanced levels of anxiety may lead to stress-induced analgesia, a possibility that is consistent with the animal literature discussed above and with evidence for stress induced analgesia in humans.[71] Thus, it is possible that different types of placebo effects can result from increased or decreased anxiety depending on the ways placebo situations/suggestions are framed and on the level of stress associated with the anxiety. Therefore, the potential mediation of placebo analgesia by either increases or decreases in anxiety needs to be explored further. This can be done by studies that separately and reliably measure pain sensation intensity, pain unpleasantness, and anxiety.

However, it is unlikely that anxiety mediates all placebo analgesic effects. A study by Montgomery and Kirsch[72] demonstrates that placebo analgesia can be induced on a specific area of the body, such as the index finger. This rules out the possibility that placebo effects consist of nothing more than a reduction in anxiety or some other global mechanism that would affect the entire body. Instead, this result supports the idea that highly specific response expectancies mediate placebo analgesia.

## Release of endogenous opioids

The question of how the above mentioned psychological factors influence the opioid system has yet to be answered. However, recent studies by Benedetti and his colleagues[73,74] have started to explore this subject. Benedetti *et al.* have corroborated the finding that placebo analgesia can be mediated by endogenous opioids in humans[75–79] and they have extended this area of research by examining the relation between psychological factors and the endogenous opioid system. Amanzio and Benedetti[73] investigated whether conditioning and expectancy are related to an endogenous opioid mediated placebo effect. The experiment employed a tourniquet pain procedure and used measures of pain tolerance. Conditioning was achieved by repeated injections of either morphine or the non-opioid ketorolac. Another experimental condition included open injections of saline combined with the instruction that the injected substance was a potent analgesic, an instruction that was presumed to have produced expectations of pain reduction. The study showed that placebo analgesia obtained by the verbally induced expectancy was reversed completely by naloxone whereas placebo analgesia obtained by conditioning was reversed by naloxone, only if the conditioning had been carried out with the opioid substance, morphine. Interestingly, conditioning with the non-opioid drug, ketorolac, produced an analgesic effect that was *not* naloxone reversible.

Benedetti *et al.*[74] followed up this elegant study with one that, inspired by Montgomery and Kirsch,[72] tested the hypothesis that placebo analgesia develops as a result of a highly specific response expectancy and is mediated by endogenous opioid mechanisms. In this study, pain was produced simultaneously in four limbs by intradermal capsaicin injections and placebo cream was applied to only one of the four sites. Placebo analgesia developed only in the site that was treated, and this specific placebo effect was completely antagonized by naloxone. These results are consistent with the theory of highly specific placebo effects and they indicate that somatotopic representation may be the link between expectancy on one hand and the opioid system on the other. However, a distinct limitation to the studies by Benedetti and his colleagues[73,74] is that the subjects were never asked about their level of expectancy. It was simply assumed that the expectancy manipulation had the intended effect of producing an expectation of pain reduction. Furthermore only the dimension of pain sensation intensity was measured.

A study by Price *et al.*[62] corroborated and extended both the results of Montgomery and Kirsch[59,72] and Benedetti *et al.*[74] They applied two "strengths" of placebo creams, A (strong placebo) and B (weak placebo) as well as a control agent (C) to three adjacent areas on the forearms. Similar to the study of Montgomery and Kirsch,[59] they conditioned participants by combining these treatments with varying degrees of surreptitious lowering of intensities of painful skin temperature stimuli. Thus, in comparison to the pretreatment baseline condition, participants presumably experienced no reduction, a small reduction, and a large reduction in areas C, B, and A respectively. When stimulus strength was then raised back to equal levels in all three areas and subjects were again tested, the assessed placebo effects were graded in proportion to the extent to which stimulus strength had been secretly lowered during manipulation trials. Since these three areas were immediately adjacent, the results provide even further evidence for somatotopic specificity of the placebo effect than had been demonstrated by Montgomery and Kirsch[72] and Benedetti *et al.*[74] Second, these effects were strongly associated with participants' *expected* levels of pain within each area, expectations that were assessed just prior to trials for which placebo effects were assessed. The combination of these results demonstrates that expectations directed toward highly specific body locations can mediate placebo analgesia under at least some circumstances. Under clinical circumstances, specific expectations of patients can also be potently influenced by the expectations of the clinicians that treat them.[80]

Therefore, under at least some conditions, placebo analgesia depends on highly specific response expectancies and opioid mechanisms. However, one must keep in mind that an opioid mechanism is highly unlikely to be a common mechanism for all placebo phenomena (for example, immunological and cardiac responses) or even for all types of placebo analgesia.

## Memory distortion

Not all placebo analgesic effects relate as easily to interactions between psychological and biological factors. The same study by Price *et al.*[62] demonstrates that the method used to assess pain relief also contributes to the magnitude of placebo analgesia. Placebo analgesic effects were assessed both concurrently with placebo trials as well as several minutes after all pain trials had terminated. Placebo effects were modest when assessed concurrently with placebo trials, 0·5 to 1·3 visual analogue scale (VAS) unit differences on a 10 unit scale. However, when the same participants rated pain and pain reduction based on *remembered* pain intensities, placebo effects were three to four times larger than those assessed *during* placebo trials, 2·0 to 4·3 visual analogue scale unit differences. The main reason for these differences was that participants remembered the untreated pain as being much more intense and unpleasant than it actually was. Finally, participants' ratings of remembered pain intensities were similar to ratings of expected pain levels prior to placebo trials and were strongly associated with them ($r = 0{\cdot}5–0{\cdot}6$). Expectations and memory distortions mediate large placebo effects based on retrospective ratings of pain or pain relief. Large placebo effects based on memory distortion may not demonstrate potent anti-nociceptive effects but rather potent psychological influences.

The selective exaggeration of remembered pain intensity and the consequent enhancement of apparent placebo analgesia are consistent with a previous study showing that memory distortion of pretreatment pain contributes to an exaggeration of self reports of pain relief.[81] They found that pain relief scores based on memory were over three times higher than those based on pretreatment minus present pain VAS ratings, consistent with the results of Price *et al.*'s study.[62]

Patients' reports of relief following treatment are often used to establish the effectiveness of treatments.[81] To the extent that such measures are used in clinical studies of pain treatments, estimates of magnitudes of analgesic effects from both placebo and active treatments are likely to be significantly enhanced with retrospective reports. One has to openly wonder about the extent to which commonly quoted magnitudes of placebo analgesia[82–84] as well as reported magnitudes of analgesia from active treatments were based on retrospective judgments of pain relief.

## Future directions

To be able to present evidence that placebo analgesic effects constitute more than mere bias or changes resulting from patients' compliance, it is essential to examine how psychological factors interact with biological factors in placebo analgesia. A better understanding of this interaction may have theoretical and empirical, as well as clinical implications. At a theoretical level, it may contribute to an interdisciplinary comprehension of placebo effects that will make it possible to study different biological, psychological and cultural aspects of placebo effects within the same framework. At an empirical level, it may lead to more advanced ways of measuring and controlling for placebo effects that will improve the scientific evaluation of pain treatments in general. Finally at an applied level, an expanded understanding of how psychological manipulations of placebo administration bring about biological changes is likely to illuminate some of the factors that are generally effective in pain relieving treatments. These factors could be utilized to facilitate the efficacy of analgesic treatments. In order to reach a more refined understanding of the interaction between the psychological and the biological factors in placebo effects, it is important to clarify some of the possible biological and psychological mechanisms in placebo analgesia.

Placebo analgesia clearly depends on different psychological and neurological processes and psychological factors interact with biological mechanisms to give rise to both opioid and non-opioid mediated placebo analgesic effects. Therefore, it seems plausible that multiple types of placebo analgesic effects can be produced depending on the ways placebo suggestions and circumstances are framed. Thus, it may be that expectancy and release of opioids mainly characterize some forms of placebo effects, while anxiety reduction or memory distortion characterizes others.

Investigations of interactions between psychological and biological factors are in the early stages. Until now, the main strategy for examining whether placebo analgesia is opioid mediated has consisted of antagonizing the analgesic effects with a narcotic antagonist, such as naloxone, or measuring plasma or CSF levels of opioid peptides. The test of naloxone reversibility is a powerful and feasible approach to determining involvement of endogenous opioid systems. Naloxone is fairly specific for opiate receptors and is subjectively undetectable when given on a double blind basis. However, a major limitation to this approach is that one cannot determine the exact central nervous system sites at which these opioid-related mechanisms take place. Several recent technologies and experimental approaches have been developed whereby neural mechanisms of analgesia can be studied more directly in human participants. These include functional imaging methods such as positron emission tomography or functional MRI and measures of spinal nociceptive reflexes. For example, the R-III is a spinally mediated withdrawal reflex that can be non-invasively measured in human volunteers and it correlates well with reported pain intensity. Inhibition of this spinal reflex during placebo analgesia would support the hypothesis that a brainstem-to-spinal pathway was involved in the mechanism of this type of analgesia. One or several of these measurements can be interfaced with valid measures of expectancy and desire for pain relief, as well as with reliable measurement of pain intensity and pain unpleasantness. Such an approach would make it possible to simultaneously examine how the placebo analgesic effect is expressed at different levels. For example, one could determine whether nociceptive spinal reflexes, pain sensation intensity, and pain unpleasantness are reduced simultaneously. If so, then placebo administration leads to a reduction in the pain signal at early stages of processing and reflects an anti-nociceptive effect. This approach has been shown to be useful in hypnotic analgesia studies.[85]

Advancement in measurement of placebo analgesia will not only contribute to a more refined understanding of the mechanisms in placebo analgesia, but it is also likely to contribute to a more precise determination of the magnitude of placebo analgesia. A strategy can be developed whereby it is possible to assess most or all of the relevant mediating factors that contribute to placebo effects. This strategy is based on two considerations. The first is that expectancy and desire for pain relief could be measured and integrated within the designs of analgesic studies. If, as shown by several studies of experimental pain, one or both of these parameters can account for most of the variance in placebo effects, then they could be incorporated into clinical analgesia studies. Their measurement could provide an important adjunct or substitute means of assessing the contribution of placebo effects. The inclusion of measures of expectation and desire in analgesic studies would allow assessments of the "blindness" of studies. After all, if pain patients of double blind analgesia studies cannot subjectively distinguish active from placebo treatments, then their levels of expectation and desire for relief should be the same across both types of treatment. Alternatively, if they can subjectively distinguish the two treatments, it would be very important to understand the contribution of desire for relief and expectation to pain relief.

A second consideration would be that of designing the pain measurements in a manner that takes into account the confounding influences of memory distortion and natural history in assessment of the placebo effect. Thus, it would be far better to assess analgesia concurrently rather than retrospectively and it would be important to take into consideration the natural history of the pain to be analyzed.

The possibility of a refined analysis of placebo effects within studies has far reaching scientific and medical implications.[60,86] Our present limited capacity to ascertain, measure, and control for placebo effects is at the heart of complex and difficult questions about pharmacological therapies for pain as well as many non-pharmacological therapies, particularly those related to surgery, hypnosis, electrical stimulation, and "alternative medical treatments".

## References


1 Helmstetter FJ, Tershner SA. Lesions of the periacqueductal gray and rostroventral medulla disrupt antinociceptive but not cardiovascular aversive conditional responses. *J Neurosci* 1994;**14**:7099–108.

2 Fanselow MS. Shock-induced analgesia on the formalin test: effects of shock severity, naloxone, hypophysectomy, and associative variables. *Behav Neurosci* 1984;**98**:79–95.

3 Fanselow MS. The midbrain periacqueductal gray as a coordinator of action in response to fear and anxiety. In: Depaulis A, Bandler R, eds. *The Midbrain Periacqueductal Gray Matter*. New York: Plenum Press, 1991:151–73.

4 Watkins LR, Mayer DJ. Involvement of spinal opioid systems in footshock-induced analgesia: antagonism by naloxone is possible only before induction of analgesia. *Brain Res* 1982;**242**:309–16.

5 Watkins LR, Young EG, Kinscheck IB, Mayer DJ. The neural basis of footshock analgesia: The role of specific ventral medullary nuclei. *Brain Res* 1983;**276**:305–15.

6 Reynolds DV. Surgery in the rat during electrical analgesia induced by focal brain stimulation. *Science* 1969;**164**:444–5.

7 Mayer DJ, Wolfle TL, Akil H, Carder B, Liebeskind JV. Analgesia from electrical stimulation in the brainstem of the rat. *Science* 1971;**174**:1351–4.

8 Mayer DJ, Manning BH. The role of opioid peptides in environmentally-induced analgesia. In: Tseng LF, ed. *The Pharmacology of Opioid Peptides*. Chur, Switzerland: Harwood, 1995:345–95.

9 Tsou K, Jang CS. Studies on the site of analgesic action of morphine by intracerebral micro-injection. *Sci Sinica* 1964;**13**:1099–109.

10 Satoh M, Takagi H. Effect of morphine on the pre- and postsynaptic inhibitions in the spinal cord. *Eur J Pharmacol* 1971;**14**:150–4.

11 Samanin R, Valzelli L. Increase of morphine-induced analgesia by stimulation of the nucleus raphe dorsalis comment. *Eur J Pharmacol* 1971;**16**:298–302.

12 Mayer DJ, Hayes R. Stimulation-produced analgesia: development of tolerance and cross tolerance to morphine. *Science* 1975;**188**:941–3.

13 Akil H, Mayer DJ, Liebeskind J. Comparaison chez le rat entre l'analgesie induite par stimulation de la substance grise periaqueducale et l'analgesie morphinique. *C R Acad Sci* 1972;**274**:3603–5.

14 Akil H, Madden J, Patrick RL, *et al.* Stress-induced increase in endogenous opiate peptides: Concurrent analgesia and its partial reversal by naloxone. In: Kosterlitz HW, ed. *Opiates and Endogenous Opioid Peptides*. Amsterdam: Elsevier, 1976:63–73.

15 Hughes J. Search for the endogenous ligand of the opiate receptor. *Neurosci Res Prog Bull* 1975;**13**:55–8.

16 Hiller JM, Pearson J, Simon EJ. Distribution of stereospecific binding of the potent narcotic analgesic etorphine in the human brain: predominance in the limbic system. *Res Commun Chem Pathol Pharmacol* 1973;**6**:1052–62.

17 Pert CB, Snyder SH. Opiate receptor: demonstration in nervous tissue. *Science* 1973;**179**:1011–13.

18 Terenius L. Stereospecific interaction between narcotic analgesics and a synaptic plasma membrane fraction of rat cerebral cortex. *Acta Pharmacol Toxicol* 1973;**32**:317–20.

19 Pert CB, Snowman AM, Snyder SH. Localization of opiate receptor binding in synaptic membranes of rat brain. *Brain Res* 1974;**70**:184–8.

20 Pert CB, Kuhar MJ, Snyder SH. Autoradiographic localization of the opiate receptor in rat brain. *Life Sci* 1975;**16**:1849–54.

21 Manning BH, Mayer DJ. The central nucleus of the amygdala contributes to the production of morphine antinociception in the rat tail-flick test. *J Neurosci* 1995;**15**:8199–213.

22 Takagi H, Doi T, Akaike A. Microinjection of morphine into the medial part of the bulbar reticular formation in rabbit and rat: inhibitory effects on lamina V cells of spinal dorsal horn and behavioral analgesia. In: Kosterlitz HW, ed. *Opiates and Endogenous Opioid Peptides*. Amsterdam: Elsevier, 1976:191–200.

23 Takagi H. The nucleus reticularis paragigantocellularis as a site of analgesic action of morphine and enkephalin. *Trends Pharmacol Sci* 1980;**1**:182–4.

24 Azami J, Llewelyn MB, Roberts MHT. The contribution of nucleus reticularis paragigantocellularis and nucleus raphe magnus to the analgesia produced by systemically administered morphine, investigated with the microinjection technique. *Pain* 1982;**12**:229–46.

25 Zorman G, Belcher G, Adams JE, Fields HL. Lumbar intrathecal naloxone blocks analgesia produced by microstimulation of the ventromedial medulla in the rat. *Brain Res* 1982;**236**:77–89.

26 Oley N, Cordova C, Kelly ML, Bronzino JD. Morphine administration to the region of the solitary tract nucleus produces analgesia in rats. *Brain Res* 1982;**236**:511–15.

27 Yaksh TL, Rudy TA. Chronic catheterization of the spinal subarachnoid space. *Physiol Behav* 1976;**17**:1031–6.

28 Delfs JM, Kong A, Mestak Y, *et al.* Expression of mu opioid receptor mRNA in rat brain: An in situ hybridization study at the single cell level. *J Comp Neurol* 1994;**345**:46–8.

29 Atweh SF, Kuhar MJ. Autoradiographic localization of opiate receptors in the rat brain. II. The brain stem. *Brain Res* 1977;**129**:1–12.

30 Fields HL, Heinricher MM, Mason P. Neurotransmitters in nociceptive modulatory circuits. *Ann Rev Neurosci* 1991;**14**:219–45.

31 Fields HL, Price DD. Toward a neurobiology of placebo analgesia. In: Harrington A, ed. *The placebo effect: an interdisciplinary exploration*. Cambridge, Massachusetts: Harvard University Press, 1997:93–115.

32 Hayes RL, Bennett GJ, Newlon PG, Mayer DJ. Behavioral and physiological studies on non-narcotic analgesia in the rat elicited by certain environmental stimuli. *Brain Res* 1978;**155**:69–90.

33 Hayes RL, Price DD, Bennett GJ, Wilcox GJ, Mayer DJ. Differential effects of spinal cord lesions on narcotic and non-narcotic suppression of nociceptive reflexes: further evidence for the physiologic multiplicity of pain modulation. *Brain Res* 1978;**155**:91–101.

34 Watkins LR, Cobelli DA, Mayer DJ. Opiate vs non-opiate footshock induced analgesia (FSIA): descending and intraspinal components. *Brain Res* 1982;**245**:97–106.

35 Faris PL, Komisaruk BR, Watkins LR, Mayer DJ. Evidence for the neuropeptide cholecystokinin as an antagonist of opiate analgesia. *Science* 1983;**219**:310–12.

36 Watkins LR, Kinscheck IB, Mayer DJ. Potentiation of opiate analgesia and apparent reversal of morphine tolerance by proglumide. *Science* 1984;**224**:395–6.

37 Wiertelak EP, Maier SF, Watkins LR. Cholecystokinin antianalgesia: safety cues abolish morphine analgesia. *Science* 1992;**256**:830–3.

38 Emson PC, Corder SJ, Ratter S, *et al.* Regional distribution of proopiomelanocortin-derived peptides in the human brain. *Neuroendocrinology* 1984;**38**:45–50.

39 Pittius CW, Seizenger BR, Pasi A, Mehraein P, Herz A. Distribution and characterization of opioid peptides derived from proenkephalin A in human and rat central nervous system. *Brain Res* 1984;**304**:127–36.

40 Grevert P, Baizman ER, Goldstein A. Naloxone effects on a nociceptive response of hypophysectomized and adrenalectomized mice. *Life Sci* 1978;**23**:723–8.

41 El-Sobky A, Dostrovsky JO, Wall PD. Lack of effect of naloxone on pain perception in humans. *Nature* 1976;**263**:783–4.

42 Buchsbaum MS, Davis GC, Bunney WEJ. Naloxone alters pain perception and somatosensory evoked potentials in normal subjects. *Nature* 1977;**270**:620–1.

43 Levine JD, Gordon NC, Bornstein JC, Fields HL. Role of pain in placebo analgesia. *Proc Natl Acad Sci USA* 1979;**76**:3528–31.

44 Gracely RH, Dubner R, Wolskee PJ, Deeter WR. Placebo and naloxone can alter post-surgical pain by separate mechanisms. *Nature* 1983;**306**:264.

45 Richardson DE, Akil H. Pain reduction by electrical brain stimulation in man. Part I: Acute administration in periaqueductal and periventricular sites. *J Neurosurg* 1973;**47**:78–183.

46 Young RF, Feldman RA, Kroening R, *et al.* Electrical stimulation of the brain in the treatment of chronic pain in man. In: Liebeskind JC, Kruger L, eds. *Advances in Pain Research and Therapy: Neural Mechanisms of Pain.* New York: Raven Press, 1984:289.

47 Duncan GH, Bushnell MC, Marchand S. Deep brain stimulation: a review of basic research and clinical studies. *Pain* 1991;**45**:49–59.

48 Adams JE. Naloxone reversal of analgesia produced by brain stimulation in the human. *Pain* 1976;**2**:161–6.

49 Hosobuchi Y, Adams JE, Linchitz R. Pain relief by electrical stimulation of the central gray matter in humans and its reversal by naloxone. *Science* 1977;**196**:183–6.

50 Hosobuchi Y. Tryptophan reversal of tolerance to analgesia induced by grey stimulation. *Lancet* 1978;**2**:47.

51 Price DD, Mayer DJ. Evidence for endogenous opiate analgesic mechanisms triggered by somatosensory stimulation (including acupuncture) in humans. *Pain Forum* 1995;**4**:40–3.

52 Laska E, Sunshine A. Anticipation of analgesia: a placebo effect. *Headache* 1973;**1**:1–11.

53 Voudouris NJ, Peck CL, Coleman G. Conditioned placebo responses. *J Per Soc Psychol* 1985;**48**:47–53.

54 Voudouris NJ, Peck CL, Coleman G. Conditioned response models of placebo phenomena: further support. *Pain* 1989;**38**:109–16.

55 Voudouris NJ, Peck CL, Coleman G. The role of conditioning and expectancy in the placebo response. *Pain* 1990;**43**:121–8.

56 Rescorla RA. Pavlovian conditioning: It's not what you think it is. *Am Psychologist* 1988;**43**:151–60.

57 Kirsch I. Response expectancy as a determinant of experience and behavior. *Am Psychologist* 1985;**40**:1189–202.

58 Kirsch I. *Changing expectations: a key to effective psychotherapy*. Pacific Grove, CA: Brooks/Cole, 1990.

59 Montgomery GH, Kirsch I. Classical conditioning and the placebo effect. *Pain* 1997;**72**:107–13.

60 Price DD, Fields HL. The contribution of desire and expectation to placebo analgesia: implications for new research strategies. In: Harrington A, ed. *The placebo effect: an interdisciplinary exploration*. Cambridge, Massachusetts: Harvard University Press, 1997:117–37.

61 Jospe M. *The Placebo Effect in Healing*. Lexington, Mass: Lexington Books, 1978.

62 Price DD, Milling LS, Kirsch I, Duff A, Montgomery GH, Nicholls SS. An analysis of factors that contribute to the magnitude of placebo analgesia in an experimental paradigm. *Pain* 1999;**83**:147–56.

63 Jensen MP, Karoly P. Motivation and expectancy factors in symptom perception: a laboratory study of the placebo effect. *Psychosom Med* 1991;**53**:144–52.

64 Price DD, Barrell JJ. Some general laws of human emotion: interrelationships between intensities of desire, expectation, and emotional feelings. *J Pers* 1984;**52**: 389–409.

65 Price DD, Barrell JE, Barrell JJ. A quantitative-experiential analysis of human emotions. *Motivation and Emotions* 1985;**9**:19–38.

66 Gryll ST, Katahn M. Situational factors contributing to the placebo effect. *Psychopharmacology* 1978;**57**:253–61.

67 Evans FJ. Expectancy, therapeutic instructions, and the placebo response. In: White L, Tursky B, Schwartz GE, eds. *Placebo: Theory, Research and Mechanisms*. New York: The Guilford Press, 1985.

68 Hashish I, Hai HK, Harvey W, Feinmann C, Harris M. Reduction of postoperative pain and swelling by ultrasound treatment: a placebo effect. *Pain* 1988;**33**:303–11.

69 Gracely RH. Psychophysical assessment of human pain. In: Bonica JJ, Liebeskind JC, Albe–Fessard DG, eds. *Advances in Pain Research and Therapy Vol. 3*. New York: Raven Press, 1979.
70 Price DD, Barrell JJ. Mechanisms of analgesia produced by hypnosis and placebo suggestions. *Prog Brain Res* 2000;**122**:255–71.
71 Pitman RK, van der Kolk BA, Orr SP, Greenberg MS. Naloxone-reversible analgesic response to combat-related stimuli in post-traumatic stress disorder. A pilot study. *Arch Gen Psychiatry* 1990;**47**:541–4.
72 Montgomery GH, Kirsch I. Mechanisms of placebo pain reduction: an empirical investigation. *Psychol Sci* 1996;**7**:174–6.
73 Amanzio M, Benedetti F. Neuropharmacological dissection of placebo analgesia: expectation-activated opioid systems versus conditioning-activated specific subsystems. *J Neurosci* 1999;**19**:484–94.
74 Benedetti F, Arduino C, Amanzio M. Somatotopic activation of opioid systems by target-directed expectations of analgesia. *J Neurosci* 1999;**19**:3639–48.
75 Levine JD, Gordon NC, Fields HL. The mechanism of placebo analgesia. *Lancet* 1978;**ii**:654–7.
76 Grevert P, Albert LH, Goldstein A. Partial antagonism of placebo analgesia by naloxone. *Pain* 1983;**16**:129–43.
77 Levine JD, Gordon NC. Influence of the method of drug administration on analgesic response. *Nature* 1984;**312**:755–6.
78 Benedetti F, Amanzio M, Giuliano M. Potentiation of placebo analgesia by proglumide. *Lancet* 1995;**346**:1231.
79 Benedetti F. The opposite effects of the opiate antagonist naloxone and the cholecystokinin antagonist prolumide on placebo analgesia. *Pain* 1996;**64**:535–43.
80 Gracely RH, Dubner R, Deeter WD, Wolskee PJ. Clinicians expectations influence placebo analgesia. *Lancet* 1985;**1**:43.
81 Feine JS, Lavigne GJ, Dao TT, Morin C, Lund JP. Memories of chronic pain and perceptions of relief. *Pain* 1998;**77**:137–41.
82 Beecher HK. The powerful placebo. *JAMA* 1955;**159**:1602–6.
83 Beecher HK. *Measurement of Subjective Responses: Quantitative Effects of Drugs*. New York: Oxford University Press, 1959.
84 Turner JA, Deyo RA, Loeser JD, von Korff M, Fordyce WE. The importance of placebo effects in pain treatment and research. *JAMA* 1994;**271**:1609–14.
85 Kirnan BD, Dane JR, Philips LH, Price DD. Hypnotic analgesia reduces R-III nociceptive reflex: further evidence concerning the multifactorial nature of hypnotic analgesia. *Pain* 1995;**60**:39–47.
86 Wall PD. The placebo and the placebo response. In: Wall PD, Melzack R, eds. *Textbook of Pain*. New York: Churchill Livingstone, 1994.

# *Section 4:*
# Use of placebo groups in clinical trials – methodological and ethical issues

# 10: Placebo controlled trials and active controlled trials: ethics and inference

ROBERT J TEMPLE

## Summary

The use of a placebo group in clinical trials raises two issues, one ethical, the other inferential. The ethical question is when, if ever, a placebo group can be used in a trial when there is known effective available therapy. The other is whether, and when, an active control equivalence or non-inferiority study can be used, instead of a placebo controlled or other superiority trial, to document effectiveness. Although some, supported by a recent revision of the *Declaration of Helsinki*, argue that placebo controls should never be used in the face of an existing effective agent, others, supported by a recent international guideline, say that acceptability of placebo depends on the consequence to the patient of not receiving the known therapy. A placebo cannot be used if doing so would harm the patient (for example, by increasing risk of death or irreversible injury). In contrast, informed, autonomous patients can agree to be in a trial in which they could receive placebo instead of a symptomatic treatment. The inferential issue is important because an active control equivalence trial is a valid way to demonstrate effectiveness only if a trial can be shown to have "assay sensitivity", i.e. the ability to distinguish effective from less effective treatments. Unfortunately, for many effective treatments, a significant proportion of apparently well designed studies fail to distinguish drug from placebo, so that assay sensitivity cannot be assumed and an active control equivalence trial cannot demonstrate effectiveness.

## Introduction

There are two distinct but related aspects of the use of a placebo group in a clinical trial. First, there is the ethical question: when, if ever, is it ethically acceptable to use a placebo group in a clinical trial when there is existing effective, available therapy for the condition being studied? My answer is that this depends entirely on the consequences to the well informed subject of the trial of omitting or delaying the effective treatment. Second, there is the inferential question: when can an active control trial, the usual alternative to a placebo controlled trial, in which the goal is to show similarity (or lack of a difference of a certain size) of a new drug to a known active control, provide reliable evidence that a new drug is effective? Active control trials in which the goal is to show *superiority* of the new drug to the active control, like trials that show superiority to placebo or a lower dose of the drug – all *difference-showing trials* – do not raise an inferential question. Success in such trials, that is, superiority to the control, constitutes clear evidence of effectiveness. Trials in which the goal is not to show superiority but to *show* lack of a difference, however, have a less straightforward interpretation. Such trials must be known to have *assay sensitivity*, the ability to distinguish between effective and ineffective treatments, if they are to provide reliable evidence about the effectiveness of the new drug.

The need for assay sensitivity is widely recognized and is inherent in the logic of an equivalence/non-inferiority trial.[1,2] The only real issues are how to:

- support the assumption of assay sensitivity when it is not directly measured in the absence of a placebo
- choose an appropriate non-inferiority margin (how much less effective than the control the new drug can be and still be considered to have a positive effect)
- analyze the data to determine whether an effect of the new drug has been shown.

Unfortunately, in many situations, active control trials cannot be known to have assay sensitivity and are therefore uninformative about the effectiveness of the test treatment. These questions have recently been considered at length in two published papers and an international guidance document.[2,3,4]

## Ethical issues: the *Declaration of Helsinki*

A recent change in the *Declaration of Helsinki* forcefully raises the ethical issue. The new Declaration seems to be far less ambiguous than the previous version in asserting that when there is an effective existing therapy, a placebo cannot be used under any circumstances. The history of the Declaration, and its interpretation, are pertinent here.

### The 1975 Declaration and its meaning

In 1975 the following sentence was added to the Declaration: "In any medical study, every patient – including those of a control group, if any – should be assured of the best proven diagnostic and therapeutic method."[5] The question is, what did this mean? Some, like Rothman and Michels,[6] have argued that the Declaration's meaning was straightforward and that the Declaration must be read literally: no placebo controlled trial can be carried out when there is an existing effective therapy, no matter what condition was being treated. Thus, there could be no placebo controlled trials in baldness (as there is available minoxidil and finasteride), in allergic rhinitis (there is loratadine and fexofenadine), in headache (ibuprofen, aspirin), in constipation or diarrhea, in heartburn, in insomnia, in anxiety, etc.

It is clear that the medical community, regulators, and ethicists have not been reading the Declaration this way, and thousands of placebo controlled trials in symptomatic conditions have been conducted, published, and utilized in evaluating new drugs. Why was the Declaration not read as Rothman and Michels insisted it should be? There were probably three reasons.

- The literal words of the Declaration, which made no specific reference to placebos, would bar *all* trials when there was existing therapy, as people given the new drug would not be receiving the "best proven … therapeutic method". Surely the framers could not have meant to bar all trials of new agents when there was an existing treatment. It was easy to conclude the Declaration did not intend to bar placebo controlled trials either.
- In describing the history of its revisions in 1985, the World Medical Association gave as its reason for the 1975 change the intent to reinforce the idea that the physician-patient relationship "must be respected just as it would be in a purely therapeutic situation". The issue of placebo controlled trials was not even mentioned, which seemed to undermine the idea that the added words were meant to bar placebo controls.[7]
- Even ethical statements, which always involve judgment, need to display logic and consistency.[8] It simply does not make sense to assert that it is unethical to *invite* a fully informed person to participate in a placebo controlled study in which a symptomatic treatment will be deferred or omitted if no harm (perhaps including excessive discomfort) is involved. There is no impact on the patient's underlying health in such studies and patients are always free to leave a trial without penalty and receive standard treatment. The trial is easily explained; that is, it is easy to make it very clear that the usual therapy will not be given and that some patients will be randomly assigned to a placebo. (Whether this is always properly done is an important, but different, question.) There thus should be no confusion between patient care and the experiment being conducted – the so-called therapeutic misconception. (That misconception actually seems a far greater problem in a setting of serious illness.)

For these reasons it was widely believed that the Declaration did not in fact mean what Rothman and Michels said it did; certainly, as noted, investigators, regulators, institutional review boards (IRBs) and journals behaved as if that were the case.

## The 2000 revision of the Declaration

If the 1975 Declaration was ambiguous, a change made in October 2000[9] seemed to remove all doubt and place the World Medical Association squarely in the Rothman and Michels camp. Indeed, Rothman and Michels had, just a few months earlier, called for precisely the change that was made.[10] In the 2000 revision, the following section was added: "The benefits, risks, burdens, and effectiveness of a new method should be tested against those of the best current prophylactic, diagnostic, and therapeutic methods. This does not exclude the use of placebo, or no treatment, in studies where no proven prophylactic, diagnostic, or therapeutic method exists". Although the first sentence could be read as a statement of scientific preference (study what is important), the second sentence conveys the idea that if there *is* proven treatment it must be the only comparator.

## The role of the patient and autonomy

The new Declaration seems unambiguous, yet it still fails to provide a clear ethical argument for its newly revised principle. It fails to explain *why* an informed and uncoerced patient cannot make, in entering a placebo controlled trial, the kind of decision to forgo symptomatic therapy that patients make every day, deciding *not* to treat headache, dental pain, anxiety, social phobia, obsessive compulsive disease, depression, seasonal allergies, benign prostatic hypertrophy, erectile dysfunction, baldness, etc. Rothman and Michels do address this issue, at least to some extent, and clearly believe that, even with properly informed consent, patients should not be allowed to make such decisions in the context of a clinical trial.[6,10] The reasons they give will be considered below. On its face, however, their view seems to be at odds with the fundamental requirement for, and assumption of, autonomy in participants in clinical studies. Indeed, if patients are not able, and cannot be trusted, to make the decision to defer symptomatic treatment of a condition they are usually very familiar with, they are no better prepared, ethically, to participate in an active control trial (giving up assured standard therapy in favor of a less tested new agent); in fact, when such trials involve serious illness, where lack of equal effectiveness of the test drug could be medically important, they might be considered less prepared to do so.

Rothman and Michels, and the framers of the 2000 Declaration, by simply barring all trials when there is available effective therapy, do not need to consider how one might distinguish situations in which a placebo control could be acceptable from those in which it would not be. If we do not accept such an absolute bar to use of placebos, a different ethical principle is needed, one that takes into account the potential adverse consequences of avoiding or delaying use of a standard effective treatment.

## ICH-E10 – choice of control group and related issues

Recently, the International Conference on Harmonization, in a guidance document on choice of control group in clinical trials, concluded the following, distinguishing between available therapy that prevents serious harm and available therapy that treats symptoms:

> In cases where an *available* treatment is known to prevent serious harm, such as death or irreversible morbidity in the study population, it is generally inappropriate to use a placebo control.
>
> In other situations, where there is no serious harm, it is generally considered ethical to ask patients to participate in a placebo controlled trial, even if they may experience discomfort as a result, provided the setting is non-coercive, and patients are fully informed about available therapies and the consequences of delaying treatment … Whether a particular placebo controlled trial of a new agent will be acceptable to subjects and investigators when there is known effective therapy is a matter of patient, investigator, and IRB judgement, and acceptability may differ among ICH regions. Acceptability could depend on the specific trial design and population chosen.

This position is based on the idea that the ethics of a placebo controlled trial depend on the consequences of non-treatment. Thus, it is plainly not acceptable to conduct new placebo controlled trials of new thrombolytics, long-term antihypertensive treatment, or new angiotensin-converting enzyme inhibitors in patients with impaired ventricular function and heart failure, because these available therapies are life-saving. The ICH statement also recognizes that all parties to the trial will inevitably also consider other "practical" matters, such as how much discomfort they are willing to accept/allow (always assuming an informed patient). Thus, although it may be ethical to invite a patient to participate in a trial in which he will be uncomfortable, even very uncomfortable, IRBs, investigators, and, of course, patients, may not want to participate. Whether they do could depend on many factors, such as:

- the design of the trial. Building in an "early escape" mechanism,[11] for example, so that only a single episode of symptoms, or attainment of a particular level of symptom, even briefly, would be experienced by a patient, may make a trial acceptable when a planned several week observation period might not be
- the importance of the new therapy. Patients, investigators, and IRBs could consider whether the value of a possible new treatment was "worth" the discomfort.

It has been suggested that, beyond a certain point, patient discomfort should be considered harm and placebo controlled trials unacceptable.[12] An example cited on several occasions is placebo controlled trials of anti-emetics in patients receiving emetogenic chemotherapy.[12] But this example is confounded as it is argued both that the placebo control was unethical because it caused too much discomfort and available therapy would have prevented this harm, and also that the placebo control was unnecessary because active control comparisons would have been valid.[12] If the latter is correct, there would usually be no need for a placebo control here (except perhaps where it was important to examine the effectiveness of lower, less effective, doses to mitigate toxicity). The ethical question arises principally when an equivalence or non-inferiority study using the active control cannot be informative. Suppose the effect of current anti-nausea therapy, while real, was not so satisfactory and large, and that a placebo controlled trial was needed to evaluate a new agent. Would it then be unreasonable and unethical to use a placebo control design, perhaps one where patients in the trial were treated with an active drug after a single vomiting or severe nausea episode? In fact, in situations less emetogenic than the first day of highly emetogenic chemotherapy, such as postsurgical settings, current therapy is not so easily distinguished from placebo, with about a third of studies failing to do so.[13] A recent study used, and needed, a placebo control group to study the effect of ondansetron and dexamethasone on the second day of moderately emetogenic chemotherapy in patients who tolerated the first day well.[14]

While the principle set forth in E-10 is reasonably straightforward, there will be cases in which it is not clear whether patients given placebo might be harmed, even if the available therapy does not have a well-documented effect on mortality or irreversible morbidity. Some of these situations have been discussed recently.[3]

In a recent publication, Rothman and Michels give three reasons for disagreeing with the approach taken in the E-10 guidance and for believing the Declaration should bar, absolutely, the use of a placebo control when there is existing therapy, and for not agreeing that placebo controls can be used when informed patients agree to defer symptomatic treatments.

- The position puts scientific arguments, "right or wrong", before ethical concerns, demanding placebo controls even where effective treatment is available and equipoise is impossible.
- Quoting Nicholson in the January 2000 Hastings Center Report of an international workshop, this approach "also puts the interests of society before the interest of the research subject, which is prohibited by the Declaration, and the physician fails in his duty to do his best for the patient".
- Researchers "should be given zero latitude *to decide* how much additional risk or discomfort a patient should endure" (emphasis added). "This sharp boundary would protect society from rogue

investigators … No investigator or regulatory official has the right to decide how much sacrifice in terms of risk or discomfort a patient should endure in the name of science".

- "Informed consent is not enough" because the rest of the Declaration still applies.

None of these arguments is sound or persuasive. First, the view that patients can volunteer to delay symptomatic treatment does not place scientific arguments over ethical concerns because it is based on the view that it is not unethical to ask a fully informed patient to volunteer to delay such treatment; if this is true, there is then no competition between science and ethics. If one were to argue that patients could be denied available life-saving treatment to establish some useful scientific point, that position would, in contrast, represent placing science ahead of ethics; but no one is proposing such a position.

Second, the societal interest is not placed above the patient's interest. The patient, in agreeing to participate, is *expressing* his or her interest, and whether participation is based on the hope of finding new drugs for the patient's condition, altruism, enjoyment of clinical trial participation, or some other reason, that participation represents the declared, independently reached, interest of the patient.

Third, researchers never *decide* on the risk or discomfort a patient should endure – the patient decides whether the risk and discomfort are acceptable. The entire clinical trial enterprise depends on appreciation of, and belief in, patients' ability to understand their interests and to make an informed, independent decision about participation. This belief in informed autonomy is critical to any trial, placebo controlled or not.

Reference to the "rogue investigator" suggests another, perhaps more critical, reason for Rothman and Michel's absoluteness – fear of a "slippery slope". Slippery slope arguments, while perhaps understandable, substitute rigid, not necessarily sensible, dicta for reasoned judgment; they can be seriously misleading, as they require arguing for a ban on *all* when the real objection is to *some*.

An apparent modification of the absolute bar to placebo controls[6] has been suggested by Rothman[10] previously and at this conference, namely, that a distinction should be made between patients with a condition or illness who come to a physician for treatment and "healthy volunteers" who agree, *while well*, to participate in a placebo controlled trial of, for example, their next headache. The full basis for and nature of this distinction is not made clear. For example, would a patient with a chronic condition such as osteoarthritis or hypertension, not currently seeking new treatment from the doctor, but still not well, be a "healthy volunteer" for this purpose? In fact, studies of many, perhaps most, symptomatic treatments do enrol subjects while "well", so that many placebo controlled trials could be acceptable under this modification. It does, however, seem to be a distinction without a real difference. What is critical is that the *treatment* of patients be plainly distinguished from the *study* of patients. Although this is perhaps easier when the invitation to participate is by internet, it does not seem unduly difficult even when initiated in the presence of a patient, so long as the role of the physician is made clear.

An interesting question, perhaps, is whether it would be helpful to think more generally of people with symptoms or signs treated only briefly, even if the illness is long term, as "normal volunteers" with a characteristic of interest (angina, mild hypertension, erectile dysfunction) who are not being "treated" by the study any more than volunteers in a phase 1 study are treated. The symptomatic treatment of osteoarthritis or erectile dysfunction for a month, or a short-term study of response to a new antihypertensive or lipid-lowering drug, after which long-term treatment must be resumed or initiated (that is the actual treatment) should probably be distinguished from outcome studies in which the long-term treatment itself is under study or short-term studies of serious illnesses where outcome is critical (for example, sepsis). Here one is in fact delivering patient care, or at least potential patient care, and available effective treatment cannot be denied.

## Usefulness of active control trials in assessing effectiveness: the problem of assay sensitivity

### Fundamental difference between difference-showing (superiority) and non-inferiority trials

The ethics of placebo controlled trials would not be a critical issue if active control equivalence or non-inferiority trials could regularly be used to demonstrate the effectiveness of new treatments.[1,2,3] The problem is that in many situations such trials, even if successful in showing equivalence or non-inferiority of a new treatment to a control, do not demonstrate effectiveness of the test drug. Trials that seek to show a difference between treatments (superiority of a test drug to a placebo, a lower dose of test drug, or an active drug) have inferential properties that are fundamentally different from trials in which the goal is to show a lack of difference, or, in practice, lack of difference greater than a specified size. There are two principal problems.

- In the equivalence trial, there is a critical, but untested (in the trial) assumption, namely, that the trial could have distinguished between an effective and an ineffective treatment. This ability to distinguish treatments is called "assay sensitivity". Because assay sensitivity is not measured in the trial (unless superiority to a treatment is shown or there is an additional placebo group to serve as an "internal standard"), its presence must be deduced from historical experience and analysis of the present trial.
- The goal of showing no difference between treatments creates a lack of incentives to assure study excellence.

## Assay sensitivity

There are two distinct ways to show that a new treatment is effective. One is to show that it is better than some other treatment. This directly proves that the new treatment is effective so long as the control treatment is not harmful. The second is to show that the new treatment is just as good as, that is, equivalent to, or not significantly worse than, a treatment known to be effective. Then the known effectiveness of the control treatment is attributed to the new, indistinguishable treatment. The naïve equivalence study of the past simply compared two treatments, found no significant difference between them, and declared the "equivalence" and the effectiveness of the new treatment. This approach is now recognized as inadequate because too small a study, with a large variance, will not allow even a sizable difference to be detected and will always lead to "success". The remedy for the variance problem is the non-inferiority study.[15] This design specifies as a null hypothesis that the new drug (T) is inferior to the control (C) by at least some amount, the non-inferiority margin (M):

$$\text{Ho is } C - T \geq M$$
$$\text{Ha is } C - T < M$$

Where Ho is the null hypothesis and Ha is the alternative hypothesis.

If a degree of inferiority of M or greater is ruled out (that is, if the upper bound of the 95% confidence interval for $C - T$ is $< M$), the new treatment is declared non-inferior to the control. But non-inferiority does not necessarily demonstrate effectiveness. The choice of M is obviously critical. In order to assure that a finding of non-inferiority demonstrates some degree of effectiveness, M can be no larger than the entire effect the active control can reliably be expected to have in the study *compared to a placebo*. In that case, as long as $C - T$ is smaller than M, the study would show that the test drug has at least some (greater than zero) effect. If M is larger than the effect of the control drug in that study, then ruling out a difference greater than M would not demonstrate any effect at all. The non-inferiority design solves the problem of the naïve equivalence trial. If the study is simply too small, the 95% confidence interval of $C - T$ will be wide and its upper bound will exceed M, so that the inferiority hypothesis (Ho) will not be rejected. The study will thus not, on the basis of small size alone, wrongly declare non-inferiority. This design does not, however, solve the assay sensitivity problem.

Any non-inferiority study raises the question: did the active control have an effect of at least the size expected (M) in the trial that was carried out? That is, did *this* trial have assay sensitivity, the ability to show a difference of a specified size (M) between treatments if such a difference exists? Put yet another way, if the test agent had an effect equal to a placebo, would the upper bound for the difference $C - T$ have exceeded M? If the trial could not have detected a difference of at least M (the entire effect of the control) then even the most powerful demonstration of non-inferiority would be meaningless, as the study would lack the ability to distinguish ineffective from effective test treatments. As will be explained below, unless the trial also has a placebo arm, one must rely on information external to the trial to conclude that the trial, as designed and conducted, could have distinguished between active drugs and placebo.

Superiority studies also need assay sensitivity to be fully informative, of course, but superiority studies and non-inferiority studies lacking the ability to distinguish effective from ineffective treatments yield importantly different conclusions, albeit both erroneous ones. A placebo controlled (superiority) trial of an effective drug with assay sensitivity will document the effectiveness of the drug by rejecting the null hypothesis of no effect. The demonstration of superiority also documents the assay sensitivity of the trial. If the study lacks assay sensitivity, it will incorrectly show no effect of the drug, an error that could cost us effective therapy, but not one that could put an ineffective treatment into the world. In contrast, an active control trial of an ineffective drug, if the trial lacks assay sensitivity, could demonstrate non-inferiority successfully and support the erroneous conclusion that the drug is effective, potentially leading to the marketing of an ineffective agent. To summarize:

Superiority = efficacy
Non-inferiority ≠ efficacy
(unless assay sensitivity is present)

It might seem curious that there could be doubts about the ability of a well designed clinical trial to distinguish between active and inactive drugs. In fact, many apparently excellent and adequately sized trials of symptomatic and other treatments fail to distinguish known effective drugs from placebo. The reasons for this are not usually apparent in particular cases, but presumably involve the study population (its ability to respond to the treatment) and many aspects of study quality (see below); it is also clear that assay sensitivity is a problem in settings in which drug effect size is modest and the response in a placebo group is relatively large compared to drug effect size. This problem has long been recognized. Writing in 1979, Lasagna[16] pointed out that:

> … a comparison between new drug and standard … is convincing only when the new remedy is superior to standard treatment. If it is inferior, or even indistinguishable from a standard remedy, the results are not readily interpretable. In the absence of placebo controls, one does not know if the 'inferior' new medicine has any effect at all, and 'equivalent' performance may reflect simply a patient population that cannot distinguish between two active treatments that differ considerably from one another, or between active drug and placebo. Certain clinical conditions, such as serious depressive states, are notoriously difficult to evaluate because of the delay in drug effects and the high rate of spontaneous improvement, and even known remedies are not readily distinguished from placebo in control trials.

## Establishing assay sensitivity

As assay sensitivity is not measured in a non-inferiority trial, its presence must be deduced (unless there is a third placebo arm to provide an internal standard and allow direct assessment of the presence of assay sensitivity, a very useful study design). Establishment of assay sensitivity has four components.

- Establishment of "historical evidence of sensitivity to drug effects", an abstract conclusion (not related to the current trial), generally based on past placebo controlled trials of the control drug (and perhaps closely related drugs), that in a setting like the present study, appropriately designed, sized, and conducted trials reliably show an effect of a particular size on a specified endpoint.
- Designing a new active control trial that is very similar (population, entry criteria, concomitant therapy, endpoints, run-in periods) to the trials for which historical evidence of sensitivity to drug effects has been established. Changes in these design features can undermine the historical conclusion and change, or even eliminate, the effect of the control and thus the appropriate non-inferiority margin.
- From historical experience, and considering the possibility of changes in practice that may affect the effect size of the control, choosing an appropriate non-inferiority margin, that margin being no larger than the effect the control can be reliably presumed to have had in the study. Note that a smaller margin than one representing the entire effect of the control can be chosen if, on clinical grounds, it were considered important to retain a particular fraction of the control agent's effect. Pocock suggests[1] that one would usually want the margin to be much smaller than the active control's superiority margin over placebo, but although a reasonable desire, this will often prove impractical. Experience with thrombolytics, where the effect of the control agents was well established, showed that attempting to assure preservation of even 50% of the survival effect of the control, the level of assurance FDA in the end asked for, led to sample sizes of over 15 000 patients for a drug that was actually of equal effectiveness. Similarly, the margin cannot be chosen to exclude a "clinically meaningful difference" if that difference is larger than the assured effect of the control in the study.
- Conducting the study in such a way that the assay sensitivity is not undermined by poor quality, such as poor compliance or excessive concomitant therapy. (See below, *Incentives toward study quality in active control trials*, and Pocock.[1])

As the statement by Lasagna indicates, there are many settings in which historical evidence of sensitivity to drug effects cannot be established (Box 10.1). The difficulties associated with depression trials have been well discussed. Leber[2,17] examined all six three-arm studies comparing nomifensine, imipramine, and placebo. The trials varied in size from

**Box 10.1 Settings in which historical evidence of sensitivity to drug effects is not established**

Depression
Anxiety
Dementia
Symptomatic congestive heart failure
Angina pectoris
Seasonal allergies
Pain
Gastro-esophageal reflux diseases (motility-modifying drugs)
Post-infarction β blockade
Asthma prophylaxis (non-steroid treatments)

7–8 per group to 30–39 per group and all measured the change in the Hamilton Depression Scale from baseline at 4 weeks, a standard assessment in depression. The comparison between imipramine and nomifensine showed no differences, with five of the six trials giving on-treatment values within one point of each other, two slightly favoring nomifensine, two slightly favoring imipramine. The sixth study had only 7–8 patients per group, and favored nomifensine by 2·2 points, a trivial difference in so small a study. Certainly these trials seemed to represent a strong "equivalence" showing. Five of the six trials, however, had no capacity to distinguish active from inactive therapy, as imipramine and placebo also differed little, in five of the six studies by 0·1–2 points, with two studies favoring placebo, two imipramine, and one tied. Only the sixth study (again, the one with just 7–8 patients per group) could distinguish the active from inactive treatments, with a 14 point, statistically significant, difference between both active drugs, and placebo.

This is not an isolated finding in depression. Over many years about one half to one third of apparently well designed depression studies have been unable to distinguish known active drugs from placebo, even as sample sizes have moved to 40–80 per group and larger (Laughren T, unpublished observation).

There is little doubt that angiotensin-converting enzyme inhibitors (ACEIs) are effective treatment for symptomatic congestive heart failure. Nonetheless, when Dr Milton Packer, recent chair of FDA's Cardiovascular and Renal Drugs Advisory Committee, examined results of large (generally 100 patients per group, or more) trials of four ACEIs and one other effective agent in heart failure, using results of FDA reviews, he found that these effective drugs could demonstrate this effectiveness only about half the time on any given measure, with the most "objective measure", exercise testing, proving most difficult (Table 10.1).

Table 10.1 Results of controlled trials in symptomatic heart failure.

| Drug | ET | Sympt | NYHA | Global |
|---|---|---|---|---|
| | Benefit shown (yes/total studies) | | | |
| ACE 1 | 1/2 | 2/2 | 1/2 | 2/2 |
| ACE 2 | 1/2 | 1/2 | 2/3 | 1/1 |
| ACE 3 | 1/3 | 2/3 | 2/3 | 0/2 (QOL) |
| ACE 4 | 2/4 | 3/4 | 2/4 | - |
| Drug 5 LD | 2/3 | 0/2 | 2/2 | - |
| HD | 0/3 | 0/3 | 0/2 | - |

ET = exercise testing
NYHA = change in New York Heart Association congestive heart failure class
LD = low dose
HD = high dose
QOL = Quality of Life scale

As noted earlier, Tramer[13] reported a failure rate of about one third in placebo controlled trials of ondansetron in nausea and vomiting after surgery, perhaps because in many of the studies the placebo emesis rate was too low to improve. Similarly, in some depression trials, the improvement on placebo is quite dramatic, perhaps leaving little "upside sensitivity".

In many other symptomatic settings, similar difficulties arise and historical evidence of sensitivity to drug effects cannot be established (Box 10.1). It is tempting to believe that these inconsistent results are simply a matter of sample size and that there must be some study size in which effective agents will regularly be able to show their effectiveness. Indeed, Rothman and Michels[12] chide the FDA for not insisting that studies be of sufficient size to establish the effects of approved drugs precisely enough for them to be used as active controls. (This seems at odds with the view of Rothman and Michels that placebos cannot be used when there is established effective therapy. If large and numerous studies could in fact define effect size as they suggest, the later studies, or the late stages of the very large studies needed, would be randomizing patients to placebo long after effectiveness had been established.) It is surely possible that the inconsistency is in part a matter of sample size, but that really begs the question. Even if there really is *some* effect in most or all studies, one that could be detectable with much larger studies, what seems to be present is a treatment effect by study interaction, with considerable differences in treatment effect, larger than would be expected due to chance, in different studies, some of which seem to show no effect at all. Note that in all these cases there is no doubt of the effectiveness of the treatment. Even if only one half to two thirds of antidepressant trials succeed in distinguishing drug from placebo, that is well beyond what would occur by chance.

## Incentive toward study quality in active control trials

As Pocock[1] and others[4] point out, many kinds of study defects (Box 10.2) decrease the likelihood of showing a difference between treatments, a potential problem where such a lack of difference is the desired outcome of a non-inferiority trial. The inconsistent results of placebo controlled trials of many therapies occur even when trial sponsors and investigators are trying as hard as possible to assure the assay sensitivity of the trial, so that the trial will demonstrate effectiveness. In those settings, trialists undertake in many ways to avoid the kinds of defects listed in Box 10.2. Lead-in periods, for example, are used to eliminate placebo responders/spontaneous remissions. Rigorous diagnostic criteria are used to ensure that patients really have the disease under study. Patients whose measurements are too variable (for example, on treadmill tests) are excluded prior to randomization.

**Box 10.2 Study defects that undermine assay sensitivity**

Poor compliance
Non-protocol crossover
Spontaneous improvement in the population
A poorly responsive population
Concomitant medication that obscures effect
Poor diagnostic criteria (patients lack disease)
Insensitive (inappropriate) measures of drug effect
Poor quality of measurements
Mixing up the treatments

All of the defects in Box 10.2 have the effect of decreasing differences between treatments; that is, they introduce a bias toward a finding of no difference. Although these defects can be fatal to a trial designed to show a difference, lack of a difference is the *desired* outcome of a non-inferiority trial. Moreoever, although the defects listed in Box 10.2 minimize treatment effects, they do not have major (or in some cases, any) effects on variance, so they generally do not interfere with the showing of non-inferiority by widening the confidence interval for C–T.

It seems apparent that the non-inferiority setting does not create the same incentives for study excellence as the difference-showing trial setting does. This is particularly worrisome given the failure even of placebo controlled trials to show assay sensitivity in many cases.

## Comparing therapies

Rothman and Michels[6] have argued that results of placebo controlled trials are not really of interest, and that once effective drugs exist, what is interesting is how a new drug compares with the established drug. An implication of this is that drugs no more effective than available drugs are of no value. In fact, many important advances (new antidepressants, new antipsychotics, non-sedating antihistamines) are not more effective than their predecessors. Comparisons with placebo that are needed to show effectiveness are therefore still useful. Moreover, even if the main purpose of a trial were to compare two therapies, and not to establish effectiveness, a valid showing of equivalence still requires assay sensitivity, the ability to distinguish more and less effective treatments. All the caveats described above for effectiveness trials therefore remain applicable. A three-arm study is again a useful design, perhaps with larger sample sizes in the active control groups.

## Using active control non-inferiority trials

**Box 10.3 Active control non-inferiority trials considered credible**

Most bacterial infections
Thrombolytics (where angioplasty is not used)
Many stages of HIV infection
Treatment of responsive tremors where treatment affects survival or other accepted endpoint
Anesthetic agents
β-agonists in bronchospasm

There are, of course, many settings in which active-control non-inferiority trials are reliable. Some of these are shown in Box 10.3. In general, these are cases where the difference between drug and a placebo is large and it is easy to distinguish the effect of the treatment from the natural history of the disease. In some cases, detailed analyses of previous trials have allowed definition of a plausible non-inferiority margin. Analysis of placebo controlled thrombolysis trials revealed a regular ability to distinguish treatment from placebo and it was possible to set a non-inferiority margin based on effect size (reduced by 50% to preserve the established effect of the control). It is of interest, however, as acute angioplasty is moving toward becoming standard care in many centers in the United States for acute infarction, that the magnitude of the effect of a thrombolytic when added to angioplasty is uncertain, so that non-inferiority trials of new thrombolytics in the United States would become difficult to interpret in the presence of a high rate of angioplasty.

An important area of future research in clinical trial methodology is how to use available data, where placebo controlled trials are no longer possible, to choose a non-inferiority margin that is sufficiently conservative to ensure that a non-inferiority showing translates into real evidence of effectiveness, yet not so conservative that it becomes excessively difficult to utilize the non-inferiority design.

## Designing clinical trials to solve ethical and practical problems

In many cases, modifications of study design can overcome ethical problems or satisfy the desires of investigators and patients to minimize patient discomfort. These have been discussed previously.[2,11]

### Add-on studies

Not all placebo controlled trials leave patients untreated. In many cases, where existing therapy cannot be omitted because it is life-saving or prevents irreversible injury, a new treatment can be studied as add-on therapy. In an add-on study all patients receive either specified or "physicians' choice" therapy and then are randomized to added new treatment or added placebo. This design is usual in studies of cancer, congestive heart failure, and epilepsy, where omitting standard treatment would not be acceptable. Although this design leaves some uncertainty as to the value of the baseline treatments in the presence of the test drug, it does establish the value of the addition.

### Randomized withdrawal; early escape

Although it is, I believe, ethical to ask a patient to participate in a placebo controlled trial that may lead to discomfort, that does not mean indifference to patient discomfort is appropriate. One way to minimize discomfort is to define a failure criterion that triggers "early escape" from the trial for patients whose symptoms reach a defined intensity. Then time to failure, or frequency of failure, can become part of the study endpoint; any patient experiencing such failure is removed from the study.

A similar approach would be to use time-to-event measures as study outcomes; for example, some anti-epileptic drug trials have used time to first seizure (or first several seizures) as the study endpoint, so that patients do not have increased seizure rates for a prolonged period. Many trials in atrial fibrillation prevention have also used a time-to-recurrence endpoint, rather than number of recurrences per year.

The randomized withdrawal design was specifically proposed by Amery[18] as a way of limiting exposure to placebo in patients with angina pectoris. In this design, patients are given open-label drug initially. After a period of time, they are randomly assigned to continued drug or placebo. Effectiveness can be measured as time to return of symptoms or as overall symptoms during a defined period. This design can also be used to establish long-term effectiveness, when a long-term placebo controlled trial would not be acceptable; it is now the standard method for studying maintenance therapy (long-term effectiveness) of antidepressants and other psychotropic drugs.

## Conclusions

Placebo controlled trials and active controlled trials raise important ethical and inferential issues; it is important to keep the two distinct. There are many situations in which an active control trial showing equivalence/non-inferiority of a new drug to a control is uninformative as to the effectiveness of the new drug. That is not an ethical statement, but a statement about inference. Given the potential uninformativeness of an active control trial, whether a placebo control can be used in a given situation then becomes a critical ethical question, one that may determine whether it is possible to develop new agents in a particular therapeutic area. The ethical and inferential questions are not weighed against each other and do not represent competing values. A trial must be both ethical and informative if it is to be conducted, and the need for a placebo controlled trial to establish effectiveness does not make it acceptable to conduct one if the trial is unethical. It may simply be necessary to recognize that the showing of effectiveness cannot be accomplished. On the other hand, if placebo controlled trials are needed to establish effectiveness, their use should not be discouraged as unethical on spurious grounds, and it is important to remember that a study of no value, such as an uninformative active control trial, is also ethically doubtful.[9] It is therefore important to consider clearly, in those cases where an active control trial is not informative, whether a placebo controlled trial can be conducted. As a general matter, an independent, well-informed patient can agree to defer or omit established effective therapy when the consequence of deferral or omission is development or persistence of symptoms but not permanent damage. Such deferral or omission is similar to choices patients regularly make and can be well understood by patients. Patients must always be able to leave a study if they are dissatisfied with the treatment received.

## References


1 Pocock SJ. The pros and cons of non-inferiority (equivalence) trials. This volume, chapter 12.

2 Temple R, Ellenberga SS. Placebo controlled trials and active-control trials in the evaluation of new treatments. Part 1: Ethical and scientific issues. *Ann Intern Med* 2000; **133**:455–63.

3 Ellenberg SS, Temple R. Placebo controlled trials and active-control trials in the evaluation of new treatments. Part 2: Practical issues and specific cases. *Ann Intern Med* 2000;**133**:464–70.

4 International Conference on Harmonization: Choice of control group in clinical trials. *Federal Register* 2001;**66**:24390–24391.

5 World Medical Association. Declaration of Helsinki. Recommendations guiding physicians in biomedical research involving human subjects. *JAMA* 1997;**277**:925–6.

6 Rothman KJ, Michels KB. The continued unethical use of placebo controls. *N Engl J Med* 1994;**331**:394–8.

7 World Medical Association. *Summary History of the World Medical Association Declaration of Helsinki.* Ferney-Voltaire, France: World Medical Association, 1985.

8 Clouser KD. Medical ethics: some uses, abuses, and limitations. *N Engl J Med* 1975; **293**:384–7.

9 World Medical Association. Declaration of Helsinki. Ethical principles for medical research involving human subjects. *JAMA* 2000;**284**:3043–5.

10 Rothman KJ, Michels KJS, Baum M. Education and debate for and against: *Declaration of Helsinki* should be strengthened. *BMJ* 2000;**321**:422–5.

# 11: When is it appropriate to use a placebo arm in a trial?

KENNETH J ROTHMAN, KARIN B MICHELS

## What a placebo arm offers

Scientifically, there are many reasons to want to use a placebo in an experiment, and there is no reason not to use one. That is not to say that there is no virtue in using active comparison groups in trials. They are useful as well. But placebo comparisons are unquestionably desirable from the scientific point of view. Let me summarise the main reasons, some of which also apply to other control groups.

### A placebo comparison facilitates random assignment

Random assignment is one of the most desirable features of an experiment, and is considered nearly a hallmark of a proper experiment. The purpose of random assignment is to prevent confounding – that is, an imbalance between the compared study groups – by other factors that affect the outcome under study. Random assignment is not the only way to prevent confounding. Restriction – limiting the eligibility criteria to a single value of a factor that would affect the outcome – is another technique that is in fact much more effective than randomization, since it absolutely prevents confounding. Randomization, however, while less certain to prevent confounding than is restriction, achieves its goal for all variables simultaneously, whereas restriction must be employed separately for each identified factor that might affect the outcome. Furthermore, randomization is effective even for unidentified variables, whereas restriction cannot be employed for unidentified variables. It is possible and indeed routine to combine restriction for some variables with randomization to prevent confounding by other variables.

To implement random assignment, it is necessary to have two or more groups in the experiment. If there are two, typically one is the study group, or arm that receives the new intervention, and the other is a comparison group. To prevent biases from entering the study because patients are treated differently in the study and comparison group, it is helpful at least to simulate the offering of a treatment for the comparison group. Offering a placebo treatment accomplishes this goal and thus facilitates random assignment.

### A placebo group facilitates blinding

Knowledge of the treatment may affect the behavior of patients, the decisions of investigators, and of the determinations of the evaluators of the study outcome. Many study decisions that might affect the study results could be affected by knowledge of the treatment assignment. One example would be a decision to discontinue a patient's intervention because of adverse effects of treatment. A large worry is that knowledge of the treatment assignment would affect a patient's classification with respect to the study outcome. The extent to which this knowledge can distort the study result depends on the type of outcome. For example, if the outcome is death, it is unlikely to be recorded incorrectly even with knowledge of the treatment assignment. If the outcome is death from a specific cause, however, there is more room for judgment in determining the cause of death and thus a potential benefit from keeping the evaluator ignorant of the treatment assignment. The need for blinding increases as the outcome measure becomes more subjective.

Blinding is often impossible or unfeasible, because the nature of the treatment itself precludes keeping the treatment assignment unknown. For example, the treatment may have characteristic side effects or a unique administration. In many cases, however, the feasibility of blinding is improved by offering a placebo treatment to the comparison group. The placebo can be administered as a simulated treatment that improves the feasibility of keeping the actual assignment unknown to patients and the evaluators of the outcome.

### Offering a placebo enables the investigator to control for the "placebo effect"

The placebo effect is a real therapeutic effect that comes from the offering of a treatment.[1] The magnitude of the placebo effect varies with the nature of the disease, the type of patient, and the way in which the placebo is administered. Without offering a placebo treatment for the comparison group, the placebo effect will be experienced by those receiving the study intervention but might otherwise not be experienced by the comparison group. Thus, the observed treatment effect would then be a mixture of the placebo effect of offering the new treatment plus the actual treatment effect. By offering placebo treatment to the comparison group, the non-placebo component of the effect of the new intervention can be separated from its placebo effect.

It is possible to control for the placebo effect without a placebo group. In fact, offering any treatment, placebo or non-placebo, to the comparison group will control for the placebo effect in any comparison between the treatment arms of the study, because any observed difference cannot be explained as a placebo effect. Thus, it is not necessary to use a placebo comparison to control for the placebo effect.

## The arguments against placebo

The reason not to use a placebo arm in an experiment is straightforward: in many circumstances, offering a placebo is unethical. Why? It is unethical to conduct a trial that deprives participants of the level of care for their condition that they would have received if they were not participants in a trial. This principle is part of the *Declaration of Helsinki*, the ethical standard adopted by the World Medical Association to safeguard from ethical abuses patients who participate in medical experiments: "The benefits, risks, burdens and effectiveness of a new method should be tested against those of the best current prophylactic, diagnostic, and therapeutic methods. This does not exclude the use of placebo, or no treatment, in studies where no proven prophylactic, diagnostic or therapeutic method exists".[2]

The ethical principle that underlies this prohibition is that of equipoise, which is a state of genuine uncertainty regarding which of two or more treatments is preferable.[3] Unless equipoise prevails with respect to the treatments evaluated in a given study, the investigators will be offering a treatment to some patients that they believe is inferior. Doing so violates a basic maxim embodied in the *Declaration of Helsinki*, which states that "In medical research on human subjects, considerations related to the well-being of the human subject should take precedence over the interests of science and society".[2]

Without this maxim, there would be little reason, and little constraint, to avoid placebo controls in any experiment. Scientifically, there is no question that we usually have better information in a trial if we can include a placebo arm. Nevertheless, the scientific advantages of a placebo group are often exaggerated. Here I list the main scientific arguments offered in defense of placebo, along with a concise critique of each argument.

### Scientific arguments

*A placebo arm is a needed reference point*

If a placebo effect is considered the baseline from which other biologic effects are measured – and it is debatable whether it should be – then a placebo arm in a trial is a key reference point from which to measure the effect of the new treatment. While having this reference point is undeniably advantageous, it is not crucial. A reasonable case can be made that the best available treatment – setting aside for the moment how "best" ought to be defined – would make a better reference point, despite the fact that it is a moving target. With a placebo reference point, one might find a new treatment to be better than placebo but it might be considerably inferior to the best available treatment. Of course, one solution to that problem is to have both a placebo and an active treatment comparison group with which to compare the new treatment, an approach that has been recommended by Temple.[4] Nevertheless, if a single reference point is needed from which to gauge a new treatment, why not use the current best remedy, rather than a placebo? Doing so will reveal how well the new treatment does in relation to the best now available, a more interesting question than assessing how well the new treatment does in relation to the placebo effect by itself. It is important to remember that any comparison group that involves the offering of treatment will control for the placebo effect; if the current best treatment is used for comparison, the treatment effect in that comparison group is actually a combination of the placebo effect plus the non-placebo therapeutic effect of the treatment.

A common misconception that feeds enthusiasm for the placebo comparison is that the placebo effect is a constant reference point. In reality the placebo effect varies greatly with the nature of the disease, the characteristics of the patient, and the manner in which the treatment is offered. It may be that the placebo effect is much more variable than the non-placebo effects that are intended to be measured in the typical medical experiment.

*In an equivalence trial, neither treatment may be effective*

Both Temple and Pocock emphasize that without a placebo as an anchor point, it is difficult to know whether the new treatment and an active control are equally effective or equally ineffective.[4,5] According to this argument, a placebo group is necessary to determine whether equivalence actually implies effectiveness. The problem with the argument is that it is circular: trials designed to show that a new treatment is better than placebo need not be very large if the new treatment is any good. The trial may show that the new treatment is more effective than placebo, but if it is a small study, it will lack precision and there will not be much information on exactly how effective the new treatment is. Suppose, however, that large studies were conducted instead. Then we would have good precision measuring the effect of new treatments, and when these new treatments were compared with newer treatments later, there would be much less doubt about the benchmark. The uncertainty in equivalence trials stems in large part from the lack of information that exists on the comparator treatments in the first place.[6]

Note that this argument can be refuted by the actual practice of regulatory agencies, who rely on equivalence trials rather than placebo comparisons, to evaluate certain classes of new treatments, such as antibiotics or cancer therapy. No new antibiotic will be compared with a placebo, for ethical reasons that few would contest. Yet do we really believe that new antibiotics are approved that are completely ineffective, because they have been compared with an old antibiotic that has mysteriously lost its efficacy?

*Statistical significance is a useful decision tool, but there is no such test for an equivalence trial*

The drawback of using statistical significance as a decision tool has been pointed out on many occasions.[7] Put simply, statistical significance is a terrible method on which to base any decision. It is ironic that in the application of decision theory, one does not encounter tests of statistical significance, but outside of decision theory, one sees the use of statistical significance touted as an important decision tool. About the only thing about significance testing that facilitates decision making is that often both the decision and the significance test are dichotomous. That argument, however, works equally well for flipping a coin. The basic problem with statistical significance testing is that the process, along with the p values on which it is based, conflate study size with strength of effect.[8] The goal in assessing the effectiveness of a new treatment should be obtaining an unbiased estimate of the magnitude of the effect, along with its precision. Statistical significance simply does not accomplish this goal. If measurement is the goal, it can be achieved with respect to any baseline that is well characterised. Placebo is one, but a precisely measured comparator such as might be used in an equivalence trial is another.

*Many errors in a trial tend to reduce differences, a tendency that works against a new treatment in a placebo comparison, but works in favor of it in an equivalence trial*

The worry is that sloppy study design and execution will be rewarded in equivalence trials. Although this is a real problem, it is not a new issue: it is a feature of any epidemiologic study that shows an absence of effect. If a large study of electromagnetic fields and cancer occurrence shows no increased cancer risk, it may be that a real effect has been obscured by inaccurate measurement. Epidemiologists deal with this problem routinely by examining individual sources of error and by conducting sensitivity analyses to assess the extent to which a study's findings are dependent on specific sources of error.[9] Again, if this problem is important, it prompts the question of how equivalence trials can be accepted by regulatory bodies for some classes of treatments (such as antibiotics and cancer therapies) and yet be rejected for others.

*Equivalence trials require considerably more patients than placebo controlled trials*

The more information that you collect, the more you will know. Small placebo controlled studies offer much less information than large studies about the magnitude of the effects being evaluated. This argument only points out how little is now being learned about treatment effects in small studies that compare effective agents against placebo.

*Identifying the best treatment for comparison is not always easy*

If placebo comparisons are disallowed when a better treatment exists, how does one judge what is the proper comparison? A treatment can be judged better on many different scales, from cost to quality of life. How does one integrate into the calculation the risk of specific but rare adverse outcomes, for example? These are legitimate questions that must be answered to choose the appropriate comparison group. Just because the decision about which comparison to use is challenging is no reason to choose a less effective treatment.[10]

*Placebo is sometimes used in conjunction with standard therapy*

One argument that has been used in defense of placebo is that placebo is often combined with additional therapy, with the combination representing the standard of care. The new treatment is offered over and above the standard of care and contrasted with placebo to see if the addition to standard therapy makes a difference. The ethical objection to using placebo does not apply in this instance, if it is true that the standard of care is being offered to all arms of the trial. It is only when placebo treatment displaces a treatment known to be preferable to placebo that there is any ethical objection to the use of placebo in human experiments.

## Ethical arguments

*The greatest good for the greatest number*

Should any of the above scientific arguments be weighed against an ethical directive? Many people place ethical concerns ahead of pragmatic concerns. There is one argument, however, along utilitarian lines, that attempts to weigh the ethical concerns against the scientific concerns. According to this argument, the interests of patients in a trial are superseded by the need to accumulate scientific results, because these results will benefit many more people than the few who are participating in the trial. As noted above, the *Declaration of Helsinki* takes a clear stand against the utilitarian argument, stating that the wellbeing of the human subject takes precedence over the interests of science and society. Why should this principle prevail over the inclination to do the greatest good for the greatest number? The *Declaration of Helsinki* is a descendant of the *Nuremberg Code*, which broadly sought to establish guidelines to elevate the rights of individuals over the forces of a society that might subordinate those rights in favor of its own interests. In a word, the Declaration provides protection.

*Informed consent is sufficient*

Some have argued that informed consent is not merely necessary but is also sufficient for an ethical study: the claim is that we do not need to protect patients from that to which they consent voluntarily.[11–13] For example, Levine states the concern that "subjects might be exploited to serve the interests of industry or of investigators … can be minimized by the establishment of standards requiring informed consent and equitable selection of subjects".[12] Temple and Ellenberg state that "placebo-controlled trials may be ethically conducted even when effective therapy exists, as long as patients will not be harmed by participation and are fully informed about their alternatives".[13] According to this view, it is paternalistic to prohibit placebo controlled studies when better treatments exist, because doing so intrudes on autonomy. Of course, it is not unusual for autonomy to be in conflict with other ethical principles. Perhaps most important, however, is the realization that informed consent is a legal fiction, never actually achieved.[14] Furthermore, even idealised informed consent does not offer the patient the option to participate in a trial of any design other than what the investigator has already chosen. Informed consent does not typically inform the patient what treatments will be foregone by consenting to participate in the trial. The *Declaration of Helsinki* addresses the inadequacy of informed consent as a justification for offering inadequate treatment as follows: "The responsibility for the human subject must always rest with a medically qualified person and never rest on the subject of the research, even though the subject has given his or her consent … When obtaining informed consent for the research project the physician should be particularly cautious if the subject is in a dependent relationship with the physician or may consent under duress".[2]

*IRB approval is sufficient*

Another argument is that Institutional Review Boards provide a sufficient safeguard against the investigator who goes too far in denying adequate treatment to his or her research subjects. Unfortunately, this view is another fiction. IRBs carry heavy workloads; their members are not always sufficiently trained in the issues that bear upon their decisions; they are often swayed by FDA preferences (a study blocked by an IRB will often just be conducted elsewhere, representing a loss for the institution); and the applicants are often colleagues of the IRB members.[15–17]

## When is a placebo arm appropriate?

The above discussion relates to ethical concerns regarding patients. The *Declaration of Helsinki* distinguishes carefully between therapeutic research and research on healthy volunteers. This distinction is important, because patients depend on medical advice from their physician, who may also be the investigator who is soliciting the patient for a research study. With research on healthy volunteers, however, the absence of this dependence provides greater latitude. The distinction between patients and volunteers may be difficult in some cases. I believe that it should be based on whether the individual is currently seeking relief or treatment for a problem. Thus, a patient who is seeking relief of a headache should not be offered a placebo under any circumstances, whether in a trial or otherwise, because many effective headache remedies exist. On the other hand, a person prone to headaches could, with informed consent, volunteer for a study in which a placebo might be assigned instead of effective treatment for the next headache that the individual develops. The difference is that the individual has volunteered to participate in a trial that is not intended to treat a current problem, and thus is a healthy volunteer.

With respect to experimentation on patients, I have summarised both the scientific arguments and ethical arguments that have been raised in defense of using placebo controls. I propose that regardless of merit, the scientific arguments should be disregarded, because the rights of the individual supersede the rights of society. This principle is not universal: it is reasonable to consider the rights of society above those of the individual when society faces grave risks from the individual. Thus, it may be ethical in some situations to impose a quarantine on individuals or to impose mandatory vaccination to protect the public's health. In the area of medical experimentation, however, the *Declaration of Helsinki* asserts the primacy of individual rights over those of society. If one accepts this assertion, then the scientific arguments in favor of placebo when better treatments are available are all moot. Perhaps much of the debate about the use of placebo when better treatments are available can be focused into a debate on this principle.

If the goals of science are weighed against the rights of the individual to receive the best treatment, there is little hope for the patient to have any rights at all. The potential value of knowledge in terms of the number of present and future people who could benefit will be essentially infinitely greater than the value to the participant in the study of getting a better treatment, because the number of people who can benefit from the knowledge is unbounded. If we reject this comparison, do we condemn a vast multitude to inferior treatments because we have chauvinistically placed the rights of a few individuals ahead of so many others? Not really. Scientists are creative in finding ways to learn, and the knowledge is apt to be accumulated one way or another, even if it takes longer and costs more to do so. As discussed above, the scientific arguments against the use of placebo can be rebutted. But in any event, I propose that they should not even be entertained, given the acceptance of the general principle that the right of patients who volunteer for medical experiments takes precedence over the interests of science and society, as the *Declaration of Helsinki* states.

What of the argument that an absolutist stance will impede knowledge when the risk to the patient is minimal? This is an argument that denies the principle that the rights of the patient come first, and eases into the pragmatics of allowing a debate to proceed about how much risk of adversity or pain the physician should allow the patient to sustain for the purposes of the physician's research. Can the patient with a headache be offered a placebo? The adversity in that instance is surely minuscule. But as soon as the line is moved from the absolute position that the patient with a problem should be offered the best treatment available, with no exception, the underlying ethical principle has been vacated and there remains no ethical constraint at all beyond the conscience of the investigator. Avoiding that situation is the reason to have ethical codes.

## References


1 Shapiro AK and Shapiro E. The placebo: is it much ado about nothing? Chapter 1 in Harrington A, ed. *The Placebo Effect. An Interdisciplinary Exploration*. Cambridge, MA: Harvard University Press, 1997.
2 World Medical Association. Declaration of Helsinki. http://www.wma.net/e/policy/17-c_e.html
3 Freedman B. Equipoise and the ethics of clinical research. *N Engl J Med* 1987; **317**:141–5.
4 Temple RJ. Placebo controlled trials and active controlled trials: ethics and inference. This volume, chapter 10.
5 Pocock SJ. The pros and cons of non-inferiority (equivalence) trials. This volume, chapter 12.
6 Rothman KJ. Placebo mania. (Editorial) *BMJ* 1996;**313**:3–4.
7 For discussion and further references, see Rothman KJ, Greenland S. *Modern Epidemiology*, 2nd ed. Philadelphia: Lippincott Williams & Wilkins, 1998.
8 Lang J, Rothman KJ, Cann CI. That confounded P-value (Editorial). *Epidemiology* 1998; **9**:7–8.
9 Greenland S. Basic methods for sensitivity analysis and external adjustment. In: *Modern Epidemiology*, 2nd ed. Rothman KJ, Greenland S, eds. Philadelphia: Lippincott Williams & Wilkins, 1998.
10 Rothman KJ, Michels KB. The continuing unethical use of placebo controls. *N Engl J Med* 1994;**331**:394–8.
11 Lasagna L. The Helsinki Declaration: timeless guide or irrelevant anachronism? *J Clin Psychopharmacol* 1995;**15**:96–8.
12 Levine RJ. Should the *Declaration of Helsinki* be revised? *N Engl J Med* 1999;**341**:1853.
13 Temple R, Ellenberg SS. Placebo-controlled trials and active-control trials in the evaluation of new treatments. Part 1: Ethical and scientific issues. *Ann Intern Med* 2000;**133**:456–64.
14 Laforet GG. The fiction of informed consent. *JAMA* 1976;**235**:1579–85.
15 Savulescu J, Chalmers I, Blunt J. Are research ethics committees behaving unethically? Some suggestions for improving performance and accountability. *BMJ* 1996;**313**: 1390–3.
16 Denny WF. The continuing unethical use of placebo controls (letter). *N Engl J Med* 1995;**332**:61–2.
17 Department of Health and Human Services, Inspector General. *Institutional review boards: a time for reform*. Washington, DC: Department of Health and Human Services, 1998.

# 12: The pros and cons of non-inferiority (equivalence) trials

STUART J POCOCK

## Introduction

The term "non-inferiority trial" is commonly used to refer to a randomized clinical trial in which a new test treatment is compared with a standard active treatment rather than a placebo or untreated control group. A prior judgment is made that for the new treatment to be of merit it only needs to be as good as the active control as regards appropriate outcome measure(s) of response. While superiority of new treatment over active control would be an added (perhaps unrealistic) bonus, the clear demonstration of non-inferiority in one or more specific criteria of patient response is the desirable goal which motivates such a trial. The term "equivalence trial" is sometimes used in this context but does not reflect so well the (usually) one-sided nature of this non-inferiority question, and is implicitly dismissive of the desirable option that the new treatment could actually be superior to the active control treatment. So the more appropriate term "non-inferiority" is used hereon.

The aim of this article is to present a balanced view of the role of non-inferiority trials in the development of safe and effective new treatments. This involves a mix of ethical, scientific, statistical and practical considerations. This article elucidates some of the pros and cons of non-inferiority trials and offers some pointers on how to enhance their public health value. The desirability (or not) of a non-inferiority trial strategy will depend on the particular circumstances. While general guidance can be given, the relative merits of non-inferiority active control trials or placebo controlled trials aimed at demonstrating superiority for evaluating any specific new treatment rests on a complex of issues requiring wise judgments and continued open debate.

## Choice of control group: active versus placebo

One starting principle is that no patient be denied a *known* effective treatment by entering a clinical trial. An equally important principle is that the degree of scientific rigor adopted in the evaluation of a new treatment is sufficient to prevent any ineffective, unsafe or inferior treatments obtaining regulatory approval or gaining widespread use. Both principles highlight the ethical responsibility of a society and its medical researchers to facilitate the best possible health care both now and in the future.

The first principle is more easily grasped because it relates immediately to the individual rights of the next patient. Of importance here is the distinction between a treatment *known* to be effective, and one *thought* to be effective, *hoped* to be more effective, *believed* to be effective or *in widespread use* without evidence of effectiveness. Arguments against the use of placebo controls are put forward because treatment practice involves other active treatments. The question is how convincing is the evidence that such active treatments are better than placebo in aspects that genuinely benefit patient welfare. While one needs to consider the understandable wish to do something positive for every patient, one needs to draw a clear distinction between desire for benefit in a supposedly active potential control treatment and hard evidence of benefit from previous clinical trials.

So what is the extent of evidence? Is it "proof beyond reasonable doubt" of patient benefit derived from several large studies generalizable to the relevant patient population or is it just one or two statistically significant results, perhaps on short-term studies of limited size studying surrogate endpoints rather than overall patient benefit. Remember $p < 0{\cdot}05$ for a treatment difference in a clinical trial does not equate with proof of effect.

Even the relevance of a highly statistically significant treatment difference can be questioned on several grounds.

- Might the trial have been biased in some aspect of its design or analysis?
- Were the patients, the delivery of treatment, the outcome measure used and the length of follow up sufficiently relevant to normal clinical practice and patient benefit?
- Was the absolute magnitude of benefit sufficiently large taking account of any adverse side effects of a treatment?
- How many trials were performed and on how many patients?

That is, in sizing up the evidence that a pre-existing active treatment is superior to placebo one needs to exercise one's constructive critical faculties when appraising its clinical trial evidence for internal validity, external validity, overall patient benefit and extent of research.

Should the overall evidence for patient benefit on a pre-existing active treatment be less than totally convincing, then the dangers of exclusively adopting that treatment as an active control group (instead of a placebo control group) for the evaluation of other new treatments are substantial. In certain areas this problem is tackled by having both an active control group and a placebo control group, so that non-inferiority compared to the former and superiority over the latter can be evaluated within the same trial, or set of trials.

It is important to recognize that approval of a drug by regulatory authorities as being safe and effective for a specific condition does not in itself imply that the use of that drug as an active control without a placebo group would provide a reliable basis for a non-inferiority trial of a new drug. [See Further Reading: Temple and Ellenberg (2000)]

This ongoing dilemma for clinical trials research can be summarized by the wish to avoid two types of error.

- *Type 1 error*

This would be the *acceptance of a useless treatment* into widespread use, and one needs to consider the increased risk of this error occurring by not using placebo controls and instead pursuing a non-inferiority (equivalence) trial design with an active control group. The consequences of such an error will depend on the nature of the treatment and disease. If the ineffective treatment has substantial side effects then great harm could ensue, if it is expensive then it detracts from more fruitful use of health care costs, if it is a safe, useless, cheap "placebo" for a minor condition then perhaps not much harm is done.

Even if there is an effective active control treatment, there can still be problems in the design, conduct, analysis and interpretation of a non-inferiority trial that could lead to such a Type 1 error. Such problems are outlined in the rest of this article.

- *Type 2 error*

This is the *failure to use an effective active control treatment* by adopting a placebo control group instead. As expressed above, the degree of certainty with which such an error occurs depends on the extent of prior knowledge that the active control is truly effective. Also, the severity of this error will depend on particular circumstances. At one extreme it would be absolutely intolerable to deny a known effective agent that reduces mortality in a rapidly progressing life-threatening condition. However, in a more minor ailment in which recovery often happens on placebo or no-treatment, the denial of a known active agent in a short-term placebo controlled trial, after which all patients can go on to receive active treatment, has much less serious consequences for patient welfare.

In many trials, having a placebo control group does not mean such patients receive no active intervention. Often, all randomized patients undergo normal accepted care, including other active drugs as appropriate, but the addition of a new treatment is compared with addition of a placebo. It is often debated whether such ancillary care and supplementary drugs should be according to a fixed protocol or pragmatically left to individual clinical judgment as in routine clinical practice. It is also relevant to ask would the patient have got the active control treatment if they were not included in a clinical trial. In some circumstances the answer is "no they would not" in which case there appears a perverse twist in the ethical argument whereby trialists are required to adopt more stringent ethical standards than regular treating physicians.

Thus, every time one chooses between active controls or placebo controls in planning a randomized trial, one has to consider the above risks of Type I and Type 2 error, taking account of the likelihood of them occurring and the severity of the consequences. The consequent decisions are not easily taken: neither passionate one-sided ethical arguments against placebo controls in general nor scientific pleas for mandatory up front demonstration of new treatment superiority over placebo should dominate our thinking and planning. Rather one aims for an ethical balance of the genuine needs of the next patient in a trial to receive good care and the longer term public health need to only allow marketing approval and widespread use of treatments that actually work.

## Types of non-inferiority trial

There are many different circumstances that may lead to undertaking a non-inferiority trial design. The *simplest case* is where one wishes to demonstrate (if true) that the efficacy of a new drug is the same as an existing active drug, and one is not anticipating any other differences. This will be particularly plausible if the drugs are of the same class, in which case such a "me too" drug development could lead to an additional marketable product but not a substantial improvement in therapeutic care. The merits of such a narrow diversity of products within a specific drug class may appear rather small, except as regards company profits. However, even if the average benefits and safety profiles of two drugs in a class appear identical, it is possible that individual patients may benefit more from one drug than the other.

Either before or after marketing approval, there is sometimes a need for a large randomized controlled safety study to evaluate a concern that may have arisen from observational adverse event reporting. For instance, the POINT study evaluated in 11 302 patients undergoing surgery the safety of one non-steroidal anti-inflammatory (NSAID) pain relief drug ketorolac compared with two others, diclofenac and ketoprofen, this non-inferiority safety study being motivated by concerns in the European regulatory authority, the Committee for Proprietary Medicinal Products (CPMP).

A *more complex and interesting scenario* arises when the aim is to demonstrate equivalence (non-inferiority) of a new treatment to an active control, while knowing or suspecting that the two treatments will differ in some other important respects.

Possibilities here are:

- *The new treatment has less side effects*

  For instance, low dose aspirin versus anticoagulation following thrombolysis after a myocardial infarction may be equivalent as regards recurrence of infarct or cardiac death, but the former produces less bleeding complications. Aspirin is hardly a new drug! However, in the context where anticoagulation had become the norm it was a new alternative strategy.
- *The new treatment is less invasive*

  Carotid endarterectomy is a surgical procedure for patients at high risk of a stroke. If carotid stenting could be demonstrated as equally efficacious, for many patients it might be the treatment of choice, being less invasive. This is the motivation behind a proposed NIH-funded trial comparing these two intervention strategies.
- *The new treatment is cheaper*

  An analogous situation concerns the relative merits of bypass surgery and coronary angioplasty for patients with angina. Trials have shown that the prognosis, i.e. death and/or myocardial infarction, appears similar for both intervention strategies, the former provides better symptomatic relief initially but is more invasive. However, any health care strategy must take costs and cost-effectiveness into account, and much interest in these trials has focused on the reduced initial costs of an angioplasty and whether that gain is maintained over several years' follow up.

The complexity of these situations arises from the fact that one is looking at a trade-off between efficacy and other issues regarding side effects, patient acceptability and costs. Although such trials are often presented as non-inferiority (equivalence) trials it is possible that some modest reduction in efficacy may be acceptable alongside the other benefits of a new treatment. One example of this may be the acellular pertussis vaccines, which have come to be used in preference to whole cell pertussis vaccines because of fewer adverse events, even though their efficacy may be somewhat lower.

Another issue is whether any particular trial comparing a new treatment with an active standard treatment should be formulated as a non-inferiority trial or not. Given the relative state of ignorance with which one starts any new study, one is often unsure whether to optimistically pursue the prospect of demonstrating a new treatment's superiority or whether to settle for demonstrating non-inferiority on the basis that that will be still good enough to make the new treatment of some value. Though the statistical power calculations differ somewhat for these two scenarios (i.e. the latter reverses the roles of null and alternative hypotheses), the underlying statistical and scientific intent is unaltered. What one wants is a sufficiently large and unbiased study so that the true magnitude of treatment difference is estimated precisely. That is, when the trial is completed the point estimate and confidence interval for the appropriate measure(s) of treatment difference contain all the relevant evidence on which to hang claims of non-inferiority or superiority.

Rigorous adherence to a single prespecified criterion of non-inferiority, except for the convenience of planning the size of a trial, may not necessarily be the most sensible way of interpreting a trial's results. Nevertheless, formulating one's realistic goals, and hence the required number of patients, is an important feature of any non-inferiority trial's planning and the next section is devoted to this topic.

## Appropriate goals and sample sizes for non-inferiority trials

First it is essential to realize that failure to demonstrate a statistically significant difference between two treatments does not allow one to assert that the two treatments are equivalent, or even similar, in their efficacy. Obviously, the fewer patients there are in a trial the less power to detect any meaningful difference so that non-significance in a conventional test of a null hypothesis is a hopeless criterion for inferring non-inferiority. It would actually encourage the pursuit of smaller trials!

Instead, the most widely accepted approach to determining the required size of a non-inferiority trial is to first define the smallest true magnitude of inferiority that would be regarded as *unacceptable*, assuming one has already chosen a primary outcome measure of response for this purpose. Anything truly that bad or even worse needs to be detected reliably so that any claim of non-inferiority for the new treatment can then be ruled out. However, one is prepared to accept more minor differences from true equivalence as being "good enough".

The logical basis here is that even if one carries out an extremely large clinical trial, one never fully proves that two treatments are truly identical in their efficacy. The confidence interval for the treatment difference gets smaller and smaller as the sample size increases, but proof of equivalence would require a confidence interval centered on zero and with zero width. An impossible task!

In a spirit of achievable compromise one sets out to arbitrarily choose this minimum clinically relevant difference, commonly called delta ($\delta$), which if true would deny any claim of a new treatment's non-inferiority. We then choose a sample size sufficiently large such that if there is true equivalence of new and control treatments there is a high probability that the confidence interval for treatment difference will be wholly to one side (the good side!) of this "$\delta$".

The simplest case to quantify is for a binary response (success or failure). Let $\pi$ be the anticipated percentage of successes on each treatment if true equivalence exists. Let $\delta$ be the "minimum clinically relevant difference". Suppose results will be expressed as an estimated percentage of treatment difference with a 95% confidence interval around it. Also, suppose one wants to be 90% sure that if treatments are truly identical then the confidence interval will exclude $\delta$, in a more favorable direction of course.

A simple commonly used formula in this instance is that the required sample size is

$$2n = \frac{4 \times 10{\cdot}5 \times \pi\,(100 - \pi)}{\delta^2}$$

More complex refinements exist and alternative but similar formulae exist for other types of outcome data, such as comparison of risk ratios or means of a quantitative measure, but this formula will adequately illustrate the problems of choosing the size of a non-inferiority trial.

The difficulty lies in choosing appropriate values for $\pi$ and $\delta$, especially the latter. For example, consider a non-inferiority trial comparing a new drug with omeprazole for treatment of *H. pylori* infection. The binary response is eradication of infection (yes or no). From past experience with omeprazole, $\pi$ = 85% was the anticipated eradication rate. For trial planning $\delta$ was set at 15%. This means that the new drug would be regarded as non-inferior provided that the possibility of its eradication rate being 15% worse than omeprazole could be ruled out (in the sense that the 95% confidence interval for the treatment difference in eradication rates would not include a 15% inferiority relative to omeprazole).

Hence the trial required $2n = \dfrac{4 \times 10{\cdot}5 \times 85 \times 15}{15^2} = 238$ randomized patients.

Leaping ahead to the actual results of this trial, the observed eradication rates on new drug and omeprazole were 109/126 (86·5%) and 110/129 (85·3%) respectively. The 95% confidence interval for the treatment difference was −7·5% to + 9·8%. A difference of −15% is clearly ruled out of consideration, and on that basis the trial data support the new drug's non-inferiority relative to omeprazole. Of course, one still cannot claim with certainty that the new drug is identical in efficacy to omeprazole. After all, the confidence interval for treatment difference does go beyond 5% in both favorable and unfavorable directions. But according to the predefined goal, adequate evidence of non-inferiority is deemed to have been achieved.

Now just suppose that the new drug had had an eradication rate of 99/126 (78·6%) instead of the above 109/126. In that case, the 95% confidence interval for the treatment difference would have been from −16·1% to + 2·7%. This would have been a most unhelpful result since one could neither claim non-inferiority (since the confidence interval would include −15%) nor could one rule out equivalence of the two treatments (because the confidence interval includes no difference).

Fortunately, this did not happen in reality, but it illustrates the inconclusiveness that can easily arise if non-inferiority trials are conducted with fairly modest sample sizes. It seems quite fashionable to choose $\delta = 15\%$ in non-inferiority trials. Indeed the regulatory authority did approve such a choice for the above trial, and there are more general regulatory guidelines for choice of $\delta$ in such anti-infective trials. But it is hard to come up with an objective reasoning behind this apparently arbitrary oft used choice. Why not $\delta = 10\%$ instead? That would require $2n = 535$ patients, more than twice as many. On the basis that only the slightest possible inferiority of the new drug should be allowable, $\delta = 5\%$ might seem a plausibly tight safety margin, but that requires nine times as many patients, a staggering $2n = 2142$ patients.

These calculations are all based on 95% confidence and being 90% sure of ruling out non-inferiority. More generally if one requires 100 $(1 - \alpha)\%$ confidence and wants 100 $(1 - \beta)\%$ surety, then one requires

$$4 \times (z_{\alpha/2} + z_{\beta})^2 \times \frac{\pi(100 - \pi)}{\delta^2}$$

patients where $z_{\alpha/2}$ and $z_{\beta}$ are standardized normal deviates associated with one-tail probabilities $\alpha/2$ and $\beta$ respectively.

For instance, with a 90% confidence interval and only 80% surety each of the above sample sizes is reduced by 40%. However, with the tougher demands set by a 99% confidence interval and being 95% sure of rejecting a difference $\delta$ and claiming non-inferiority when equivalence truly exists, each of the above sample sizes increases by 70%.

For those more used to power calculations for trials aimed at detecting differences, it is worth noting that the above formulae have reversed the usual concepts of null and alternative hypothesis, and type 1 and 2 errors $\alpha$, $\beta$. For a non-inferiority trial, $\alpha/2$ is the probability that the 100 $(1 - \alpha)\%$ confidence interval excludes $\delta$ when the null hypothesis, treatment difference $= \delta$, is in fact true. $\beta$ is the probability that the confidence interval includes $\delta$ (or worse) when the alternative hypothesis of no treatment difference is in fact true.

In practice, there seems a pragmatic acceptance by trialists and regulatory authorities that fairly generous choices of $\delta$, $\alpha$ and $\beta$ are allowed in order not to demand inordinately large numbers of patients in non-inferiority trials. Should we be concerned therefore that the adoption of non-inferiority designs with generously large choices of $\delta$ could be permitting treatments with more modest but important extents of inferiority to be falsely accepted as non-inferior? This is an inherent weakness of non-inferiority trials as currently performed. We do take a sizeable risk that some truly inferior treatments will slip through the net.

Perhaps one could draw a distinction between 1) trials comparing two drugs in the same class where there may exist a high prior belief that treatments truly should be equally efficacious, and 2) trials comparing quite contrasting treatments, for example, drugs of differing types, or radically differing intervention strategies where there are no firm grounds on which to anticipate non-inferiority. A generous $\delta$ leading to a smaller required sample size seems more permissible in the first instance (as was the case from the above *H. pylori* example). Perversely, the more contrasting the treatments the harder it often is to recruit patients, but that is just the instance when large sample sizes are needed in order to be confident of true non-inferiority.

The appropriate choice of $\delta$ is particularly important when a non-inferiority trial versus active control is taking place because it is considered unethical to proceed with a placebo control group. The worst that could happen is that the non-inferiority margin is set so wide that a new treatment not much (if at all) better than placebo gets accepted as "non-inferior" on such an unduly loose criterion. Hence, it is useful to infer, preferably from past placebo controlled trials, the magnitude of superiority of the active control over placebo. The choice of $\delta$ both for planning trial size and interpreting results of the new trial needs to be substantially smaller than this estimate for several reasons:

1 The magnitude of superiority of active control over placebo may well be an overestimate. The placebo controlled evidence may be limited, past trials may have some biases present and to carry forward one (perhaps lucky) active treatment's possibly exaggerated effect into future planning reflects a lack of scientific caution.
2 Without a direct comparison with a placebo control group one is using an indirect argument via a comparison with active control to infer that a new treatment is worthwhile. For a whole variety of reasons discussed in the next section (for example, patient selection, non-compliance) the circumstances of the non-inferiority trial may be sufficiently different from the placebo controlled trials to cast doubt on the appropriateness of the active treatment's apparent magnitude of superiority over placebo. A safety margin of less ambitious efficacy may be in order.
3 Any new treatment needs to have a certain minimum magnitude of efficacy compared to placebo in order to be worthwhile, especially if other considerations (side effects, costs, inconvenience) come into play. Thus, even supposing issues 1 and 2 above did not apply (they usually do though!), one would still want $\delta$ to be much smaller than the active control's superiority margin over placebo.

These issues are linked to the earlier arguments concerning the choice between placebo and active controls. The ideal circumstance for a non-inferiority trial is when the superiority of active control compared to placebo is irrefutable and well documented, the non-inferiority trial can be conducted in very similar conditions and the choice of $\delta$ is small enough to convince one that any new treatment passing such a non-inferiority test is truly of therapeutic value.

Fundamentally, many non-inferiority trials are not large enough to satisfy these requirements, meaning that the risk of a Type 1 error (as discussed in section 2 above), false acceptance of a useless treatment, is often greater than it should be.

## The potential inferiority of non-inferiority trials

For conventional clinical trials aimed at exploring the potential superiority of a new treatment over standard treatment (whether placebo or active) many of the pitfalls that can arise operate in the direction of making it harder to detect a genuine treatment difference. Such conservatism leads to the observed treatment difference being a dilution of the true effects under ideal conditions. This is often seen as an appropriate pragmatism, whereby the attempted unbiased comparison of new and standard treatment policies in a practical setting where strict adherence to protocol inevitably does not always happen, means that the real-life benefit of a new treatment is seen for what it really is. That is, a new treatment has to fight its way through the hiccups, failings, frailties and unpredictability of human beings (both trialists and patients), in order to demonstrate its superiority over standard care.

The great difficulty with non-inferiority trials is that their very motivation is to demonstrate the similarity of new and standard treatments, so that all these same problems work towards achieving this goal even if it is not true. The anti-conservatism of a poorly designed and poorly conducted non-inferiority trial can greatly enhance the risk of a Type 1 error, the adoption of a useless treatment whose inadequacies could not be detected.

One could argue that the unscrupulous investigator has every incentive to undertake a sloppy non-inferiority trial. For instance, with selection of inappropriate patients, poor compliance with intended treatments, use of non-discriminatory outcome measures, inconsistencies between observers, too short a follow up and a substantial amount of missing data, it would not be surprising if the results were closely comparable even if the real treatments properly given to the right patients were substantially different in real patient benefit.

So in non-inferiority trials it is especially important to adhere to a well-defined relevant study protocol, and also to document that such adherence is successfully achieved. Some of the principal difficulties to bear in mind are as follows.

- *Selection of patients*

  It is important to select the type of patient for whom the efficacy of the active control treatment has been clearly established. For instance, were one to deviate, even in part, from the patient population in whom superiority over placebo had previously been demonstrated, then any claim regarding a new treatment's merits could not well distinguish between genuine non-inferiority or inappropriate selection of patients. Informative generalizability depends on a representative patient sample of the same kind as had previously demonstrated efficacy for the active control.

- *Treatment compliance*

  The first requirement is that one chooses a genuinely efficacious active control treatment, and that it be given in the same form, dose and quality as was previously used to demonstrate that efficacy. One then requires that for both new and active treatment groups a satisfactorily high level of patient compliance is achieved, and that appropriate measures of such compliance are recorded. Any reasons for alteration or discontinuation of treatments need documenting. Also, use of concomitant non-randomized treatments needs documenting (and possibly standardizing) since any differential use of other efficacious treatments could conceivably mask the inferiority of a new treatment.
- *Outcome measures*

  One needs to choose outcome measures that reflect genuine patient benefit (i.e. surrogate markers may well not suffice), and which were previously used to demonstrate the efficacy of the active control treatment. Each such measure (or endpoint) needs consistent well-defined criteria, with appropriate steps to reduce observer variation or bias. In addition, rigorous, objective reporting of adverse events is an important issue, since any non-inferiority needs to concern safety as well as efficacy.
- *Duration of treatment and evaluations*

  In any non-inferiority trial, the randomized treatments need to be given for long enough and the patient response evaluated over a long enough period so that any potential treatment differences have a realistic opportunity to reveal themselves. Due attention needs to be given to the durations of treatment and follow up in previous trials demonstrating efficacy of the active control treatment, and also the intended duration of treatment in future clinical practice.
- *Statistical analysis issues*

  Any non-inferiority trial requires a well-documented statistical analysis plan. There will often be a single primary outcome measure with a predefined non-inferiority criterion and method of analysis, but this should not preclude appropriate secondary analyses of other outcome measures, which could become important if they exhibit any signs of the new treatment's inferiority or if interpretation of the primary outcome findings is not clear cut.

In major Phase III trials aimed at detecting treatment differences, *analysis by intention to treat* is routinely highlighted. That is, one analyses the complete follow up results for all randomized patients regardless of their compliance with intended treatment in a spirit of comparing the treatment policies as actually given. Although this may dilute any idealized treatment differences under (unrealistic) circumstances of 100% compliance, that is generally considered wise pragmatism compared with any potential exaggerations of efficacy that could arise from focusing on treatment compliers only. The dilemma for non-inferiority trials is that faced with non-negligible non-compliance, analysis by intention to treat could artificially enhance the claim of non-inferiority by diluting some real treatment difference. More weight may instead be attached to per protocol analyses (which focus on patient outcome amongst compliers only or up until compliance ceases in each patient) in the hope that they may reveal undesirable treatment differences. But this in turn has problems since compliers are a select group of patients who may give a favorably biased view (for example, if the treatment is not helping, you drop out). These difficulties become particularly problematic if compliance differs between treatment groups. Thus, for non-inferiority trials there is no single, ideal analysis strategy in the face of substantial non-compliance or missing data, and both analysis by intention to treat and well-defined per protocol analyses would seem warranted. Such non-compliance will inevitably lead to a degree of concern over any affirmative claims of non-inferiority, which feeds back to the need to minimize any such protocol deviations.

In general, statistical considerations in the design, monitoring and analysis of non-inferiority are less well established than for superiority trials, making it a fruitful area for further methodological research.

## Concluding remarks

The most important advantage of a non-inferiority trial is that faced with clear evidence of efficacy for an existing standard treatment, it would be ethically unacceptable to proceed with a placebo or inactive control group in the evaluation of a new treatment for the same condition. In any particular circumstance an important reservation before jumping to that conclusion is that such evidence of efficacy really is strong enough to warrant exclusion of placebo controls. Too lax an acceptance of non-inferiority trials, with a less than convincing active control treatment, could potentially lead to the adoption of more and more ineffective treatments, and this would be a misguided over-reaction to the ethical concerns in conducting randomized controlled trials.

So when one has made the right judgment to undertake a non-inferiority trial with an active control treatment, all necessary steps need to be taken to ensure that any failings in the trial design, conduct or analysis could not artificially dilute out any real treatment differences. That is, false claims of non-inferiority need to be avoided.

Inevitably one can never prove that two treatments are identical, and hence some degree of compromise is required so that realistically achievable but adequately large numbers of patients are randomized in a non-inferiority trial. Thus, any clinically important treatment difference can be demonstrated not to exist with reasonable confidence. One suspects that in too many instances sample size determination for non-inferiority trials is based on too generous a criterion of what constitutes a minimum clinically important treatment difference, and this increases the risk that some inferior treatments may gain regulatory approval and widespread use.

So placebo controls may rightly need to be ruled out in certain areas of clinical research, but it would be wrong to rush too enthusiastically into more widespread use of non-inferiority (equivalence) trials without full consideration of their inherent problems.

## Further reading

Blackwelder WC. "Proving the null hypothesis" in clinical trials. *Control Clin Trials* 1982; **3**:345–53.

Farrington CP, Manning G. Test statistics and sample size formulae for comparative binomial trials with null hypothesis of non-zero risk difference or non-unity relative risk. *Stat Med* 1990;**9**:1447–54.

Garbe E, Röhmel J, Gundert-Remy U. Clinical and statistical issues in therapeutic equivalence trials. *Eur J Clin Pharmacol* 1993;**45**:1–7.

International Conference on Harmonisation. Choice of Control Group in Clinical Trials. *Federal Register* 1999;**64**:51767–77.

Jones B, Jarvis P, Lewis JA, Ebbutt AF. Trials to assess equivalence: the importance of rigorous methods. *BMJ* 1996;**313**:36–9.

Roebruck P, Kühn A. Comparison of tests and sample size formulae for proving therapeutic equivalence based on the difference of binomial probabilities. *Stat Med* 1995;**14**:1583–94.

Senn S. Inherent difficulties with active control equivalence studies. *Stat Med* 1993;**12**: 2367–75.

Senn S. Active Control Equivalence Studies. Chapter 15 in *Statistical Issues in Drug Development*. Chichester: Wiley, 1997.

Snapinn SM. Noninferiority trials. *Curr Control Trials Cardiovasc Med* 2000;**1**:19–21.

Temple R, Ellenberg SS. Placebo-controlled trials and active-control trials in the evaluation of new treatments. *Ann Intern Med* 2000;**133**:455–70.

# 13: Use of placebo in large-scale, pragmatic trials

ROBERT M CALIFF, SANA M AL-KHATIB

## Introduction

The need for clinical trials to distinguish modest, but clinically meaningful, treatment effect differences is increasing due to the proliferation of biologically powerful therapeutic options and the attention to aggregate health care finances. In addition, examples of therapies used in patients that were thought to be effective, but were later found to be useless[1] or detrimental,[2] have highlighted the necessity for a greater understanding of "evidence-based medicine." This need for large-scale clinical trials to produce definitive results about therapeutic outcomes reflects society's growing expectation that medical therapies be grounded in empirical evidence of a tangible benefit.

At the same time, the number of potential therapies exceeds our ability to use them in many common diseases. Widely prevalent diseases such as coronary heart disease and heart failure have over six beneficial pharmacological therapies that are all prescribed simultaneously. Additionally, health care delivery systems can view their expenditures in aggregate, leading to increasing concern about the cost of using therapies of unknown clinical benefit. The benefits and risks of therapeutics are important to determine not only in the context of new therapies, but also when evaluating multiple alternatives within a "class" and in different combinations of therapies. Since most therapeutics have only a modest benefit and other potential therapies could be more useful, the methodology used to assess the effect of treatment must be able to detect small differences. In order to inform clinical practice, trials have to effectively identify clinically meaningful treatment effect differences, which are often small. It is in this context that the placebo issue will be evaluated.

This evident need for large clinical trials also raises concern about the appropriate methodology for conducting such trials, and the use of placebo is one such critical methodological issue. Considerable evidence points to the necessity for placebo controls when no difference or only a modest treatment difference is expected between therapies being compared. Separating bias from a true treatment effect demands attention to methodological detail; a small error in the estimate of treatment effect that occurs throughout a trial cannot be later compensated for by a large sample size. On the other hand, placebo controls may be unnecessary, depending on the methodology and classification of the clinical trial.

## General classification of trials

Clinical trials are designed for one of two primary reasons. *Explanatory* or *scientific* trials bring understanding about a biological or psychological mechanism of disease activity or therapeutic intervention. These trials are sized to allow definitive acceptance or refutation of a hypothesis. Typically, a relatively small sample size and detailed collection of data are required. The inclusion and exclusion criteria for patient participation are usually constructed to exclude patients with confounding conditions and to maximize the ability to measure differences with respect to the outcome of interest. Economies of scale are normally not an issue in explanatory trials.

*Pragmatic* or *evaluative* trials inform health care patients, providers, and payers about the preferred diagnostic or treatment strategy when comparing alternatives. Since these trials are designed to educate the clinical practice, the selection of endpoints is determined by outcome qualities that would allow patients and providers to make rational decisions about which strategy to choose and allow payers to determine which strategies should be paid for.

Experience with pragmatic trials has demonstrated that there is no substitute for measuring the outcomes most important to patients: living longer, feeling better, spending less money, and avoiding unpleasant experiences. These trials must make an effort to enrol a patient population reflective of the patients who would actually receive the treatment rather than a "pristine" population free of confounding problems. When the treatment is designed to prevent major negative clinical outcomes or long-term manifestations of a disease, a large sample size is frequently needed. This review focuses on the use of placebo in such large, pragmatic trials.

## Two circumstances of placebo use

In placebo controlled trials, a matching placebo (or sham procedure) is made for the active treatment. The placebo looks and tastes like the active treatment, and it is administered in the same fashion. In active control trials, a "double dummy" procedure is often used. In this procedure, matching placebo is made for each active treatment, so that the patient receives four treatments (each active treatment and its placebo). This technique allows masking of the assigned treatment.

Table 13.1 Criteria for use of placebo in pragmatic trials.

| Less likely to use placebo | Criterion | More likely to use placebo |
|---|---|---|
| Objective, particularly mortality | Type of endpoint | Subjective |
| Different ancillary therapy required in each arm of trial | Medical and behavioral context | No interactions with other complex regimens |
| No concerns about strong investigator preference | – | Charged environment regarding treatment |
| Alternative treatment already proven effective | Ethical context | No proven effective treatment for the disease |
| Placebo use would make study too expensive | Cost to the study | Tolerable |
| Allow alternative design | Attitude of regulator | Placebo required |

## Deciding whether to use a placebo

Using placebo in large clinical trials creates logistical, financial, and methodological difficulties, but the major arguments for placebo are twofold. First, the use of placebo allows the treatment assignment to be masked, thereby preventing bias on the part of the patient or the investigators. Second, when a matching placebo is used in a pharmacological trial or a sham procedure for a device evaluation, both treatments reap the outcome consequences of the placebo effect. Ideally, in a large, placebo controlled trial, the difference in outcomes in the two randomized groups reflects equal influence of placebo effect in each group. As a result, the difference in outcome between the comparison groups is simply due to the treatment itself.

Unfortunately, almost no empirical research exists to allow quantification of the decision criteria for using placebo, so in the end a subjective judgment is made. For pragmatic trials, the decision process may include a series of considerations that can be evaluated formally (Table 13.1). The following considerations also are involved in evaluating the need for placebo in a specific clinical trial.

### Type of endpoints

Two characteristics of the type of endpoint may be considered: its measurability by independent observers and its objectivity. Less bias will be present when endpoints are measured by observers who are independent of the patients and investigators and blinded to the patients' treatment assignments. Therefore, the use of independent observers presents a strong argument for not requiring placebo. For example, in the measurement of the endpoints of myocardial infarction (MI), stroke, or severe recurrent ischemia, clinical events committees[3] have become the usual accepted practice, even in blinded trials. These committees review data documenting suspected events in a blinded fashion, leading to uniform criteria for event classification. Similarly, when an imaging endpoint is critical as in studies of fractures, a blinded imaging core laboratory can provide objectivity even when placebo is not used.

Large clinical trials often are oriented toward the measurement of objective, irreversible endpoints. Placebo is less valuable with highly objective endpoints than with subjective endpoints, since subjective bias in the assessment of an objective endpoint is less likely. The most objective, unarguable endpoint is death; this outcome is seldom disputed even with knowledge of the treatment assignment (although the availability of organ transplantation and mechanical organ assist devices has made this more complex[4]). Thus, when time to death is the critical endpoint measurement, bias in the endpoint's ascertainment by the investigators is unlikely. Even patients who are otherwise lost to follow up can be accounted for eventually using the National Death Index.[5]

Furthermore, while substantial documentation exists about the impact of the placebo effect on subjectively perceived outcomes, little data exist about its impact on mortality. As such, if the outcome of interest is death, using placebo may not be required. However, if the outcome of interest is death from a specific cause, there is potential for subjective bias in determining the cause.[6] This bias may be best prevented by using placebo to avoid any risk that those classifying the event would allow knowledge of the treatment assignment to impact their judgment.

Discrete non-fatal clinical events can be defined in a relatively objective manner, although most diagnostic algorithms are less objective than commonly believed. When investigators judge whether or not a non-fatal MI has occurred in trials of acute coronary syndromes, the number of events is consistently underestimated, although a relatively objective standard is used.[7] Similarly, the diagnosis of stroke can be difficult, even with brain imaging.[8] In addition, the investigator's discretion regarding the timing of laboratory measurements or of the patient's admission into the hospital allows many patients to have missing data or fragments of data that are suggestive, but not conclusive. While conscious bias is highly unlikely in a pragmatic clinical trial and one would have to postulate a large conspiracy in multicenter trials to entertain the notion of biased assessment, subconscious bias in ascertainment of the endpoint is always a worry. Placebo takes care of this concern.

The most troublesome outcomes with regard to subjective bias are symptoms and quality of life. Patients and providers who are aware of the treatment assignment may be more likely to report subjective improvement or side effects expected from the treatment. Furthermore, the placebo effect may have a significant impact on subjectively perceived outcomes. Thus, investigators should use placebo to prevent subjective assessment of these outcomes and to control for the placebo effect.

### Medical and behavioral context

The second important point in considering when to use placebo focuses on the medical and behavioral context of the trial. When clinical behavior changes as a result of the insertion of a placebo into a trial, scientific concerns may exist about using placebo. For example, these concerns may be present in trials investigating infused antithrombotic medications (or other therapies) when additional therapy should be different as a result of the initial randomization. When a patient is in a blinded study, it is likely that the investigator will infuse the study drug at a lower threshold than if the treatment is known, since uncertainty about an experimental treatment leads to anxiety about the potential outcome. Similarly, as combinations of therapies become more common, circumstances will increase in which coadministration of a second treatment with one of the experimental drugs (but not the other) is relatively contraindicated. In these situations, employing placebo would lead to less than the best practice pattern for patient care.

It is also important to factor the motivation of study participants into the equation. Patients, investigators, or both can have strong biases for or against particular therapies. When a strong bias exists for the benefit of a treatment, placebo is particularly important. This argument can be illustrated by recent studies of two mechanical approaches developed to relieve angina in patients with refractory angina pectoris: transmyocardial laser revascularization (TMR)[9] and percutaneous myocardial laser revascularization (PMLR).[10,11] Both procedures create channels in the myocardium using a laser, but TMR requires open chest surgery while PMLR uses a percutaneous device.

Initial studies of TMR did not use a sham procedure. In one of the first major device trials, the primary endpoint was angina status, a subjective endpoint that was assessed by surgeons who had performed the procedures or by their co-ordinators. The trial was markedly positive, although many of the participating surgeons had an equity interest in the company that developed the device. A subsequent trial using a percutaneous method of myocardial laser revascularization used a sham laser treatment in the randomized controls. The results of this trial showed an improvement in angina status in both groups with no difference in outcomes between the groups.*

---

* Leon MB. A randomized blinded clinical trial comparing percutaneous laser myocardial revascularization (using biosense LV mapping) vs placebo in patients with refractory coronary ischemia. Presented at: Annual Meeting of the American Heart Association, New Orleans, LA, November 13–16, 2000.

## Ethical context

While ethics are not purely separable from any particular component of a clinical trial in deciding whether or not to use a placebo control in a clinical trial, one must ask if using a placebo is ethical for that specific trial. In many instances, the answer is clear. If a treatment with proven effectiveness exists for the disease to be studied, randomizing patients to placebo is generally not ethical, whenever doing so would risk harm to the patients.[12] However, proven effectiveness is a relative term, and the extent of evidence supporting this effectiveness must be scrutinized. For example, if the proof is derived from large, randomized clinical trials applicable to the relevant patient population, it constitutes solid evidence and precludes the use of placebo in the study in question. If the proof is derived from poorly designed or poorly conducted clinical trials or from retrospective analyses, it does not constitute solid evidence and use of placebo in that setting is permissible.

Even if equipoise (uncertainty about which treatment is better) is present regarding the treatments to be compared, placebo use is questionable if it entails known increased risk of harm to research subjects. In trials of fibrinolytic therapy, concern exists about the delays in treatment time induced by the use of double dummy placebo infusions. Although a recent analysis indicated that this delay may be as short as 10 minutes, the ethical constraint is important since delay in treatment clearly increases the risk of death.[13] Similarly, the use of sham device procedures is a complex issue because of the risk associated with the procedure itself with no opportunity for patient benefit.

However, placebo controls, when appropriate, are preferred to active controls due to the scientific uncertainty inherent to equivalence (non-inferiority) trials.[14,15] Accordingly, it has been argued that if research subjects are not likely to be harmed by receiving placebo and they give voluntary informed consent, administering placebo could be permissible in some studies despite the existence of a known effective therapy.[16]

On the other hand, the likelihood of no harm is often assumed rather than proven, which raises concerns about the use of placebo in many clinical trials including short-term clinical trials of peptic ulcer disease, diabetes, and hypertension.[17–19] Thus, it is essential to prove that the use of placebo in such trials is safe. In that regard, we conducted a meta-analysis of short-term, placebo controlled clinical trials of hypertension to assess the safety of placebo use.[20] Indeed, a short period of placebo in patients with mild hypertension was found to cause no discoverable increase in clinical events. Similar analyses may help provide safety data essential in making informed decisions about the appropriate selection of controls.

## Cost to the study

In almost every situation, a placebo controlled trial is more costly to implement than a trial comparing usual care without a placebo. Not only is there a cost to manufacturing the placebo, but its distribution and accounting can induce an additional substantial cost, at both the clinical site and the co-ordinating center. Furthermore, the use of placebo may induce expenses in the context of the protocol since extra personnel will be required and extra procedures may be needed to monitor therapy in a blinded fashion.

In large trials, the placebo's manufacturing and packaging can be considerably expensive. The placebo may be difficult or impossible to make or buy. Typically, the manufacturer of an active drug also is contracted to make the placebo, and in some cases this manufacturer is the only entity with a placebo formulation for the active drug. Thus, when the manufacturer is not interested in the study, the placebo may not be available, and making new placebo is an expensive endeavor.

In addition, the cost of manufacturing and packaging will rise in trials involving an infusion or multiple titration steps. The trial also would pay for the logistical requirements needed to account for the placebo at the clinical site and the co-ordinating center. In trials of intravenous treatment of acute illnesses, this task often results in the hanging of an additional double dummy infusion at a different rate of infusion with different mixing instructions. This burden can double the cost of the trial at the clinical site due to the extra nursing and pharmacy time required. In pharmacological trials evaluating long-term therapy, the situation can become complex when the active treatment needs to be monitored and the dose adjusted or titrated. In one ongoing trial, an active control trial with a double dummy involves thrice daily pills with active control and allowance for both up titration and down titration depending upon blood pressure.[21]

In some cases, sham titrations of the placebo are required. For placebo controlled trials of oral anticoagulation, the coagulation status is typically monitored in a blinded fashion, and control patients are randomly titrated to a different dose of placebo at a rate consistent with the titration requirements of the actively treated group.

As a result of these financial issues, when the choice for the control is between placebo and usual care, investigators may have to decide between using placebo with a marginal sample size or not using placebo but having an adequate sample size. On the other hand, when choosing between a placebo control and an active control when either is appropriate, a placebo controlled trial generally requires a smaller sample size and costs less.

**Attitude of regulators**

Most large clinical trials are either completely or partially funded by the medical products industry, and therefore the conduct of such trials is under the purview of the medical products regulatory authorities. In the current environment, the decisions made by regulators have a major influence on decisions about all aspects of the conduct of international trials. Most of the industry takes a conservative posture with regard to regulatory advice as a result of the high cost of completing a trial and having it invalidated by the regulators because of the claims needed for marketing medical products. Given the legal requirements' stringency for product marketing, the regulators also have a tendency to be conservative. As discussed in Chapter 10, regulators are driven by these requirements to focus on distinguishing active treatment from no treatment rather than comparing active treatments.[22]

The advent of the International Conference on Harmonization (ICH) has been helpful in establishing general approaches to controls in clinical trials.[23,24] The ICH guidelines even leave room for not using placebo in constructing a randomized or a non-randomized control group. It has been possible, as described in the following examples, to effectively use these opportunities for flexibility in the design of large, pragmatic trials with the goal of obtaining regulatory approval for product marketing.

*Large, simple mortality trials*

Fibrinolytic therapy is a medical approach to the opening of a coronary artery completely occluded by a thrombus. The cardinal manifestation of this problem is ST segment elevation on the electrocardiogram (ECG) associated with typical symptoms. MI heralded by elevation of the ST segment of the ECG carries a mortality of 6–10% at 30 days in patients eligible for clinical trials.[25,26]

The Global Utilization of Streptokinase and Tissue plasminogen activator for Occluded coronary arteries (GUSTO-I) trial[27] was mounted to compare the mortality effects of an accelerated administration of alteplase compared with a standard administration of streptokinase. The study was conducted in a highly charged medical environment in which claims had been made about both treatments, and the press had developed a fascination with the topic. The infusion regimen of each agent was different, as was the likely need for supportive therapy during the infusion. Furthermore, the use of other anticoagulation (intravenous versus subcutaneous heparin) was different by protocol.

A precedent had been set in this field by previous trials of fibrinolytic therapy. The Second International Study of Infarct Survival (ISIS-2) study[28] compared streptokinase with usual care, while the companion Gruppo Italiano per lo Studio della Sopravvivenza nell'Infarto Miocardico (GISSI-2) study[29] compared streptokinase with placebo. Each study found a significant benefit of streptokinase with a similar order of magnitude.[30]

After consideration of the relevant issues, it was decided to conduct GUSTO-I as an open-label, comparative study. The primary endpoint was mortality at 30 days, and all participants were comfortable that this endpoint could not be altered based on perceptions by the patients or investigators. A key secondary endpoint was non-fatal stroke, a more subjective component. A brain image was required for every patient with a focal neurological deficit, and these scans were read by a blinded committee in conjunction with a summary of the clinical scenario.[31] The medical logistics to conduct a blinded study with these regimens would have been unacceptable, and the cost would have made the study impossible to conduct. When presented with a proposal on study conduct, the regulators demonstrated considerable flexibility in allowing this study to be unblinded with quantitative documentation of the quality of the study conduct at all levels, including the stroke events review committee.

In the Global Utilization of Strategies To Open occluded coronary arteries (GUSTO-III) trial,[32] a genetically modified t-PA, reteplase, could be administered by a double bolus rather than an infusion. The primary endpoint was mortality, and the critical secondary endpoint was stroke that was adjudicated by a stroke assessment committee. The medical environment was quite different from the GUSTO-I study; there was no reason to believe that investigators would be biased toward one treatment over the other. Again, with the agreement of the regulators, a decision was made to conduct the study as an open-label study without placebo for each active agent, permitting it to be conducted with a larger sample size and a budget allowing the study to be done.

The Assessment of the Safety and Efficacy of a New Thrombolytic agent (ASSENT-2) trial[33] had the same issues as GUSTO-III. Tenecteplase is a biologically modified t-PA with a longer half life and greater fibrin specificity. The goal of ASSENT-2 was to conduct a non-inferiority trial with 30-day death as the primary endpoint. Although blinding had all of the logistical difficulties as in GUSTO-III, the sponsor of the trial was willing to bear the extra cost of blinding. In this case, the same sponsor owned t-PA (the standard) and tenecteplase (the experimental agent). ASSENT-2 was done as a blinded, double dummy trial.

*Complex outcomes in trials investigating acute coronary syndromes*

When the epicardial vessel is not occluded but the patient has symptoms of acute myocardial ischemia, the patient may have a non-ST elevation acute coronary syndrome.[34] This syndrome has a lower mortality risk in the acute phase compared with ST elevation MI, making mortality reduction an unlikely target for therapy. Therefore acute therapies are expected to improve a broader array of clinical outcomes.

In the Global Use of Strategies To Open occluded coronary arteries[35] (GUSTO-IIa) and the Platelet Glycoprotein IIb/IIIa in Unstable Angina: Receptor Suppression Using Integrilin Therapy[36] (PURSUIT) trials, antithrombotic agents were given either in comparison with heparin[35] or in addition to aspirin and heparin.[36] The primary endpoint in both studies was a composite of death or non-fatal MI. Key secondary endpoints included time until revascularization, stroke, and cost. The medical environment was not highly charged on the best treatment, and no reason for bias was evident. While cost was an issue in both trials, in neither case did the commercial sponsor balk at the additional cost to ensure blinding, and it was the expectation of the regulators that both trials would be blinded.

GUSTO-IIa[35] used a double dummy technique in which patients were treated with heparin and placebo infusion or hirudin and placebo infusion. In addition, MI and stroke endpoints were adjudicated by an independent data and safety monitoring committee. The blinding was made easier because both infusions were monitored with the activated partial thromboplastin time (aPTT) with similar therapeutic ranges. Dose adjustments were made using a prespecified algorithm.

The PURSUIT[36] trial used a placebo control versus experimental agent on top of standard therapy. The medical environment was conducive, although a major logistical issue arose when patients were referred for either surgery or percutaneous coronary intervention. In the case of surgery, serious concerns about bleeding led to the need for a rapid system to allow unblinding. With percutaneous intervention, a member of the class of drugs being evaluated (glycoprotein IIb/IIIa inhibitors) was already available for clinical use to improve the outcomes of percutaneous intervention.[37] At the time of PURSUIT, the use of glycoprotein IIb/IIIa inhibitors was not widespread enough to have a major impact on the trial. However, later trials with orally administered glycoprotein IIb/IIIa inhibitors[38] required a double dummy second administration of oral antiplatelet therapy, which added complications.

*Placebo effect in trials with biological therapies*

Patients with major depression can be treated with a variety of biological therapies, some of which are regulated by the FDA and some of which are not. The placebo effect is substantial, and the subjective bias can be a major factor in the assessment of outcomes. The behavioral research community has developed sophisticated methods to deal with these issues, including an adamant adherence to the use of placebo controls and multiple measurements prior to enrolment to reduce the regression to the mean phenomenon.

In an ongoing trial coordinated by the Duke Clinical Research Institute (DCRI), the manufacturer of one of the active comparators refused to provide placebo for the trial until extreme pressure was exerted. When the steering committee added titration steps to the protocol, the financial impact on the packaging and distribution was not considered until it became evident that the study budget was inadequate. Furthermore, the packaging facility for the study had to return the initial batch of placebo because it was contaminated. Eventually all of these logistical issues were resolved, and the study is currently nearing completion.

As discussed in the section on TMR and PMLR, interest in growth of new blood vessels has been intense. The Phase II studies with intravenously administered growth factors showed an improvement in anginal symptoms and exercise capacity in treated patients, but no control groups were used.[39,40] The medical environment favoring an improvement in these subjective endpoints was clear. To be eligible for the early trials, patients were required to have refractory angina with no other options. When a placebo controlled trial was done with one of the growth factors,[41] both groups improved in exercise time and anginal status, and no significant difference was found between groups. Subsequent trials have used placebo controls with the concurrence of the investigators, sponsors, and regulators.

*Percutaneous coronary intervention*

In the setting of percutaneous coronary intervention, the adjunctive pharmacology used before, during, and after the procedure is an integral part of achieving procedural success. The glycoprotein IIb/IIIa platelet inhibitors were developed for this purpose and have established substantial success in preventing death and MI.[37] The most effective agent in this class of drugs has been abciximab, a chimeric Fab fragment of a monoclonal antibody against the glycoprotein IIb/IIIa receptor; abciximab is expensive, but it meets the general criteria for cost-effectiveness, with a cost per year of life saved of under $15 000.[42] Cost considerations, however, led many interventional cardiologists to implant coronary stents without the protection of the glycoprotein IIb/IIIa inhibitor. Indeed, less than half of patients treated with coronary stenting were being treated with adjunctive glycoprotein IIb/IIIa inhibition.

Eptifibatide is a less expensive glycoprotein IIb/IIIa inhibitor that, initially, did not have results as profound as those shown with abciximab in clinical trials,[43] but further pharmacokinetic analysis revealed that the dose administered in these trials may have been inadequate. Thus, a decision was made to conduct a more definitive trial to demonstrate eptifibatide's efficacy. Because the study involved a somewhat subjective endpoint of myocardial necrosis and the subject area was associated with highly charged emotions and strong clinical opinions, it was decided to design the trial as placebo controlled. The situation was complex because of the definitive evidence that the *class* was beneficial, with resultant labeling by the US Food and Drug Administration (FDA) reflecting this benefit. In extensive discussions with the clinical community, many prominent cardiologists strongly believed that a placebo controlled trial was necessary because the cost of the proven effective treatment made it prohibitive for routine treatment. These discussions also included some debate about the clinical importance of reduction in markers of myocardial damage.

The FDA initially ruled that the proposed trial did not meet ethical standards, but based on input from independent ethicists and extensive surveys assessing the views of the clinical community, the decision was made to proceed with a placebo controlled trial (JE Tcheng, MD, unpublished data, 2000). The surveys showed that a glycoprotein IIb/IIIa inhibitor was used in less than 25% of cases: 90% of cardiologists surveyed believed the cost was "too high" and 58% were not convinced of the drug's cost-effectiveness. The trial was undertaken and was stopped early by the Data and Safety Monitoring Committee because of a clear benefit.[44] The result was accepted by the clinical community, but questions have been raised by the European regulatory authorities about whether the trial should have been stopped prematurely. This trial points out the complexity of decisionmaking about placebo in pragmatic trials and the difficulties that may arise as a function of those decisions.

## Needed research

Surprisingly little research has been done on the use of placebo in large, clinical trials. Indeed, such research would seem to be a critical component of improving the current methodology of clinical trials, given the cost and the societal implications associated with failure of a large, pragmatic trial to provide a correct or definitive answer to a clinical question. Since these trials have a profound impact on treatment choices for large numbers of patients, this area deserves focused attention.

Do the results of trials with "hard" outcomes differ when placebo controls are used? The potential for bias to impact the assessment of subjective endpoints is self-evident, and empirical findings support the importance of the use of placebo in these situations. However, we have less reason to believe that placebo would provide a more objective test in a mortality trial. It would be useful to conduct more mortality trials with placebo control in half the patients and usual care without placebo in the remainder.

Does the placebo effect extend beyond subjective endpoints to hard endpoints of survival and clinical events? Separately from the question of bias in the assessment of endpoints, the question of whether the placebo effect is relevant for clinical events remains unanswered. The above described trial, in which half of a trial has a placebo control and the other half has a usual care control, would provide insight into whether a patient treated with placebo has a lower risk of dying or experiencing a stroke or MI than a patient not receiving placebo.

Because of the increasing push for adequately sized trials and the rising cost of placebo use, there is an urgent need to develop a better understanding of the impact of placebo on the results of pragmatic trials. In an increasing number of cases, a critical issue in a trial's design will hinge on the question of whether the trial can be done at all or after careful consideration is made of the trade-off between using placebo and having an adequate sample size.

In conclusion, large, pragmatic trials have become a necessary and vital part of the societal mandate for the practice of evidence-based medicine.

Whereas every large trial involving placebo is subjected to great scrutiny, many trialists are unaware of the complex logistical and cost issues derivative of the choices made about placebo. Furthermore, almost no empirical research exists to influence the choices that are made. While the research imperative is clear, in the interim, a set of trial and endpoint attributes can be used to make a reasonable decision regarding the use of placebo.

# References

1 Cairns JA, Gent M, Singer J, *et al.* Aspirin, sulfinpyrazone, or both in unstable angina. Results of a Canadian multicenter trial. *N Engl J Med* 1985;**313**:1369–75.

2 The Cardiac Arrhythmia Suppression Trial (CAST) Investigators. Preliminary report: effect of encainide and flecainide on mortality in a randomized trial of arrhythmia suppression after myocardial infarction. *N Engl J Med* 1989;**61**:501–9.

3 Mahaffey KW, Granger CB, Woodlief L, Tardiff BE, Bandy S, Califf R. Centralized systematic adjudication of clinical endpoints in multicenter trials of acute coronary syndromes identifies patients at high risk for adverse clinical outcomes [abstract]. *J Am Coll Cardiol* 1996;**27**:250A–1A.

4 Shah MR, O'Connor CM, Sopko G, Hasselblad V, Califf RM, and Stevenson L. Evaluation Study of Congestive heart failure and Pulmonary artery catheterization Effectiveness (ESCAPE): design and rationale. *Am Heart J* 2001;**141**:528–35.

5 Bilgrad R. *National Death Index User's Manual.* Hyattsville, MD: US Dept of Health and Human Services, Centers for Disease Control and Prevention, National Center for Health Statistics, 1997.

6 Temple R, Pledger GW. The FDA's critique of the anturane reinfarction trial. *N Engl J Med* 1980;**303**:1488–92.

7 Mark DB, Harrington RA, Lincoff AM, *et al.* Cost-effectiveness of platelet glycoprotein IIb/IIIa inhibition with eptifibatide in patients with non-ST-elevation acute coronary syndromes. *Circulation* 1999;**101**:366–71.

8 Mahaffey KW, Granger CB, Sloan MA, *et al.* Risk factors for in-hospital nonhemorrhagic stroke in patients with acute myocardial infarction treated with thrombolysis. Results from GUSTO-I. *Circulation* 1998;**97**:757–64.

9 Cooley DA, Frazier OH, Kadipasaoglu KA, *et al.* Transmyocardial laser revascularization: clinical experience with twelve-month follow-up. *J Thorac Cardiovasc Surg* 1996;**111**:791–9.

10 Burkhoff D, Schmidt S, Schulman SP, *et al.* Transmyocardial laser revascularisation compared with continued medical therapy for treatment of refractory angina pectoris: a prospective randomised trial. *Lancet* 1999;**354**:885–90.

11 Schofield PM, Sharples LD, Caine N, *et al.* Transmyocardial laser revascularisation in patients with refractory angina: a randomised controlled trial. *Lancet* 1999;**353**:519–24.

12 Lavori PW. Placebo control groups in randomized treatment trials: a statistician's perspective. *Biol Psychiatry* 2000;**47**:717–23.

13 Newby LK, Rutsch WR, Califf RM, *et al.* Time from symptom onset to treatment and outcomes after thrombolytic therapy. GUSTO-1 Investigators. *J Am Coll Cardiol* 1996;**27**:1646–55.

14 Temple R, Ellenberg SS. Placebo controlled trials and active-control trials in the evaluation of new treatments. Part 1: ethical and scientific issues. *Ann Intern Med* 2000;**133**:455–63.

15 Pocock SJ. The pros and cons of non-inferiority (equivalence) trials. This volume, chapter 12.

16 Ellenberg SS, Temple R. Placebo controlled trials and active-control trials in the evaluation of new treatments. Part 2: practical issues and specific cases. *Ann Intern Med* 2000;**133**:464–70.

17 Peterson WL. Pharmacotherapy of bleeding peptic ulcer – is it time to give up the search? *Gastroenterology* 1989;**97**:796–7.

18 Maggs DG, Buchanan TA, Burant CF, *et al.* Metabolic effects of troglitazone monotherapy in type 2 diabetes mellitus. A randomized, double blind, placebo controlled trial. *Ann Intern Med* 1998;**128**:176–85.

19 Rothman KJ, Michels KB. The continuing unethical use of placebo controls. *N Engl J Med* 1994;**331**:394–8.

20 Al-Khatib SM, Califf RM, Hasselblad V, Alexander JH, *et al.* Placebo-controls in short-term clinical trials of hypertension. *Science* 2001;**292**:2013–15.

21 Pfeffer MA, McMurray J, Leizorovicz A, *et al.* Valsartan in acute myocardial infarction trial (VALIANT): rationale and design. *Am Heart J* 2000;**140**:727–50.

22 Temple RJ. Placebo controlled trials and active controlled trials: ethics and inference. This volume, chapter 10.

23 Dixon JR Jr. The International Conference on Harmonization, good clinical practice guideline. *Qual Assur* 1998;**6**:65–74.

24 O'Neill RT. Statistical concepts in the planning and evaluation of drug safety from clinical trials in drug development: issues of international harmonization. *Stat Med* 1995;**14**:117–27.

25 Peterson ED, Shaw LJ, Califf RM. Risk stratification after myocardial infarction. *Ann Intern Med* 1997;**126**:561–82.

26 Lee KL, Woodlief LH, Topol EJ, *et al.* Predictors of 30-day mortality in the era of reperfusion for acute myocardial infarction: results from an international trial of 41021 patients. *Circulation* 1995;**91**:1659–68.

27 The GUSTO Investigators. An international randomized trial comparing four thrombolytic strategies for acute myocardial infarction. *N Engl J Med* 1993;**329**:673–82.

28 ISIS-2 (Second International Study of Infarct Survival) Collaborative Group. Randomised trial of intravenous streptokinase, oral aspirin, both, or neither among 17 187 cases of suspected acute myocardial infarction: ISIS-2. *Lancet* 1988;**2**:349–60.

29 Gruppo Italiano per lo Studio della Sopravvivenza nell'Infarto Miocardico. GISSI-2: A factorial randomised trial of alteplase versus streptokinase and heparin versus no heparin among 12 490 patients with acute myocardial infarction. *Lancet* 1990;**336**:65–71.

30 Fibronolytic Therapy Trialists' (FTT) Collaborative Group. Indications for fibrinolytic therapy in suspected acute myocardial infarction: collaborative overview of early mortality and major morbidity results from all randomized trials of more than 1 000 patients. *Lancet* 1994;**343**:311–22.

31 Gore JM, Granger CB, Sloan MA, *et al.*, for the GUSTO-I Investigators. Stroke after thrombolysis: mortality and functional outcomes in the GUSTO-I trial. *Circulation* 1995;**92**:2811–18.

32 The Global Use of Strategies to Open Occluded Coronary Arteries (GUSTO III) Investigators. A comparison of reteplase with alteplase for acute myocardial infarction. *N Engl J Med* 1997;**333**:1118–23.

33 The Assessment of the Safety and Efficacy of a New Thrombolytic (ASSENT-2) Investigators. Single-bolus tenecteplase compared with front-loaded alteplase in acute myocardial infarction: the ASSENT-2 double blind randomised trial. *Lancet* 1999; **354**:716–22.

34 Braunwald E, Antman EM, Beasley JW, *et al.* ACC/AHA guidelines for the management of patients with unstable angina and non-ST-segment elevation myocardial infarction. A report of the American College of Cardiology/American Heart Association Task Force on Practice Guidelines (Committee on the Management of Patients With Unstable Angina). *J Am Coll Cardiol* 2000;**36**:970–1062.

35 The Global Use of Strategies to Open Occluded Coronary Arteries (GUSTO) IIa Investigators. Randomized trial of intravenous heparin versus recombinant hirudin for acute coronary syndromes. *Circulation* 1994;**90**:1631–7.

36 The PURSUIT Trial Investigators. Inhibition of platelet glycoprotein IIb/IIIa with eptifibatide in patients with acute coronary syndromes. *N Engl J Med* 1998;**339**:436–43.

37 Kong DF, Califf RM, Miller DP, *et al.* Outcomes of therapeutic agents that block the platelet glycoprotein IIb/IIIa integrin in ischemic heart disease. *Circulation* 1998; **98**:2829–35.

38 The SYMPHONY Investigators. Comparison of sibrafiban with aspirin for prevention of cardiovascular events after acute coronary syndromes: a randomised trial. *Lancet* 2000; **355**:337–45.

39 Simons M, Bonow RO, Chronos NA, *et al.* Clinical trials in coronary angiogenesis: issues, problems, consensus: An expert panel summary. *Circulation* 2000;**102**:E73–86.

40 Hendel RC, Henry TD, Rocha-Singh K, *et al.* Effect of intracoronary recombinant human vascular endothelial growth factor on myocardial perfusion: evidence for a dose-dependent effect. *Circulation* 2000;**101**:118–21.
41 Lefkovits J, Plow EF, Topol EJ. Platelet glycoprotein IIb/IIIa receptors in cardiovascular medicine. *N Engl J Med* 1995;**332**:1553–9.
42 Topol EJ, Mark DB, Lincoff AM. Outcomes at 1 year and economic implications of platelet glycoprotein IIb/IIIa blockade in patients undergoing coronary stenting: results from a multicentre randomised trial. EPISTENT Investigators. Evaluation of Platelet IIb/IIIa Inhibitor for Stenting. *Lancet* 1999;**354**:2019–24.
43 Kong DF, Califf RM. Glycoprotein IIb/IIIa receptor antagonists in non-ST-segment elevation acute coronary syndromes and percutaneous revascularisation: a review of trial reports. *Drugs* 1999;**58**:609–20.
44 The ESPRIT Investigators. Novel dosing regimen of eptifibatide in planned coronary stent implantation (ESPRIT): a randomised, placebo controlled trial. Enhanced Suppression of the Platelet IIb/IIIa Receptor with Integrilin Therapy. *Lancet* 2000; **356**:2037–44.

# 14: Placebo controls in clinical trials of new therapies for conditions for which there are known effective treatments

ROBERT J LEVINE*


## Summary

The use of placebos as controls in research designed to assess the efficacy of therapeutic or preventive agents is highly controversial. This chapter is concerned with only one part of this debate: the ethical justification of placebo controls in the evaluation of therapies for diseases or conditions for which there exists a therapy known to be at least partially effective. This analysis entails a consideration of the anti-placebo stance of the *Declaration of Helsinki* as well as the closely related position held by some commentators that use of placebo as controls rather than known effective therapy is a violation of the physician's ethical duty to provide only the best known therapy for the patient. The anti-placebo position of Helsinki was clearly established in Article II.3 of the 1996 version of the Declaration (Helsinki V). Although the most recent revision (Helsinki VI) is widely heralded as having strengthened Helsinki's anti-placebo position a careful examination of the document indicates no substantive change on this point.

In many cases, the "best proven therapeutic methods" are prohibitively expensive for use in low resource countries. These countries require the assistance of sponsors and investigators from the wealthy countries to develop inexpensive and affordable alternatives. The placebo controlled trials of the short duration regimen of AZT for the prevention of perinatal transmission


* Acknowledgement: This work was supported in part by grant number POI MH/DA 56 826–01A1 from the National Institute of Mental Health and the National Institute on Drug Abuse.

of HIV are presented as a case study which illustrates the ways in which strict adherence to Helsinki will deprive developing countries of the much-needed assistance of sponsors and investigators from wealthy countries.

A brief review of the history of Helsinki indicates that its anti-placebo position is closely related to that taken by some commentators that use of placebo controls in place of therapies known to be at least partially effective violates the fiduciary responsibility of the physician to provide only the best known therapy for the patient. A counter argument is offered. The two major flaws that provided the stimulus for the recent revision of Helsinki remain uncorrected: the distinction between therapeutic and non-therapeutic research and the excessively rigid proscription of placebo controls. I see no reason to suspect that the current iteration of these flawed articles in Helsinki VI will command any more respect than did their predecessors. This paper concludes with recommendations for criteria for the ethical justification of placebo controls in randomized clinical trials.

## Introduction

The use of placebos as controls in research designed to assess the efficacy of therapeutic or preventive agents is highly controversial. This chapter is concerned with only one part of this debate: the ethical justification of placebo controls in the evaluation of therapies for diseases or conditions for which there exists a therapy known to be at least partially effective. This analysis of this justification will entail a consideration of the anti-placebo stance of the *Declaration of Helsinki* as well as the closely related position held by some commentators that use of placebo as controls rather than known effective therapy is a violation of the physician's ethical duty to provide only the best known therapy for the patient.

The *Declaration of Helsinki* has recently been revised extensively. This revision was accomplished in response to two major criticisms:[1]

1. that the document was logically flawed as are all documents that rely on the spurious distinction between therapeutic and non-therapeutic research
2. it was alleged that its position on the ethical justification of placebos was equivocal and susceptible to differing interpretations.

Let us begin with a consideration of Helsinki's position on placebo controls as reflected in the fifth edition of the *Declaration of Helsinki* (1996). Then we shall consider the revisions in this position embodied in the most recent sixth edition (2000); these will be called Helsinki V and VI respectively.[2] This appraisal will yield the conclusions that the position on placebo was not ambiguous in the 1996 edition and that it changed very little, if at all, in the 2000 version.

## Helsinki V on placebo

In Helsinki V, Article II.3 established the "best proven therapeutic method" as the standard requirement for all patients who serve as research subjects:

> II.3 In any medical study, every patient – including those of a control group, if any – should be assured of the best proven diagnostic and therapeutic method. This does not exclude the use of inert placebo in studies where no proven diagnostic or therapeutic method exists.

The implications of this article extend far beyond the use of placebo controls in clinical trials. This article, if strictly applied, would rule out the development of all new therapies for conditions for which there are already existing "proven" therapies. One cannot evaluate a new therapy unless you withhold those that have already been demonstrated safe and effective for the same indication. Strict application of this standard would have prevented the evaluation of the effectiveness of cimetidine and other $H_2$ receptor antagonists for the treatment of peptic ulcer because the withholding of belladonna and its derivatives would have been considered an unethical withholding of the "best proven therapeutic method". Similarly, the development of new and improved antihypertensive drugs would have ceased with the establishment of the ganglionic blockers.

Article II.3 also forbids placebo controls in clinical trials in which there is virtually no risk from withholding proven therapy. Consider research in the field of analgesics and antihistamines. No experienced person would ever recommend that you are required to have an active control in the evaluation of a new analgesic. Article II.3 also rules out the use of placebo controls in clinical trials in which there is a very remote possibility of a serious adverse consequence of withholding the active drug, such as trials of new antihypertensives and of new oral hypoglycemic agents. Insisting on active controls in these areas would introduce major inefficiencies with virtually no compensating benefit; the amount of injury to research subjects that would be prevented by requiring active controls is so small that it can be and generally is considered negligible.

Placebo controlled trials of analgesics, antihypertensives and oral hypoglycemics are conducted commonly and the results are published in reputable, peer reviewed medical journals. Parenthetically, it is worth noticing that such publication is a violation of Helsinki; Article I.8 (Helsinki V) and Article 27 (Helsinki VI) hold that: "Reports of experimentation not in accordance with the principles laid down in this Declaration should not be accepted for publication".

The most controversial interpretation of Article II.3 is that it requires the provision of the best proven therapeutic method that is available in the industrialized countries even when conducting research in countries in which such therapy is not available. This interpretation provoked the most acrimonious debate in the field of research ethics since the 1970s. The debate began with the publication in the *New England Journal of Medicine* of an article that denounced as unethical the clinical trials that were being carried out in several countries to evaluate the effectiveness of the short duration regimen of AZT in preventing perinatal transmission of HIV infection.[3] The editor of the journal opined that these trials were, in certain respects, reminiscent of the notorious Tuskegee Syphilis Studies;[4] this is, in contemporary American culture, one of the most powerful metaphors for symbolizing evil in the field of research ethics. The other side of the controversy is exemplified by a statement of a physician researcher from Uganda, one of the countries in which the trials were conducted. He accused the editor of a form of "ethical imperialism" which asserts that the American vision of research ethics must dominate the conduct of research everywhere in the world.

Let us consider this clinical trial in some detail as a case study. It seems appropriate to do so since it was this controversy that served as the immediate stimulus to undertake the most recent revision of Helsinki. At the time the trial began, and indeed to this day, the standard in industrialized countries, such as the United States, for prevention of perinatal transmission of HIV is the so-called 076 regimen. The name comes from ACTG protocol number 076, the AIDS Clinical Trial Group protocol that established its safety and efficacy. The 076 regimen reduces perinatal transmission of HIV infection by about 67%; the cost of the chemicals alone for treating each infected pregnant woman was in 1997 about $800. Why can we not just provide the 076 regimen to women infected with HIV in the developing countries? First and foremost is the cost. Eight hundred dollars per woman is approximately 80 times the annual per capita health expenditure in the sub-Saharan African countries in which these trials were carried out. The cost of the chemicals is not the only problem; there are several other obstacles most of which are also related to finances. I shall name some of the others; for a more complete discussion of these problems, see Levine.[5]

Provision of the 076 regimen would also have required a revision of the host countries' customs for seeking perinatal care. In most of these countries, women simply do not consult a health care professional early enough in pregnancy to begin the regular 076 regimen. It would also have required the establishment of a capability to provide intravenous administration of AZT during delivery; in most regions of the host countries there are no facilities for the intravenous administration of anything. And finally, in the host countries for these trials, with the exception of Thailand, women breastfeed their newborn babies even when they know they are infected with HIV. The risk to the babies of providing them with any available alternatives to breastfeeding may be even greater than the risk of exposing them to infection with HIV through breastfeeding. The transmission rate of HIV infection by way of breastfeeding is about 14%.

In the regions in which the "short duration" regimen of AZT was evaluated, particularly in sub-Saharan Africa, the death rate from infant diarrheal syndromes is about 4 million per year. In these countries, there is no infant formula. We could make the infant formula available in these countries, but that would not help. One cannot mix the formula with the local water supply because it is contaminated with, among other things, the pathogens that cause the deadly infant diarrheal syndrome.

To sum up: it is clear that the 076 regimen of AZT cannot be made available to most HIV infected pregnant women in the resource poor countries now or in the foreseeable future. This is the main reason that it is essential to find methods to reduce the rate of perinatal transmission of HIV that are within the financial reach of the resource poor countries. That was the primary justification for conducting the clinical trials of the short duration regimen of AZT. The cost of the AZT in the short duration regimen was about ten per cent of that of the 076 regimen. Moreover, there was no need for intravenous therapy or administration of the drug to the babies. At the time the trials began, it seemed likely that two of the countries could afford to provide the short duration regimen if it proved effective; there was also a commitment from international agencies to assist the other resource poor countries in securing and providing the drug.

Should the best proven therapeutic method standard for a clinical trial be construed to mean the best therapy available anywhere in the world or the standard that prevails in the host country? Guidance on this point can be found in another document – the *International Ethical Guidelines for Biomedical Research Involving Human Subjects* – a document prepared by the Council of International Organizations of Medical Sciences (CIOMS) in collaboration with the World Health Organization (WHO).[6] This document, which unlike Helsinki, explicitly addresses the problems of multinational research, offers some guidelines which I believe are far superior to informed consent and other traditional protections in preventing the exploitation of people in developing countries. First, for any research that is sponsored by an agency in an industrialized country and carried out in a developing country, the research goals must be responsive to the health needs and the priorities of the host country or community. Secondly, it requires that any product developed in the course of such research be made reasonably available to the inhabitants of the host country. This then focuses multinational research on the needs of the country in which the research is carried out. No more conducting phase I drug studies in Africa simply because it is less expensive and less vigorously regulated.

In my analysis, the initiation of a research program cannot be considered the same as the establishment of an entitlement to the best therapy that is available anywhere in the world.[5] Secondly, the relevant standard is the one that prevails in the host country.[5] I think it would be improper to withhold anything that is generally available in the host country in order to do research designed to evaluate something else if such withholding presented a non-trivial risk of a serious adverse consequence.

A new ethical standard is now emerging on the international research ethics scene. This standard is called the "highest attainable and sustainable therapeutic method" standard. This ungainly name requires some explanation: "highest attainable" means that under the circumstances of the clinical trial, the level of therapy one should provide should be the best one can do. The level of therapy that is generally available in the host country should not necessarily be considered sufficient; rather, it should be considered a minimum – the least that might be considered ethically acceptable.

"Sustainable" means a level of treatment that one can reasonably expect to be continued in the host country after the research program has been completed. It is a level of treatment that the host country can reasonably be expected to maintain when the extra resources provided by sponsors from industrialized countries are no longer available.

"Sustainability", then, serves as a constraint on "highest attainable". One should provide the highest level of therapy that one can under the circumstances of the clinical trial; however, one should keep in mind that if the level of therapy is not sustainable, the results of the trial may not be responsive to the needs and priorities of the host country and the therapeutic product developed in the research program may not be reasonably available to inhabitants of the host country.

Those who insist that Helsinki must be interpreted as requiring the provision of the best proven therapeutic method that is available in industrialized countries even when research is carried out to address the needs of resource poor countries, must understand the implications of this position. To consider once again our case study – the trials of the "short duration AZT regimen" in preventing perinatal transmission of HIV – most resource poor countries cannot even afford to purchase sufficient AZT to implement the best proven therapeutic method (the 076 regimen). In order to truly provide the "best" it is also necessary to provide all of the other advantages that exist in industrialized countries that enable the 076 regimen to be effective. These include, among other things: infant formula as an alternative to breastfeeding, a water supply that is safe for infants and the facilities for intravenous administration of drugs. All of these "advantages", taken together would cost far more than the AZT.

Clearly the cost of the 076 regimen is beyond the reach of most of the resource poor countries. Insistence on this standard would accomplish nothing other than to deny to resource poor countries the possibility of developing therapies and preventions that they can afford. Moreover, it would preclude the participation of sponsors and investigators from industrialized countries in research and development programs designed to assist the resource poor countries in developing affordable treatments and preventions. (For further discussion of the "highest attainable and sustainable" standard, see Levine.[7])

Application of the "highest attainable and sustainable therapeutic method" standard is in all relevant respects a more suitable ethical standard. One of its chief advantages is that it tends to facilitate the efforts of resource poor countries to develop needed therapies and preventions that are within their financial reach. Until the imbalances in the distribution of wealth among the nations of the world are corrected, this appears to be the best we can do.

## Helsinki VI on placebo

As mentioned earlier, one of the major reasons for the most recent revision of Helsinki was to clarify its position on the ethical justification of placebo controls. I find no reason to believe that Helsinki V was either equivocal or susceptible to differing interpretations. Now let us consider whether Helsinki VI changes any aspect of its position on placebo controls. The relevant new passage is Article 29, the replacement for Article II.3:

> 29 The benefits, risks, burdens and effectiveness of a new method should be tested against those of the best current prophylactic, diagnostic, and therapeutic methods. This does not exclude the use of placebo, or no treatment, in studies where no proven prophylactic, diagnostic or therapeutic method exists.

The only improvement over Article II.3 is the removal of the proscription of the development of all new therapies for conditions for which there are already existing "proven" therapies (*supra*). And even this salutary effect is not entirely clear; it depends completely on the interpretation of the new Article 28 (*infra*).

Helsinki's absolute proscription remains intact for placebo controls in clinical trials designed to evaluate therapies for diseases or conditions for which there already exists a therapy known to be at least partially effective.

## The duty to care

Several commentators on the ethics of clinical trials have argued that the choice of a control group should be dictated by the physician's ethical obligation to provide for each patient only the best known therapeutic method. This obligation is variously known as the "duty to care",[8,9] the duty to provide "the good of personal care"[10,11] and the fiduciary obligation of undivided loyalty to the interests of the patient.[9,10]

Clinical trialists Shaw and Chalmers were among the first to comment on this point.[12] Their focus was on deciding whether any particular clinician could justify his or her collaboration in a random clinical trial (RCT).

> If the clinician knows, or has good reason to believe, that a new therapy (A) is better than another therapy (B), he cannot participate in a comparative trial of

therapy A versus therapy B. Ethically, the clinician is obligated to give therapy A to each new patient with a need for one of these therapies.

If the physician (or his peers) has genuine doubt as to which therapy is better, he should give each patient an equal chance to receive one or the other therapy. The physician must fully recognize that the new therapy might be worse than the old. Each new patient must have a fair chance of receiving either the new and, hopefully, better therapy or the limited benefits of the old therapy.

Implicit in this position is a rejection of the possibility that one could justify a placebo control in clinical trials designed to evaluate therapies for diseases or conditions for which there already exists a therapy known to be at least partially effective.

The biostatistician, Royall,[11] agrees with the lawyer, Fried,[10] that enrolment in a randomized clinical trial has a tendency to deprive the patient of the "good of personal care". In their view, this is particularly problematic when placebo controls are used rather than a known effective therapy. Royall argues that in case of such conflicts, the issue should be resolved by assigning higher priority to the good of personal care than to the needs of science. The philosopher, Schafer,[13] also recognizes the existence of a tension between the needs of science and the physician's fiduciary obligation of undivided loyalty to the interests of the patient. His proposed resolution of the dilemma is startling:

Perhaps traditional physician ethics, with its highly individualistic commitment to patient welfare needs to be modified. A more socially oriented ethic might permit RCTs to proceed with a statistically adequate sample of patient-subjects.... If the traditional ethical rules governing physician-patient interaction are to be changed, then all parties should be made aware of this fact.

The physician ethicist, Weijer, has written an excellent and comprehensive review of the major ethical considerations in the justification of placebo controls in clinical trials.[9] For Weijer, the central consideration in the ethical justification of clinical trials is the concept introduced in 1987 by Benjamin Freedman, "clinical equipoise"[8]. "Clinical equipoise" is a term used to describe a state of knowledge in the expert clinical community with regard to the relative merits of two (or more) therapies for a given condition. If the expert clinical community is genuinely uncertain as to whether therapy A is superior or inferior to therapy B for the treatment of a given condition, considering both risks and benefits, then a state of clinical equipoise exists. Clinical equipoise exists even though some members of the expert clinical community earnestly believe that one of the therapies is superior to the other. Justification of a particular clinical trial necessarily requires that there can be no third therapy C that is known to be superior to A and B that is being withheld from trial subjects.

The underlying grounding for the concept of clinical equipoise is the "duty to care" or the fiduciary responsibility of the physician to the patient.

As Weijer and Freedman each envision "clinical equipoise", it serves to enforce adherence to the duty to care in the design and conduct of clinical trials. Using this analytic tool Weijer reaches conclusions about the conditions in which placebo controls can be justified that are nearly identical with mine (*infra*). In particular, he agrees that placebo controls are justified in certain circumstances in which "effective treatment exists but is not available due to cost or short supply".

The major difference between his conclusions and mine is that I would find placebo controls ethically permissible in circumstances in which the withholding of known effective therapy would be extremely unlikely to result in an increased probability of death or of non-trivial disability. Weijer argues correctly that my discussion of this issue was based on a description of what is, rather than an analysis of what ought to be. My statement was:[5]

> It is not customary to insist on a state of clinical equipoise in placebo controlled trials unless the purpose of the active agent being evaluated is to mitigate that component of a disease process that leads to disabling or lethal complications. Thus it is not uncommon to see placebo controlled trials of new analgesics, anxiolytics, and antihypertensives that are not justified by a state of clinical equipoise.

To avoid Weijer's challenge I should have added two points.

- I was referring to studies that had been reviewed and approved by Institutional Review Boards (IRBs) and that this meant that a large number of committees that are charged with the responsibility of evaluating the ethical propriety of research had found these studies ethically justified.
- I think there should be a threshold standard for invoking the requirement for the clinical equipoise justification. Below a certain level of risk the probability of doing any lasting damage to the patient-subject is so small that special justifications such as "clinical equipoise" are unnecessary. This proposition is closely related to the law's *de minimis* doctrine; *de minimis non curat lex* or, the law does not concern itself about trifles or insignificant matters.

Weijer and some others ask: can it be said that the fiduciary duty to the wellbeing of the patient exists only when the physician is doing things that increase the patient's likelihood of sustaining a non-trivial injury? And I reply, of course not. However, we already recognize the authority of the physician to conduct research involving patients when there is no possibility of benefit to the individual patient. This recognition is explicit in US federal regulations for the protection of human research subjects even when the subjects are incapable of informed consent if the permission of a responsible relative or the legal guardian is granted. The conduct of such research is clearly not justified by the duty to care. We find it ethically acceptable to allow the physician to perform non-therapeutic procedures or interventions to serve the interests of research when the goals are of sufficient importance and the risks are reasonable in relation to the expected benefits. To be consistent, we must equally find it ethically acceptable to allow the use of placebo controls even when there is a therapy other than the one being evaluated that is known to be effective when the goals are of sufficient importance and the risks are reasonable in relation to the expected benefits.

The concept of fiduciary requires undivided loyalty to the health interests of the patient. If the physician has or even appears to have any conflicting interests these must be disclosed. The patient, then, is enabled to make a choice of whether or not to become a subject with full awareness of the potential for divided loyalty. I do not mean to claim that informed consent is the answer to all such problems. It has long been known that many patients tend to think that anything proposed by a physician either is or could be intended by the physician to benefit the patient.[14] This is the phenomenon to which Appelbaum, *et al.* gave the name "therapeutic misconception".[15,16] This does not mean that informed consent is not possible; rather it means that one should be especially careful when negotiating informed consent to complex activities such as controlled clinical trials in which there are both therapeutic and non-therapeutic components.

Many commentators have recommended that the inherent conflict between the aspirations of the medical practitioner and those of the medical researcher might best be managed by separating these two roles. One individual could serve in the role of treating physician while another could be the researcher. Most such recommendations have centered on the problem of informed consent. I have generally resisted such proposals for reasons elaborated elsewhere.[17] But now it seems to me that the potential for confusion might, in many cases, be sufficient to make such separation worthwhile. In most cases, formal clinical trials are not conducted by the patients' primary care physicians. Rather, patients are referred to specialists who are conducting clinical trials. This is almost invariably the case in developing countries where the research setting is obviously very different from the typical health care setting, particularly when the clinical trial is being conducted with sponsorship from a developed country.

In technologically developed countries, there is a common scenario, which is particularly problematic. Patients with certain chronic diseases (for example, cancer, depression) are referred to a medical center with an expectation that there they will receive expert medical advice and, perhaps, treatment. Once there, they are invited by the specialists to become subjects in controlled clinical trials. This unexpected encounter may easily lead either to the therapeutic misconception or to a feeling of intimidation; either of these can tend to invalidate the process of informed consent.

I propose that certain clinical trials should be conducted in settings that are physically removed from the patient care setting by investigators who have not previously had a therapeutic relationship with any of the patient subjects. The investigators should make it very clear to the subjects that their principal occupation is to conduct clinical research. Such arrangements should be considered for all placebo controlled trials designed to evaluate new therapies for diseases or conditions for which there are other therapies known to be at least partially effective. When withholding of the known effective therapy could result in a non-trivial adverse consequence, there should be a prima facie obligation to establish such a distinct clinical research setting. A prima facie obligation means that persons must act accordingly unless there are important ethical reasons to do otherwise.

Some participants in the contemporary debate about the ethics of placebo controls have voiced several variations of the idea of role separation. Among them are some who have opposed the physician's participation in placebo controlled trials on the grounds that this would be a violation of the fiduciary duty to care. Some of them have stated that a physician in the distinct role of clinical trialist would be sufficiently free of the customary duties of the treating physician that it would not be unethical for him or her to conduct placebo controlled trials. I find no need to enter the argument as to whether such conditions release the physicians from their fiduciary duties because I do not think that the fiduciary duties preclude participation as a researcher in placebo controlled trials.

## The history of Helsinki

Historical evidence suggests strongly that the writers of Helsinki intended the "best proven therapeutic method" as a standard of medical practice and that its construction reflected their assigning primacy to the physician's duty to care. The document that came to be known as the *Declaration of Helsinki* was drafted by the World Medical Association's Committee on Medical Ethics. In 1953, when this committee began its work, it identified:

> a need for professional guidelines designed by physicians for physicians (as opposed to the Nuremberg Code, which was formed by jurists for use in a legal trial). Moreover, it was recognized that experiments must be classified into two groups: 'experiments in new diagnostic and therapeutic methods' and 'experiments undertaken to serve other purposes than simply to cure an individual'.[18]

It is worth emphasizing that in 1953, the Committee on Medical Ethics understood as its mission the development of a document *by physicians for physicians*. The same commitment to the primacy of the values of the medical profession was expressed 11 years later in the introduction to the final draft of the Declaration:

> The Declaration of Geneva of the World Medical Association *binds the physician* with the words, 'The health of my patient will be my first consideration,' and the International Code of Medical Ethics declares that, 'A physician shall act only in the patient's interest when providing medical care which might have the effect of weakening the physical and mental condition of the patient. (*emphasis added*)'[2]

It is further worth emphasizing that a second component of its mission was to provide guidance "for *experiments in new diagnostic and therapeutic methods*" an activity that can be and should be distinguished from the evaluation of such methods. The WMA also refers to this class of activities as those "undertaken ... simply to cure an individual". Activities undertaken "simply to cure an individual" are, by definition, not research. Consider the similarity of this language to the definition of "medical practice" provided in the *Belmont Report* by the National Commission for the Protection of Human Subjects of Biomedical and Behavioral Research, viz, "activities designed solely to enhance the wellbeing of an individual patient".[19] As the Council of International Organizations of Medical Sciences (CIOMS) noted in 1993 in its *International Ethical Guidelines for Biomedical Research Involving Human Subjects*:

> The Declaration [of Helsinki] does not provide for controlled clinical trials. Rather, it assures the freedom of the physician 'to use a new diagnostic or therapeutic measure, if in his or her judgment it offers hope of saving life, re-establishing health or alleviating suffering'.[6]

In other words, the standards set forth in the *Declaration of Helsinki* for "clinical research" were designed for a category of activities that has since come to be called "compassionate use" or "treatment use" of an investigational new drug.

In 1953, when the WMA Committee on Medical Ethics began the project that culminated in the promulgation of the *Declaration of Helsinki*, it was nine years before the passage in the United States of the Harris-Kefauver Amendments to the Food, Drug and Cosmetic Act; these are the amendments that established the requirement for a demonstration of efficacy for FDA approval of a marketing permit for a new drug. Before that time all that was required was a demonstration of a new drug's safety. Although there were a few controlled clinical trials prior to 1962, they did not become a prominent feature of the clinical research enterprise until the 1962 amendments specified that the demonstration of efficacy must be based on the results of "adequate and well-controlled" clinical trials. Thus, it is not surprising that the WMA did not develop standards for the ethical conduct of the modern controlled clinical trial.

It is of further interest that Section II of the first through fifth editions of the Declaration, subtitled "Clinical research", consistently refers to the person with whom the physician interacts as the "patient". In Sections

I (Basic principles) and III (Non-clinical biomedical research) the physician (sometimes called "investigator") interacts with either "subjects", "individuals" or, in only one instance (Article III.2) "patients". According to Article III.2 patients may serve as subjects but only if they have illnesses unrelated to the "experimental design".

In the light of these considerations, I conclude that the most plausible explanation of the "best proven therapeutic method" requirement is that it is a standard of medical practice. Its appearance in Article II.3 of the *Declaration of Helsinki* then, is to serve as a reminder to physician investigators that they are not to allow the needs of science to override the values of medical practice.

## Therapeutic and non-therapeutic research

The WMA's decision to classify medical research as "experiments in new diagnostic and therapeutic methods" and "experiments undertaken to serve other purposes than simply to cure an individual" resulted in its adoption of the illogical distinction between therapeutic and non-therapeutic research as its basic organizing principle. This faulty line of thinking also gave rise to its adoption of the "best therapeutic method" standard as articulated in Article II.3, the Article that proscribes placebo controls except where there is no known effective therapy. Let us now consider briefly some of the other unfortunate and embarrassing consequences of this classification scheme.[20]

Placing one article from Section II of Helsinki V in immediate proximity to one from Section III helps elucidate the logical flaw:

> II.6 The doctor can combine medical research with professional care … only to the extent that … research is justified by its potential diagnostic or therapeutic value for the patient.
>
> III.2 The subjects should be volunteers – either healthy persons or patients for whom the experimental design is not related to the patient's illness.

Let us consider what is ruled out by this pair of articles. They rule out all research in the fields of pathogenesis and pathophysiology as well as the entire field of epidemiology. Consider, for example, a recently published study that examines the role of neurotransmitters in the pathogenesis of mental depression. This study was entirely non-therapeutic in that there were no components that could bring direct health related benefit to the individual subjects. It certainly could not be justified in terms of its potential diagnostic or therapeutic benefit to the patient. Therefore, according to the Declaration, it could only be done on normal volunteers or on patients who have some disease other than depression. This is what I mean by illogical and embarrassing.

The problems in the category of therapeutic research are equally troubling. The concept of therapeutic research is incoherent. At least some of the components of every research protocol are non-therapeutic; when they are all non-therapeutic, use of the term "non-therapeutic research" might be justified. When we evaluate entire protocols as either therapeutic or non-therapeutic, as required by Helsinki V, we end up with what I call the "fallacy of the package deal". Those who use this distinction typically classify as "therapeutic research" any protocol that includes one or more components that are intended to be therapeutic; therefore the non-therapeutic components of the protocol are justified improperly according to the more permissive standards developed for therapeutic research.

Such erroneous justifications in the recent past have included:

- in trials of thrombolytic therapy repeated coronary angiograms on patients who had clinical indications for only one
- liver biopsies performed for no reason other than to disguise treatment assignments in a double blind placebo controlled trial
- repeated endoscopies in a population of patients with peptic ulcers who had clinical indications for no more than one
- administration of placebo by way of a catheter inserted in the coronary artery.

I do not want to be misunderstood as saying that any of these procedures was unethical. Rather, they should not have been justified according to the relatively permissive standards developed for "therapeutic research".

Does the recent revision of Helsinki resolve this problem? I think not. While the language of therapeutic and non-therapeutic research has been removed from the document, the concept remains. There still is a section called "C. Additional principles for medical research combined with medical care". The first article in this section is:

> 28 The physician may combine medical research with medical care, only to the extent that the research is justified by its potential prophylactic, diagnostic or therapeutic value. When medical research is combined with medical care, additional standards apply to protect the patients who are research subjects.

As noted earlier, all research includes some components that are non-therapeutic. Helsinki VI persists in demanding that in "research combined with medical care", the entire protocol must be justified in terms of its potential prophylactic, diagnostic or therapeutic value. The door to the fallacy of the package deal remains wide open.

## Impact of the Helsinki revision

The *Declaration of Helsinki* has been violated routinely by medical researchers ever since it was first promulgated in 1964. Researchers who think about the requirements of Helsinki have noticed that their colleagues do research, for example, in the field of pathogenesis and use placebo controls in studies of new oral hypoglycemics. They have further noticed that these colleagues are not criticized as unethical. Rather, their research is rewarded by the traditional coins of the academic realm. The rewards include publication in respectable medical and scientific journals by editors who have proclaimed publicly their commitment to honor the Declaration. This includes its enjoinment against publication of reports of research conducted "not in accordance with [Helsinki's] principles."* Recognition that some articles of Helsinki are both routinely violated and widely believed to be erroneous tends to undermine the credibility and authority of the entire document. Researchers who notice that virtually everyone violates Article III.2 with impunity feel free to pick and choose among the other articles to see whether they wish to behave in accord with them.

The WMA deserves congratulations on the accomplishments reflected in Helsinki VI. Much language that was either faulty or archaic or both was replaced by more apposite wording. However, the two major flaws that provided the stimulus for this revision remain uncorrected: the distinction between therapeutic and non-therapeutic research and the excessively rigid proscription of placebo controls. I see no reason to suspect that the current iteration of these flawed articles in Helsinki VI will command any more respect than did their predecessors.

## Recommendations

The use of placebo controls in clinical trials of new therapies should be permitted in the following circumstances and given the following conditions.

1 When the new therapy is being evaluated for the treatment of a disease or condition for which there is no existing therapy known to be at least partially effective.

This should be understood as including clinical trials having as an inclusion criterion patients who have tried known existing therapies without success. It should further be understood to include patients who are aware of existing therapies and have rejected them for reasons other than a wish to enrol in a clinical trial. (For example, Jehovah's Witnesses have been enrolled in clinical trials of artificial blood substitutes after having rejected transfusions on religious grounds.)

2 When the new therapy is being evaluated for relief of symptoms and there are provisions in the protocol for allowing patient subjects to withdraw from the study at any time.

In such studies, the prospective subjects should be informed that if their reason for withdrawal is a desire to receive known effective symptomatic relief, this will be provided promptly.

* Helsinki V, Article I.8; Helsinki VI, Article 27

3 When the new therapy is designed to treat a manifestation of disease that, if untreated, could eventually lead to death or non-trivial disability, and there are existing therapies that are at least partially effective in arresting or delaying the progression to death or disability, the use of placebo controls should be limited.

There must be a demonstration that under the conditions of the trial withholding of the known effective therapy would be very unlikely to result in a serious adverse consequence. For example, studies of new antihypertensive agents employ reliable surrogate endpoints, recruit subjects with "mild" hypertension who are very unlikely to have any serious adverse consequences even if untreated and unsupervised, are closely monitored and of relatively short duration. Under such conditions the probability of a serious adverse consequence is extremely small.

4 When the new therapy is intended to be an inexpensive alternative to expensive therapies that are considered "the best proven therapeutic method" in technologically developed countries and the research is to be carried out in a developing (resource poor) country with the assistance of sponsors or investigators from one or more of the wealthy countries, the clinical trial should be responsive to the health needs and priorities of the host country and the product being evaluated should meet the "reasonable availability" and "highest attainable and sustainable" standards.

(In multinational research there are other standards that must be met by the investigators and sponsors; these are beyond the scope of this discussion.)

5 In categories 3 and 4 there should be good reasons to believe that the new therapy to be evaluated could be superior to existing and available therapies for at least some members of the patient population from which the subjects are to be recruited.

When withholding of the known effective therapies could result in a non-trivial adverse consequence, there should be a prima facie obligation to establish the clinical trial in a distinct clinical research setting. Such a setting should be physically removed from the patient care setting and the investigators should include no health care professionals who have previously had a therapeutic relationship with any of the patient subjects. The investigators should make it very clear to the subjects that their principal occupation is to conduct clinical research.

## References

1 Levine RJ. The need to revise the Declaration of Helsinki. *N Engl J Med* 1999;**341**:531–4.

2 World Medical Association Declaration of Helsinki: Ethical Principles for Medical Research Involving Human Subjects. Adopted by the 18th WMA General Assembly, Helsinki, Finland, June 1964 and amended by the 29th WMA General Assembly, Tokyo, Japan, October 1975; 35th WMA General Assembly, Venice, Italy, October 1983;

41st WMA General Assembly, Hong Kong, September 1989; 48th WMA General Assembly, Somerset West, Republic of South Africa, October 1996; and the 52nd WMA General Assembly, Edinburgh, Scotland, October 2000. *http://www.wma.net/e/policy/17c.pdf*

3 Lurie P, Wolfe SM. Unethical trials of interventions to reduce perinatal transmission of the human immunodeficiency virus in developing countries. *N Engl J Med* 1997; **337**:853–6.

4 Angell M. The ethics of clinical research in the third world. *N Engl J Med* 1997; **337**:847–9.

5 Levine RJ. The "best proven therapeutic method" standard in clinical trials in technologically developing countries. *IRB: A Review of Human Subjects Research* January/February, 1998;20(No. 1):5–9.

6 Council of International Organizations of Medical Sciences (CIOMS). *International Ethical Guidelines for Biomedical Research Involving Human Subjects.* CIOMS, Geneva, 1993.

7 Levine RJ. Global issues in clinical trials. In: *Global Dimensions of Domestic Health Issues.* Osterweis M, Holmes DE, eds. Washington: Association of Academic Health Centers, 2000:119–30.

8 Freedman B. Equipoise and the ethics of clinical research. *N Engl J Med* 1987; **317**:141–5.

9 Weijer C. Ethical challenges of the randomized clinical trial. In: Levine RJ, Gorovitz S, eds. *Biomedical Research Ethics: Updating International Guidelines: A Consultation.* Council of International Organizations of Medical Sciences (CIOMS), Geneva, 2000:57–91.

10 Fried C. *Medical Experimentation: Personal Integrity and Social Policy.* New York: American Elsevier Publishing Co., 1974.

11 Royall RM. Ethics and statistics in randomized clinical trials. *Stat Sci* 1991;**6**:52–62.

12 Shaw LW, Chalmers TC. Ethics in cooperative trials. *Ann NY Acad Sci* 1970;**169**:487–95.

13 Schafer A. The ethics of the randomized clinical trial. *N Engl J Med* 1982;**307**:719–24.

14 Levine RJ. The boundaries between biomedical or behavioral research and the accepted and routine practice of medicine. In: The National Commission for the Protection of Human Subjects of Biomedical and Behavioral Research. *The Belmont Report: Ethical Principles and Guidelines for the Protection of Human Subjects of Research.* Appendix I, 1. 1–1.44. Washington: DHEW Publication (OS) 78–0013, 1978.

15 Appelbaum PS, Roth LH, Lidz CW. The therapeutic misconception: informed consent in psychiatric research. *Int J Law Psychiatry* 1982;**5**:319–29.

16 Appelbaum PS, Roth LH, Lidz CW, Benson P, Winslade W. False hopes and best data: consent to research and the therapeutic misconception. *Hastings Center Report* 1987; **17**(2):20–24.

17 Levine RJ. *Ethics and Regulation of Clinical Research, 2nd ed.* New Haven, USA: Yale University Press, 1988.

18 Perley S, Fluss SS, Bankowski Z, Simon F. The Nuremberg Code: An International Overview. In: Annas GJ, Grodin MA, eds. *The Nazi Doctors and the Nuremberg Code: Human Rights in Human Experimentation.* New York, Oxford: Oxford University Press, 1992:149–73.

19 The National Commission for the Protection of Human Subjects of Biomedical and Behavioral Research. *The Belmont Report: Ethical Principles and Guidelines for the Protection of Human Subjects of Research.* Washington, USA: DHEW Publication (OS) 78-0012, 1978.

20 Levine RJ. International codes and guidelines for research ethics: A critical appraisal. In: Vanderpool HY, ed. *The Ethics of Research Involving Human Subjects: Facing the 21st Century.* Frederick, Maryland, USA: University Publishing Group, 1996:235–59.

# *Section 5:* Priorities for future research

# 15: The research and ethical agenda

JOAN S WILENTZ, LINDA W ENGEL

Conference participants met in six breakout groups* to develop recommendations to advance research on the placebo and explore ethical issues relating to the use of placebos in clinical practice and clinical research. The groups made recommendations within four broad areas, summarized in four parts within this chapter:

I Elucidating the nature of placebo effects
II Applying placebo effects to the patient's advantage in clinical practice
III Using placebos in clinical trials to test pharmacological and procedural interventions
IV Using placebos in clinical trials to test behavioral interventions.

## Principles guiding development and conduct of the research and ethical agenda

There was considerable overlap in the discussions and recommendations generated across the groups, with agreement on the following guiding principles.

### Principle 1

The concept of a placebo encompasses more than an intervention – a sugar pill or saline injection or sham procedure. Rather it describes a

---

* The six breakout groups addressed the following topics: (1) What research is needed to further elucidate the nature of the placebo effect? (2) The use of placebos in clinical trials to test pharmacological interventions. (3) The use of placebos in clinical trials to test procedural interventions. (4) The use of placebos in clinical trials to test behavioral interventions. (5) How can what we know about the placebo effect be used to explain the purported effectiveness of some complementary and alternative therapies and psychosocial interventions? (6) How can what we know about the placebo effect be applied to the patient's advantage in conventional medical practice? See the Appendix for the list of members.

process encompassing dynamic features of the patient–health professional interaction, including features of the setting and environment in which treatment occurs. These features operate singly and together over the course of treatment in ways that can enhance an individual's health or wellbeing, producing beneficial (placebo) effects. On the other hand, if features of this process undermine the patient's health and wellbeing, they can contribute to what has been termed a negative placebo, or "nocebo" effect. It is implicit in this principle that placebo (or nocebo) effects operate whenever patients and practitioners interact, no matter what intervention is suggested or applied – including the actual use of a placebo or in situations where no medications or other forms of therapy are given. These interactions are critical for placebo effects because they provide meanings, expectations, and/or desires for symptom changes in the patient.

**Principle 2**

Placebo effects are a subset of mind-body effects that emerge by eliciting innate healing processes and/or enabling an amelioration of symptoms. All living organisms have a capacity for self-healing. In particular, human beings are endowed with complex cells, organs, and systems that respond to threats through mechanisms designed to preserve, protect, and repair the organism, restoring balance though various homeostatic measures and feedback loops. Brain centers and pathways that affect cognition, motivation, and emotion and in this way alter the perception and meaning of illness and symptoms are included in this complex circuitry.

**Principle 3**

Given the complex and dynamic features of the placebo process, it is likely that no single model of placebo effects nor any single mechanism will be able to explain how placebo effects manifest as physiological changes in the body. The individual practitioner and patient bring to the therapeutic encounter a number of psychosocial variables (for example, cognition, conditioning, expectancy, suggestion, affective states, personality) as well as characteristics of their larger social and cultural environments. The interaction of these variables can in turn elicit the psychophysiological changes in the patient associated with placebo effects. These may employ multiple systems, including the central and autonomic nervous systems, the endocrine and immune systems, and cardiovascular and gastrointestinal processes in generating placebo effects. Specific characteristics of patients and practitioners affect how each responds in the course of illness and treatment. Research is needed to discover how these complex and interacting psychosocial variables affect psychophysiological responses from the micro levels of genes, molecules, and cells, to the macro level of pathways, organs, and systems, as well as the role of genetic, developmental, and environmental factors.

**Principle 4**

Given the multilayer interactive schema described above, basic research on the placebo process and effects requires collaborations among a broad range of disciplines and sciences, including sociology, anthropology, psychology, neurobiology, endocrinology, immunology, genetics, pharmacology, and clinical science, to address how placebo effects operate in a variety of specific conditions. Experts in study design and analysis should also be involved. Thus, psychometricians, epidemiologists, and biostatisticians are also needed. As in all research involving human participants, ethical considerations need to be taken into account at all stages of study design, implementation, and reporting. For some studies specific consultation by ethicists may be appropriate during study design. These same considerations apply both to research on the use of placebo in clinical trials and in clinical practice.

**Principle 5**

There is a need to eliminate the pejorative connotation of the word placebo as merely a sham and deceptive process and replace it with the positive meaning by which an individual's health and wellbeing can be enhanced in any therapeutic encounter. Careful consideration of Principle 1 can facilitate this transition because it shifts the emphasis of placebo away from external deceptive manipulation to interpersonal interactions and intrapersonal factors.

**Principle 6**

Studies involving placebo effects must be designed to separate actual placebo effects from various artifacts. These artifacts include investigator, observer, and patient bias, specific biological effects attributable to physical or chemical properties of the placebo (for example, hypersensitivity reactions to a coloring agent in a placebo tablet); natural history of the disorder (for example, improvement in nasal congestion due to clearing of a viral upper respiratory infection by the patient's immune response); waxing and waning of symptoms in many chronic diseases such as arthritis and multiple sclerosis; the so-called "Hawthorne" effect (the effect of being under study on the persons being studied),[1] and regression to the mean. If there is to be a "science of the placebo", it has to reflect valid study designs and measurable endpoints.

## Reference

1 Last JM, ed. *A Dictionary of Epidemiology, 2nd ed.* New York: Oxford University Press, 1988:56.

# Part I: Recommendations for research to further elucidate the nature of the placebo effect

Fabrizio Benedetti, Susan M Czajkowski, Cheryl A Kitt, Michael Stefanek, Esther M Sternberg*

To understand how placebos operate is to ask a fundamental question of how an individual's expectations, learning, reassurance, hope, beliefs, and other mental states and traits – derived in part from the larger cultural and social world – can affect the various centers and pathways of the brain and other effector systems to alter physiologic processes to improve health and wellbeing.

## Recommendation 1: study the role of classical conditioning and learning

There is strong evidence that placebo responses can in part be accounted for by classical conditioning and hence represent a form of associative learning.[1] The data have come from experiments with animals and human subjects in which active drugs have been used as the unconditioned stimulus to generate a physiological response. Following a number of training sessions subjects exhibit a physiological response to a placebo of similar appearance. These experiments also demonstrate principles associated with classical conditioning such as stimulus generalization and extinction. However, at times, the placebo response is anomalous – producing effects opposite to the active drug or giving mixed results. Further studies of conditioning to explain placebo responses are warranted, not only to determine optimal parameters for conditioning, but also to

* Members of two breakout groups contributed to these recommendations. Group 1: Robert Ader, Clarence E Davis, Gerald D Fischbach, Wayne B Jonas, Ted J Kaptchuk, Robert J Levine, Daniel E Moerman, Donald D Price, Robert M Rose, Shepard Siegel, Robert J Temple, Sabra F Woolley; Group 5: Richard R Bootzin, Margaret A Chesney, Carlo Contoreggi, Kenneth L Fox, Richard H Gracely, Anne Harrington, Ted J Kaptchuk, Donald D Price, Robert M Rose, Julian F Thayer, and John N Weinstein. See the Appendix for member information.

elucidate when and why anomalous responses occur. One hypothesis suggests that when a placebo is given to a healthy human or animal subject following an active drug, the anomalous response is the organism's means of coping with an anticipated homeostatic imbalance. Thus it has been suggested that placebo conditioning needs to be studied in pharmaco-*therapeutic* protocols in which the subjects are affected by disease (and hence already in a state of homeostatic imbalance) and are treated with placebos administered in a longitudinal design following administration of the active drug. In the real world placebos are given primarily to sick subjects and hence should be studied in them. In this context, it appears that there are few if any studies that have looked at the conditioning effect of analgesic drugs in an animal suffering pain. The clinical implication of such studies is very important. The desired outcome would be the reduction of the cumulative amount of drugs an individual takes with potentially decreased deleterious side effects while maintaining the therapeutic effects. Investigations on the role of conditioning related to the placebo effect should thus be carried out in both healthy and unhealthy subjects.

Animal studies are particularly useful in conditioning research, allowing for predictions that can be easily confirmed or not. However, studies with both humans and animals have been informative. For example, it is known that older animals and humans are slower to form conditioned responses. One might then ask whether old people show weaker placebo responses in some cases than younger people. Insofar as age-related deficits and conditioning can be partially attenuated by cholinergic manipulations one could also ask if age-related deficits in responding to placebo can be modulated by cholinergic manipulation.

## Recommendation 2: study the role of expectation, anxiety, memory distortion, the desire for relief, and other cognitive factors

Placebo effects clearly involve cognitive, motivational, and affective components. In this regard, expectations, beliefs, and memory distortion on the one hand, and anxiety and the desire for relief on the other, deserve thorough investigation. In particular, we need to understand the role these factors play in placebo (and nocebo) effects and their relationship to classical conditioning and learning. To this end, specific studies should aim at analyzing models of placebo responses where the role of both cognition and emotions can be tested and/or confirmed as mediators or moderators of placebo responses, possibly assessing the relative importance of each.

One method for investigating the role of expectancy and other cognitive factors is by examining the placebo effects of therapies such as hypnosis, psychotherapeutic interventions, and meditation, which, because they do not involve any physical intervention, provide a kind of baseline for studying the placebo effects of other therapies. Such therapies can be instrumental in enabling investigators to tease out the contribution to placebo effects of such factors as the patient's perception of the therapeutic procedure; the meaning of the therapeutic encounter for the patient; and the patient's desire or expectation for a positive outcome. These "proximate mediating factors" in turn are likely to be strongly influenced by the degree of patient-physician rapport and the clinician's confidence in the therapy's ability to help. Therapies that are rich in cues and rituals or sensory phenomena (visual, auditory, taste, touch, smell) should also be studied to determine how these factors may potentiate placebo effects and enhance healing.

Another example of a specific condition treated by a specific therapeutic approach that might reveal aspects of placebo effects is the use of mindfulness meditation as a treatment for insomnia. Such an approach is aimed not only at reducing stress per se, but with providing tools for individuals with insomnia to cope with worries about their lack of sleep. If worry is an important component of the sleep problem, meditation might be the ideal intervention, because it lets people take note of their worries and let them go. The pathways by which meditation alters effect may have important implications for understanding and applying placebo effects in clinical practice. This specific insomnia hypothesis can be tested, as can other hypotheses about mechanisms underlying specific psychological interventions for anxiety disorders, depression, and other problems.[2]

## Recommendation 3: articulate the impact of cultural, social, and behavioral environments on health and illness

Examples of fruitful areas of investigation include the mechanisms by which cultural mores influence individual experiences of treatment, pain, and side effects; the ways in which cultural and social influences determine expectations; the role of education; the effect of social inequalities and the increasing social and cultural diversity of the population; and the medical marketplace itself. These circumstances of personal history embedded in the larger social, economic, and cultural environment affect an individual's beliefs, attitudes, expectations, and behaviors, with direct and indirect effects on health and wellbeing, including how the individual responds to illness and whether interactions with health professionals potentiate or inhibit placebo effects.

Observers of placebo phenomena have remarked that there are global features of the environment that may enhance healing. This is exemplified by such phenomena as faster rates of postoperative recovery observed in patients recuperating in hospital rooms with pleasant views as opposed to comparable patients in less attractive settings.[3] Such global phenomena are important, but are challenging to study, given the lack of specificity and control over the many variables involved.

## Recommendation 4: identify the biological mediators and delineate the pathways through which placebos exert their effects

In order to document as fully as possible the mechanisms by which alterations in brain function occurring during the placebo response might affect disease expression, specific neuroendocrine, neuronal and immune intermediary pathways should be assessed. These might include neuropeptides, for example, enkephalins, endorphins, cholecystokinin, neurohormones (glucocorticoids, prolactin), and neurotransmitters (5-hydroxytryptamine, norepinephrine, dopamine), as well as second messengers (nitric oxide, prostaglandins). Furthermore, both cellular and molecular aspects of immune responses should be measured, including baseline and stimulated cytokine responses, immune cell function and trafficking, and antibody production. Finally, placebo effects on disease expression should be quantified, using objective quantitative measures specific to the illness under study.

Studies are needed to trace fully the pathways by which cognition, expectancy, personality, social learning, and social psychological interactions lead to the regulation of psychophysiological responses. Such studies should be carried out across and within multiple systems (including the nervous, endocrine, immune, cardiovascular, gastrointestinal, and other systems); across levels of analysis ranging from the molecular to population studies; using linear and non-linear systems of analysis; in both animals and humans; in both healthy and diseased subjects, and within global and disease-specific models.

There are excellent disease-specific models in which clear placebo effects occur, and where biological measurements have been tailored to the organ or body system that is being investigated. For example, there are solid empirical data establishing the legitimacy of placebo analgesia,[4,5] showing its mediation by various endogenous pain-modulating neurotransmitters and nervous system pathways. Furthermore, placebo analgesia has been shown to occur only on that part of the body where expectation of analgesia and attention are directed,[6,7] thus providing a model for studying generalized versus localized placebo effects.

The approaches applied in studying placebo analgesia should be expanded to studies aimed at elucidating the mechanisms underlying the changes in biology associated with other diseases or disease symptoms. Fruitful areas of study include hypertension-related placebo effects ($\alpha$ and $\beta$ receptor involvement),[8] depression-related placebo effects (GABA receptors or other neurotransmitters),[9] the relief of gastrointestinal symptoms[10] and asthma.[11] An additional important area of investigation is arthritis, where multiple bidirectional pathways involving central and peripheral nervous system, neuroendocrine, and immune system mechanisms are involved in the pathogenesis and relief of symptoms. In elucidating their role in placebo effects, one might ask if patients' expectations result in a reduction in pain, inflammation, or both, and if they report less pain because inflammation has been reduced.

## Recommendation 5: develop and apply investigational tools and enabling technologies

Recent advances in biomedical technology allow researchers to ask more sophisticated questions about placebo effects and to answer them in elegant ways. Placebo research could similarly advance through the development of new tools and the application of existing tools to study mind-body effects. For example:

### Mapping social and cultural influences

Just as new technologies have been critical in mapping the human genome, a program to develop instruments for mapping cultural, social, psychological, and behavioral variables would be a boon to the social and behavioral sciences. Such tools would enable the assessment of cultural contexts, social networks and influences, and psychological states and moods – the *superstructure* within which organisms live – which, interacting with the *infrastructure* of genes, cells, and molecules, affects the health and wellbeing of an individual. Research is needed to articulate the mechanisms by which, for example, personality differences influence the perception of pain or health-related behaviors, including adherence to treatment, symptom recognition, etc. As these tools are developed it may be possible to integrate them into some of the already existing technologies described below. For example, tools developed for the assessment of psychological states and moods could be integrated with neuroimaging of emotional centers of the brain.

### Neuroimaging

Methods pioneered in the fields of pain research and substance abuse can be particularly instructive in tracking the nervous system effects of placebos. Researchers have detailed the numerous neurotransmitters and pathways involved in the experience of pain and its modulation and in reward and aversive systems in the brain. In particular, the use of brain imaging through positron emission tomography (PET) and functional magnetic resonance imaging (fMRI) have yielded important information on the bidirectional networks underlying the experience of pain and in the response to a variety of mood altering drugs. In addition, there is evidence that areas of the brain where activities alter in response to pain or pleasure also respond to the anticipation of pain or pleasure, suggesting mechanisms by which response expectancies can elicit placebo effects. Further refinements in neuroimaging technology can be expected to yield critical insights into the nervous system pathways and their relationships to neuroendocrine, immune, and other effector pathways associated with placebo and other mind-body effects.

Recent imaging work in the area of emotions and feeling is similarly directed toward revealing the brain nuclei and pathways underlying positive and negative emotions. In this way neuroscientists are beginning to create behavioral maps of the brain, noting specific nuclei and pathways connecting emotional, cognitive, and motor pathways and in some cases, revealing right-left hemisphere differences. The amygdala and other limbic structures associated with emotions and feelings have also been shown to be important in expectancy, motivation, and reward, and hence are of interest in elucidating placebo effects as well as expectations associated with behavioral, pharmacological, or other interventions.

### Genomics and proteomics

Use of genomic techniques and analyses may also be useful in understanding the mechanisms through which placebos exert their effects at the genetic level. The use of microarray chip technology is a means of determining which of numerous genes are activated or suppressed in particular cells under certain conditions. For example, researchers studying placebo analgesia might use microarray technology to determine which classes of endogenous opioids or other pain-modulating neurotransmitter molecules are involved in placebo analgesia. With the sequencing of the human and other animal genomes, microarray and other genomic as well as proteomic technologies (to determine the structure and function of proteins encoded by genes) are fast becoming among the most promising tools of biomedical research in the 21st century.

## References

1 Siegel S. Explanatory mechanisms for placebo effects: Pavlovian conditioning. This volume, chapter 6.
2 Teasdale JD, Segal Z, Williams JMC. How does cognitive therapy prevent depressive relapse and why should attentional control (mindfulness) training help? *Behav Res Ther* 1995;**33**:25–9.
3 Harrington A. "Seeing" the placebo effect: Historical legacies and present opportunities.This volume, chapter 2.
4 Amanzio M, Benedetti F. Neuropharmacological dissection of placebo analgesia: expectation-activated opioid systems versus conditioning-activated specific subsystems. *J Neurosci* 1999;**19**:484–94.
5 Price DD, Soerensen LV. Endogenous opioid and non-opioid pathways as mediators of placebo analgesia. This volume, chapter 9.
6 Montgomery GH, Kirsch I. Mechanisms of placebo pain reduction: an empirical investigation. *Psychol Sci* 1996;7:174–6.
7 Benedetti F, Arduino C, Amanzio M. Somatotopic activation of opioid systems by target-directed expectations of analgesia. *J Neurosci* 1999;**19**:3639–48.
8 Antivalle M, Lattuada S, Salvaggio M, Paravicini M, Rindi M, Libretti A. Placebo effect and adaptation to noninvasive monitoring of BP. *J Hum Hypertens* 1990;**4**:633–7.

9 Brown WA, Shrivastava RK, Arato M. Pre-treatment pituitary-adrenocortical status and placebo response in depression. *Psychopharmacol Bull* 1987;**23**:155–9.

10 De Craen AJM, Moerman DE, Heistercamp SH, Tytgat GNJ, Tijssen JGP, Kleijnen J. Placebo effect in the treatment of duodenal ulcer. *Br J Clin Pharmacol* 1999;**48**:853–60.

11 Godfrey S, Silverman M. Demonstration of a placebo response in asthma by means of exercise testing. *J Psychosom Res* 1973;**17**:293–7.

# Part II: Recommendations for research on applying placebo effects in clinical practice

Ruth L Fischbach, David Spiegel*

Research to learn how to apply placebo effects to enhance the health and wellbeing of patients calls for descriptive and intervention studies. In general, these studies explore features of the therapeutic encounter, including characteristics of practitioners and patients, and propose manipulations of such encounters designed to determine "best practices" for eliciting placebo responses, an important health services research initiative. Clinical studies of placebo responses should include measurements of variables related to intervening physiology, such as heart rate and blood pressure (regulated by the autonomic nervous system), cortisol levels (as an acute measure of the stress response), and other neuroimmune and endocrine variables. Researchers should also observe disease progression and employ outcome variables, such as symptom relief of pain, anxiety, depression, and other target symptoms.

## Recommendation 1: study means of optimizing placebo effects and minimizing nocebo effects in clinical practice

The placebo has been considered a "nuisance factor" in clinical trials, when in fact it represents a powerful therapeutic ally in health care. With the goal of optimizing patients' responses to treatment, studies should be conducted to determine how modifications in expectation, drug side effects ("active placebos"), characteristics of the medical setting, and patient collaboration in treatment planning affect treatment outcomes. The interaction between a patient's expectations and adherence to a treatment regimen also warrants study. Research should be directed towards maximizing placebo effects and minimizing nocebo effects.

---

* Members of breakout group 6 contributed to these recommendations; Walter A Brown, Robert M Califf, Robert A Hahn, Anne Harrington, Halsted Holman, Irving Kirsch, Rhonda J Moore, and Howard M Spiro. See the Appendix for member information.

## Recommendation 2: study characteristics of practitioners in relation to the placebo process and responses

Health professionals vary in their ability to elicit placebo responses in patients. In some cases there may be a mismatch between the practitioner and the patient that works against the patient's improvement in health. It is important to learn what health professional schools teach about placebos and, as the state of the science advances, to determine what additional information and training may facilitate the eliciting of placebo effects in practice. At present, physicians are under great pressure to be omnipotent, regardless of their own fears of death or failure. It is important to compare the ways physicians function in situations of acute and chronic illness to determine which behavioral styles favor or inhibit placebo responses. The degree to which the practitioner communicates care about the outcome of treatment is important. The patient's understanding that whatever happens, the doctor cares and will be there to help, can have as much effect as the patient's expectation of improvement.

Studies of therapeutic variables that enhance positive placebo responses and reduce "nocebo" responses should include the time the practitioner spends with patients; the quality of their communication; the sense of caring expressed; the involvement of family or friends in treatment; patient contacts with other patients and their responses to treatment; and placebos as components of active treatment.

Several of these variables, such as empathy, listening skills, enthusiasm/commitment to the course of treatment proposed, and time available to spend with the patient reflect qualities of practitioners that can be manipulated in a series of comparative studies to determine their relative contributions and importance in generating placebo responses. Studies comparing practitioners of conventional and complementary and alternative medicine (CAM) are of particular interest. CAM practitioners often assume a "holistic" approach and focus on wellness and promotion of healing. They often view their relations to the patient as close, and as an aspect of the healing process, they try to enhance placebo effects.[1] In this regard, and given this appeal and patient satisfaction with them, CAM practitioners may provide a model to be emulated by conventional health care practitioners.

A primary goal is to learn how to operationalize the "ability to elicit placebo responses in patients" and then to identify (in a non-circular way) the characteristics of practitioners who do this well. Those two objectives could form the basis for a research program that could then be followed by studies aimed at translating the initial findings into "best practices". In turn, these best practices could be incorporated into teaching modules for medical students and residents, and finally evaluated by measuring the effectiveness of the educational program in improving health outcomes and patient satisfaction with care.

## Recommendation 3: explore the dynamics of the interaction between patients and providers, examining the roles each plays, the "props", costumes, verbal and non-verbal communication, and setting for the encounter, and how these affect the placebo process and response

In this research the doctor-patient relationship is the focus of study, with various manipulations being used to test the importance of mutually shared values, locus of control, and other variables. Some studies suggest that the rapport established at the outset – such as shared values, the patient's belief in the physician and expectation of improvement – reinforce the physician's self-confidence and enhance the potential of the patient doing well. Studies should also include research evaluating the importance of giving patients tools to participate actively in their own recovery in comparison to situations in which patients are the passive recipients of care. Patient-to-patient communication should also be studied as potentiating placebo effects. Patients given opportunities to meet with others experiencing the same disease may gain knowledge and support that can improve their coping skills and wellbeing.

An important component of the interaction is how doctors comport themselves, their bedside manner. In the old days, wearing a white coat was a powerful stimulus that triggered patient expectation of being taken care of and getting better. Diagnostic testing, including the use of the stethoscope, thermometer, blood pressure cuff, and so on, are all part of the paraphernalia of healing that empower practitioners and are likely to instil confidence in patients that their needs are being attended to.

Some studies have shown differential effects in terms of patient commitment and compliance to treatment depending on whether the clinician orally recommended the use of an over-the-counter medication or actually wrote the recommendation on a prescription pad (the latter producing greater compliance). The effects of the setting, be it private office, busy clinic, or health maintenance setting, are also factors that can positively or negatively affect placebo responses. In an increasing number of settings it is not just the physician, but also nurses who check patients in and perform ancillary tasks such as drawing blood and measuring blood pressure. These "microsystems" will also have an impact beyond the personality and actions of the health care provider.

## Recommendation 4: study the influence of culture/ethnic identity and language on the medical encounter and placebo effects

Placebo phenomena are observed in all cultures. Given the increasing diversity of the US population, it will be important to study the nature and meaning of placebos in various ethnic/cultural groups, with the understanding that features of the medical encounter will take on different saliences and meanings depending on the individual's ethnic and cultural roots. An ethnographic study of placebos in clinical trials would be useful. Levi-Strauss[2] provides a model for utilizing anthropological data to examine both synchronic (universal features across cultures) and diachronic (features specific to time and culture) elements. Placebo phenomena are observed in medical treatment throughout cultures, but some are relatively specific to certain belief patterns, the socioeconomic relationship between healer and patient, belief systems about the body and mechanisms of healing, differing patterns of religious belief, and the meaning of death and dying. Others may be more universal, involving expectation of and hope for improvement. Cross-cultural examination of common and disparate factors in placebo response could reveal both universal elements and specific means of optimizing placebo responses in a given culture.

## Recommendation 5: study the role of the spouse and family members in relation to placebo responses

The issue of patient and family involvement in the medical encounter and the placebo response is very complicated. Some practitioners are aware of and sensitive to positive and negative influences of family members in the placebo process and responses. Some practitioners are also aware of family preferences and attitudes, while other practitioners are not. For example, they may mistakenly try to involve a family in critical medical decisions when the family is not interested, or alternatively, ignore the family who wants to be deeply involved. Understanding what patients want and how their desires may or may not mesh with those of their loved ones are important considerations in the interaction between practitioner and patient and are yet other variables affecting placebo responses that need study.

## Recommendation 6: study whether it is possible for individuals to elicit placebo responses in themselves

This effort relates to the notion of the older concept of a placebo as a deceptive treatment. Insofar as the placebo concept now embodies a process by which individuals are enabled to tap into the self-healing mechanisms of the body, it would clearly be useful to study whether there are particular skills and approaches that could be taught to encourage self-placebo responses. Self-hypnosis, meditation, relaxation therapies, and other subjective interventions may be fruitful areas of investigation in terms of self-placebo effects.

## Recommendation 7: study barriers to effective placebo use

A number of barriers in the implementation of placebo use in medical practice need examination. Suggested barriers to study include: time constraints which may preclude the kinds of interactions that may facilitate placebo responses; cynicism on the part of health professionals and/or patients; mismatches between health care professionals and patients; language problems; the role of computerized or internet information; drug company advertising; and legal issues. Of particular interest is the determination of the extent to which legal obligations to inform patients about risks of medication, particularly serious or life-threatening risks, create a nocebo effect of negative expectations that could potentially influence the medical outcome. This is the "self-fulfilling prophecy" that concerns investigators and clinicians alike.

## Recommendation 8: study distinctive problems in medical practice that deserve special attention

### Antibiotics as placebos

The prescription of antibiotics as a placebo drug to treat what is typically an upper respiratory viral infection was identified as an example where use of an "active placebo" is a growing concern. The concern is real as overprescribing encourages the emergence of drug-resistant strains of bacteria. This is a different kind of placebo interaction, one that involves an active placebo, an intervention that is not appropriate for that particular disorder. Research should study how antibiotics are used as placebos in conventional medical contexts, and how physicians present them to patients. Investigators could compare the outcomes of people who are taking antibiotics for conditions judged to be viral to the outcomes of individuals told that antibiotics cannot help and could hurt them. Another suggestion is a study of how other cultures use antibiotics. In many countries antibiotics are available without prescription, providing patients with the opportunity to use antibiotics, i.e. to self-medicate, possibly generating placebo effects without any medical evaluation.[3] Study questions to pursue include:

- What are the placebo elements of this practice?
- What are the positive and negative effects of prescribing antibiotics as placebos?
- What are more creative ways we could employ to use the placebo phenomenon to its greatest effect?

### Efficacy of antidepressants

Studies to explore the relative weight of the placebo effects of antidepressants (resulting from expectation) in comparison to their pharmacologic effects would provide much needed information. Another area to study is the extensive use of selective serotonin reuptake inhibitors (SSRIs). The impact of the manner of introducing antidepressant medication can be combined with the use of suggestion techniques. One study, for example, could test whether the positive message to the patient: "you will get better by using this medication" leads to a positive outcome.

### Use of placebos in pain treatment

Research is needed, especially in situations where a placebo is provided improperly, to prove to patients that they are not really in pain, that is, where a placebo is used to invalidate their complaint. In these situations, patients experiencing pain have been given a placebo analgesic accompanied by a strong message from the physician that "this medication will reduce your pain". It is wrong to assume that if a patient responds by reporting less pain that this indicates that the patient's pain was not real. What is more likely demonstrated is that the patient is able to harness his or her own placebo response (such as the release of endogenous endorphins), thus perceiving diminished pain temporarily. Use of the placebo phenomenon to convince patients that they are not experiencing real pain is an inappropriate use of the phenomenon.

The use of placebos in chronic pain clinics also merits further research. For example, patients may be given a saline injection and be told very clearly by the physician "for some reason this therapy works for many people even though I do not know why or how it works". Expectancy can produce the effect, with the placebo injection helping patients enter a mode in which they feel that this "treatment" should benefit them, even when they are informed that the mechanism is unknown. This raises the intriguing question of whether deception is, or is not, a necessary component of the placebo response.

### Physician referral to complementary and alternative (CAM) practitioners

A final area to pursue is the effect of physician referral to CAM practitioners for treatment of pain and other disorders. The literature indicates that two-thirds of the patients who use CAM treatments also seek conventional medical care. Yet the literature also indicates that the majority of patients who use CAM treatments do not tell their doctors that they are doing so. There has been a notable positive shift in physician attitudes toward CAM treatments in the last decade. Are we better now at harnessing the placebo in CAM treatment responses simply by integrating CAM with mainstream medical care? What is the effect of making a physician referral to CAM, rather than having CAM as a source of physician–patient disagreement, or as an example of patient clandestine activity? Thus, an important issue to be studied is the interaction between utilization of CAM treatments and placebo responses in conventional medicine for treating pain and other disorders.

## References

1 Cassidy CM. Social science theory and methods in the study of alternative and complementary medicine. *J Altern Complement Med* 1995;**1**:19–40.
2 Levi-Strauss C, *Structural Anthropology* (Jacobson C, trans.) New York: Basic Books, 1963.
3 Levy SB. Antibiotic availability and use: consequences to man and his environment. *J Clin Epidemiol* 1991;**44**(Suppl 2):83S–7S.

# Part III: Recommendations for research concerning the use of placebos in clinical trials to test pharmacological and procedural interventions

David W Feigal, Jr, Kathleen J Propert, David S Wendler*

Recommendations for research on the use of placebos in clinical trials raise a number of ethical, philosophical, and statistical issues. Suggestions were made for improving clinical trial design as well as proposals urging greater attention to the ethical issues and dilemmas involving the various components of a typical randomized placebo controlled trial, such as patient referral, the informed consent process, and the role of institutional review boards (IRBs).

## Recommendation 1: further evaluate the philosophical underpinnings of the use of placebo controlled clinical trials (PCTs)

There is a need for ethical/philosophical studies to explore the nature of investigator obligations to patients or other research participants in the context of PCTs. It has been argued that investigators have an obligation *not* to treat research subjects with any interventions known to be inferior. However, investigators can and do place research subjects at risk, even those with disease, without any compensating potential for clinical benefit under certain circumstances, such as when investigators obtain tissue samples for basic research. A full account of researchers' obligations to their subjects is warranted, including a discussion of under what conditions the invitation to participate in a PCT can be consistent with an investigator's obligations to his/her subjects.

---

* Members of two breakout groups contributed to these recommendations. Group 2: Robert Ader, Robert M Califf, Robert A Hahn, Irving Kirsch, Frank G Miller, Pamela Sankar, Shepard Siegel, Robert J Temple, Charles Weijer; Group 3: Howard Brody, Clarence E Davis, Gerald D Fischbach, Robert J Levine, Daniel E Moerman, Stuart J Pocock, Kenneth J Rothman, Janet Wittes and Kimberly Wristers. See the Appendix for member information.

A primary objection to the use of placebos in clinical trials when standard treatments exist is that such use violates the principle of clinical equipoise. Roughly, the principle states that it is acceptable to include a clinical intervention, including placebo, as part of a research trial *only when it is unclear whether the intervention is clinically better than all the other interventions included in the trial and any standard interventions that exist for the disease in question.* Unfortunately, while the term "equipoise" has become standard in discussions of the ethical underpinnings of clinical trials, its meaning is not clear. First, the precise conditions which must be satisfied for clinical equipoise to be obtained are not well defined. Second, in particular cases it is often unclear whether these conditions are indeed satisfied, hence unclear whether clinical equipoise obtains. In the design and evaluation of a trial, both statistical significance and clinical significance must be considered when evaluating *how much* evidence is needed that a particular intervention is superior before equipoise no longer obtains. There is also a question of who decides whether or not equipoise obtains.

At present, many procedures (especially orthopedic surgeries) are performed without undergoing the same rigorous evaluation that drugs or other non-surgical procedures undergo prior to being put into practice. It can be argued that the use of sham (placebo) procedures would allow the same rigorous standards used in evaluating drugs to be applied to the evaluation of surgeries and other invasive procedures.

## Recommendation 2: assess the attitudes and beliefs of potential and actual research subjects

Significantly more research is needed to evaluate the views of potential clinical trial participants. For example, empirical studies should be conducted to assess the degree of risk that is acceptable to individuals considering a PCT in settings where standard treatments exist. Such studies will generally be disease-specific, since the specific risk of disease progression and the impact on overall quality of life typically are relevant considerations in determining whether to enrol in a PCT.

Even if a patient is randomized to a placebo control group, there is the possibility of clinical benefit. Indeed, it is this potential that is driving new interest in enhancing the placebo process and placebo effects in clinical settings. In the case of surgeries or other invasive procedures, proponents of the use of placebo controls suggest that these can appropriately be used and have potential benefit when the procedure is done to treat a subjective symptom or when the procedure does not cure the problem. Other criteria suggested include studies of procedures that are commonly performed, are expensive, treat problems that have the most impact on the patient's life, and pose a minimal but acceptable risk to the placebo control group.

There remain dilemmas insofar as PCTs typically regard the placebo effect as a confounding factor. This concept may conflict with whatever the participant believes about placebos and the magnitude of their effects.

## Informed consent

It is not known if the requirement for fully informed consent in the research setting may "prime" individuals to anticipate the expected side effects of a particular pharmacological intervention and thereby inhibit placebo effects. Therefore, to design research trials to assess the clinical usefulness of placebo effects it may be necessary to withhold certain information from research participants. This possibility raises a myriad of ethical issues regarding the possible need for a less than fully informed consent process. These issues should be examined both theoretically and through well-designed patient survey methodologies. Such surveys may also provide input into methods for improving the consent process in general. For example, it is expected that variations in both consent forms and the interaction between investigator and potential participant may affect willingness to participate. More research is needed to identify the ideal features of the consent process.

The risk in the case of placebo surgery can be significant so that it is essential that patients who might participate in such a clinical trial be fully informed of the risk (as well as the risk from whatever may be the standard surgical intervention). Because such patients often suffer from chronic diseases, they may be particularly desperate and vulnerable. Care must be taken to ensure that they truly understand what they are agreeing to in the trial. Further, trial design should include both short- and long-term follow up to determine whether initial outcomes change over time.

## Participants versus non-participants

There are additional questions related to patient participation in clinical trials that may be studied in the context of screening for ongoing trials. Although it is known that subjects who volunteer for trials differ from those who do not, little is known about what factors – ethnographic, psychological, medical, or other – distinguish these two populations. Similarly, it is not known whether subjects who volunteer for PCTs are different from those who volunteer for trials that do not include a placebo arm. Conducting such research presents a further difficulty insofar as the subjects of interest, namely non-participants, may not be available or agree to be studied. New methods for evaluating these populations, which will guarantee appropriate privacy protections and use of research databases, may facilitate the conduct of such research. Such studies may lead to strategies to improve recruitment of populations that are historically underrepresented in clinical research.

## Recommendation 3: assess the attitudes and beliefs of clinicians and other investigators

Clearly both patient and investigator attitudes must be considered when designing and conducting any clinical research. Within the context of a randomized clinical trial, the randomization process should ensure that there is no systematic bias in the allocation of patients to treatments. However, there may be selection biases that affect the sample of subjects actually enrolled in clinical trials. For example, some investigators may be reluctant to refer particularly sick patients for PCTs when standard treatment exists. Such biases can have a significant effect on the overall interpretation of trial results, especially regarding generalizability to community-based populations. More information is needed on the effect of investigator preferences or incentives on the mix of patients enrolling in clinical trials. There also may be institutional factors related to patient access to care or reimbursement for procedures.

Finally, the role of the investigator in the informed consent process, particularly regarding its effect on patient comprehension, needs to be better understood. Related to all of the above is the need for further study of the consistency and reliability of the decision making processes of Institutional Review Boards (IRBs).

## Recommendation 4: develop new methods or new applications of existing methods for study design and analysis to address ethical and statistical issues of both PCTs and active control trials

There is a need to develop and evaluate alternative clinical trial designs that may resolve some of the complex ethical and statistical dilemmas identified. Designs utilizing randomized withdrawal, washout periods, or "add-on" studies, in which a new therapy is given along with a standard treatment, should be considered. Attention should be given to efficient designs that minimize the length and/or frequency of treatment and follow up. Such trials would limit the potential risk or discomfort associated with participation in PCTs. For research purposes, it is also important to recognize the potential for synergistic reactions among treatments. For example, in the past it has generally been assumed that the placebo group provides baseline data that can be subtracted out to determine the true treatment effect. However, there is reason to believe that placebo responses influence active arms of a trial and even "no-treatment" groups, who nevertheless are seen by professionals, receive a diagnosis, and experience other interactions. Appropriate methodology should be used to identify such interactions. Studies of the fate of patients assigned to placebo groups – outcomes, risks, and benefits – could make use of existing databases from past clinical trials.

Related to the above are issues regarding the extent to which patients and researchers are truly masked in a PCT. Indeed, in the case of surgical interventions certain procedures would be hard to mask, for example, total knee or hip replacement; spinal fusion. One approach that has been taken to evaluating masking is to gather data on patient guesses of treatment assignment at the end of the trial and compare these to both true assignment and overall outcomes. Evaluation of the potential effects of unmasking during the trial on the assessment of outcome, especially for patient reported endpoints, would help in the interpretation of the applicability of the trial to the clinical setting where no masking is entailed.

Ongoing trials may also be used to obtain additional information about factors mediating placebo and experimental drug effects. To this end, additional data can be collected and assessed as both prognostic factors and secondary outcomes. For example, some studies have suggested that patient expectations might have a significant impact on outcomes, however this has not been fully evaluated. Methods should be developed to measure patient expectations and evaluate their effects on both clinical outcomes and patient satisfaction.

## Recommendation 5: study the processes of informed consent/assent and research participation in children and other vulnerable or special populations

All of the previous ethical and statistical issues apply in research with vulnerable populations, with a particular need for sensitivity when dealing with special populations such as children. In the case of children, the informed consent process involves a parent or parents in addition to the child, all of whom have to make a decision about whether or not to participate in the research. In some cases IRBs can waive the requirement for children's assent.

More research is needed on the views of children regarding participation in clinical research including their understanding, attitudes towards clinical trials, and views of risks. Such studies of children, appropriately targeted to specific age groups, could have a significant impact on the design of both trials and the consent/assent process. Incorporating representatives of children such as parents, teachers, or even children, into the study review and approval process should be considered. Finally, there are issues unique to the developing child that require consideration throughout the design and conduct of all clinical trials. Appropriate endpoints and trial designs in pediatric trials may differ from those for trials in adults, since there are issues of both efficacy and safety unique to growing children.

Similar issues arise in certain mental health areas such as Alzheimer's disease in which a large part of the consent process falls to a primary caregiver. We currently know little about the way these processes differ from the standard informed consent process.

## Recommendation 6: study issues related to the conduct of multinational clinical trials in developing countries

The use of placebos in multinational trials, especially in developing countries, raises an important set of ethical challenges. Much of the current debate concerns assessment of the level of care that must be ensured for research participants. Some argue that the required level of care should be assessed based on what is available within the countries where the studies are being conducted while others would claim that the standards of care should be equal across all cultural settings. There are additional issues regarding eligibility for participation. The informed consent process differs significantly across cultures. The concept of a placebo may also vary depending on the cultural context. Many of the recommendations for further study of the ethics and science of PCTs should be extended to the multicultural setting in order to elucidate these differences and identify better means for developing and testing new pharmacological interventions that may be applied in a broader range of clinical, social, and cultural contexts.

# Part IV: Recommendations for research concerning the use of placebos in clinical trials to test behavioral interventions

Thomas D Borkovec, Lisa S Onken*

To draw conclusions about which behavioral or psychosocial therapies work, and more specifically, which therapies work best to treat a particular disorder, researchers need to design studies comparing two or more therapeutic approaches. The therapies must share specific factors considered causal in improving the condition under study, but differ in other specifiable ways. By using such experimental designs investigators can conclude that the therapy that is found to be superior embodies more causal factors than the comparison therapy. The fewer specifiable ways in which the approaches differ, the more specific can be the causal conclusion.

Ideally, the determination of superiority, based on a statistically significant difference between two different therapies, requires only a sufficiently large sample size. However, the judgment of superiority in the real world often takes into consideration the interests of outside parties, for example, the public at large or third party payers, who may introduce issues tied to the degree of clinical significance of the difference and cost-benefit analyses. Nevertheless, the more specific causes of change that can be identified, the more effectively can interventions be designed to treat more people. This means specifying as precisely as possible the particular operational, theory driven elements of an intervention and of comparison interventions, including the elements considered to be related to placebo effects inherent in any active psychological or behavioral intervention. It also means linking the empirical comparison of therapies to theoretical notions of mechanisms of change. Therefore, in evaluating any between-group design, there is only one requirement from a scientific, methodological perspective: in what procedural and theoretical ways are these two interventions identical and in what ways are they different? Any

---

* Members of breakout group 4 contributed to these recommendations: Guillermo Bernal, Richard R Bootzin, Howard Brody, Louis G Castonguay, Daniel E Moerman, Nancy Petry, Stuart J Pocock, Kenneth J Rothman, and Stephen Spielberg. See the Appendix for member information.

difference in outcome can only causally be attributed to the way in which they differ.

## Problems of "placebo" behavioral interventions

In considering the use of a placebo comparison group in testing behavioral interventions, researchers face two significant challenges. First, the use of the "gold" standard placebo controlled trial (PCT) to test behavioral interventions is problematic in a number of significant ways. Conceptually, it is not possible to design psychologically inert placebos. By their very nature, behavioral interventions involve interpersonal relationships, which for the many reasons outlined throughout this volume, are not inert. Methodologically, empirical evidence indicates that because they are often not credible to clients, psychological placebos may not evoke the same level of expectancy for improvement that behavioral interventions do. It is also impossible to keep therapists (and often clients) blind as to whether the client is receiving placebo or active treatment. Ethically, because behavioral interventions often take place over a long period of time (for example, in the typical psychotherapy outcome investigation), it is difficult for therapists to continue to provide an intervention believed to be considerably less effective than the compared experimental condition.

Second, because behavioral interventions contain a large number of components and PCT designs do not distinguish among them, one can only conclude for a PCT that the experimental treatment is worthy of further investigation to identify its active components and their mechanisms of action. Yet it is knowledge of the specific components and the mechanisms by which patients improve that will allow us to design more effective treatments. To overcome these obstacles, research is needed that uses alternative designs that focus on the identification of specific causal components (see Recommendation 1) and on the elucidation of causal mechanisms.

## Recommendation 1: employ constructive, dismantling, interactive, and parametric designs in the conduct of outcome research

In constructive designs, an intervention is provided with and without an added treatment component. For example, an investigator could compare one group in which cognitive behavioral therapy is provided during the first hour of each session to another group in which cognitive behavioral therapy is provided in the first hour and interpersonal psychotherapy is administered during the second hour. In dismantling designs, a complete intervention is compared to one or more of its components. For example, cognitive behavioral therapy could be contrasted with cognitive therapy alone and/or behavior therapy alone. In interactive designs, the order in which two therapies or therapy components are provided to a client can be experimentally manipulated (for example, half of the clients receive interpersonal psychotherapy during the first hour followed by cognitive behavioral therapy during the second hour, whereas the other half receive the opposite order). Such a design allows one to determine whether the effects of two interventions merely add separately to client improvement or whether prior reception of one intervention facilitates the therapeutic effects of the other. In parametric designs, interventions that vary along a dimension can be compared. For example, an investigation could compare groups that all receive experiential therapy but vary experimentally in the depth of emotional processing that the therapist provides to the clients.

Besides specifying causal agents more precisely and providing the best methods for testing of hypotheses, these designs have the added advantage of reducing some or all of the conceptual, methodological, and ethical problems associated with the use of placebo treatments. In addition, they hold constant a greater number of technical elements across comparison conditions, and employ comparison conditions whose credibility and expectancy for improvement are more likely to be equivalent. Such designs will require larger sample sizes, given that the effect sizes for such comparisons will often be smaller than those associated with placebo comparisons. However, the gain in knowledge about specific cause-and-effect relationships far outweighs this cost, especially when contrasted with the lack of useful knowledge generated by comparing behavioral to placebo interventions.

## Recommendation 2: conduct methodological research to develop additional experimental designs and methods

Although the above designs are recommended, research should be devoted to developing additional designs that can be used to elucidate causal components and mechanisms and that minimize or eliminate the previously mentioned conceptual, methodological, and ethical problems associated with the use of placebo control groups to test behavioral interventions. It remains unclear whether future research into attempts to develop acceptable psychological placebos is likely to solve the significant problems that are inherent to these placebos.

## Recommendation 3: be wary of conclusions drawn from clinical trials in which two very different forms of intervention (for example, cognitive behavioral therapy and interpersonal therapy) are compared

Behavioral interventions, insofar as they represent fundamentally different philosophies and mechanisms of behavioral change, should not be compared in the way drugs are studied in non-inferiority trials. If such a trial were to be conducted for behavioral interventions and show equivalence, it would fail to indicate anything of value regarding cause and effect. Should such a trial show a difference in outcome, the difference sheds little light in terms of specific causal factors because the techniques of the two interventions typically vary in a large number of ways. In addition, these trials commonly use expert therapists treating clients only in their own intervention, thus destroying internal validity by confounding type of intervention with therapist characteristics.

## Recommendation 4: develop standardized protocols for behavioral interventions and their comparison groups

The therapeutic procedures used in some behavioral approaches have varied widely in past investigations. As a result, it is often not possible to replicate or compare studies. Therapy protocols need to specify carefully and precisely what the therapist does during the therapy hour in any behavioral or comparison intervention, and cumulative knowledge would be facilitated by more widespread use of protocols across studies that are more similar in their specific procedures.

## Recommendation 5: ensure that therapists provide treatments to an equal number of clients in each intervention and comparison group to eliminate any potential therapist confound in the design, and develop valid and reliable measures of the degree of competence and expertness with which treatments are administered

Unless compared treatments are equivalent in therapist characteristics (including biases and backgrounds) and in the competence and expertness with which they deliver study protocols, a significant confounding factor exists in the design. This confound needs to be eliminated by crossing therapists with treatments and by a demonstration of equivalence in competence across compared groups.

## Recommendation 6: develop and employ valid ways to measure processes associated with the moment-to-moment transactions between therapist and client within the therapy hour

Such process research would be integrated into experimental outcome designs and would focus on both measuring hypothesized mechanisms of the behavioral interventions based on their underlying theory and on hypothesized mechanisms underlying any placebo factors that may be present within the intervention. Examples of existing process measures derived from theoretical orientations include the assessment of depth and type of emotional experiencing, the strength of the therapeutic alliance, specific complementary and non-complementary behaviors of the client and the therapist during their interactions, and therapist focus on intrapersonal versus interpersonal issues. Further research should be aimed at developing additional valid and reliable measures that capture a wide range of in-session processes hypothesized by therapy theories to promote improvement.

## Recommendation 7: investigate mechanisms of improvement in outcome research studies by measuring moderator and mediator variables

Moderator variables involve factors that may correlate with the effectiveness of a therapy (for example, an intervention may be effective with one type of gender, ethnicity, therapist, or level of problem severity, but is less effective with another type). Mediator variables involve factors that are causal links between the provision of an intervention and client improvement. Examples of such factors include the nature of the therapeutic relationship, self-healing potential, client and therapist expectancy for improvement from and credibility of an intervention, suppressed emotion, and underlying cognitive beliefs.

# *Section 6:* Conclusions and future directions

# 16: Conclusions and future directions

STEPHEN E STRAUS, JOSEPHINE P BRIGGS

In the preface to this volume, we noted that we were each motivated to organize the placebo workshop by interests of our respective NIH Institutes that reflect somewhat different perspectives. That we should address these interests within the framework of a comprehensive workshop was evident. What was not completely expected, however, was just how effective the union of social and biological scientists on the one hand and clinical trialists on the other would be. The result was a conference whose total benefit, we believed, far exceeded the sum of its parts. Indeed, the meeting was noteworthy for a number of significant accomplishments.

First, the conference contributed toward the ongoing transformation of the placebo from a negative concept to one that is gaining increasing appreciation. It occurred during a time period in which the concept of the placebo effect and the larger group of mind–brain–body effects to which it belongs are overcoming the pejorative connotation they were once assigned. Yet, mind–brain–body effects, including placebo effects, are still not fully appreciated in contemporary medicine. This may be explained, in part, as a legacy of the Cartesian model that envisions the mind as being something discrete from brain and body, and by the powerful reductionist approach of the current biomedical model. Within this model, practitioners are trained to focus primarily on finding and eliminating physiologically demonstrable pathology. They are less concerned with the implications of such pathology for mind and brain, or for that matter, the potential of mind and brain to contribute to and resolve visceral pathology.

Now we are witnessing an evolution in how placebo and other related effects are perceived, facilitated by a substantial body of research that provides compelling evidence of mind–brain–body interactions. Indeed, at a subsequent meeting on mind–body interactions convened by the John D and Catherine T MacArthur Foundation Network and NIH,* distinguished

* Science of Mind–Body Interactions: An Exploration of Integrative Mechanisms. Bethesda, MD, March 26–28, 2001.

researchers reported the results of elegant studies demonstrating the many ways through which the mind can influence the brain and body at the societal, organismal, cellular, and molecular levels. The Mind–Body Interactions meeting represented to us a superb complement to the Placebo Workshop, having dealt in greater depth with the cellular and molecular, neurobiological and neuroendocrinological processes mediating these interactions than had been feasible in the context of the placebo meeting. Moreover, in dealing substantively with the biology of social interactions, it increased the breadth of the Placebo Workshop.

Second, participants in the Placebo Workshop agreed upon an expanded definition of placebo, extending its meaning beyond that of a physical pill or sham procedure to encompass clinical symbols as well as interpersonal characteristics of patient–provider interactions that can affect expectations and clinical outcomes, what Anne Harrington termed at the workshop, the dramaturgy of the therapeutic process, for example, the white coat, the bedside manner, the verbal and non-verbal communication, the setting.

Third, conference participants outlined a multicomponent model to explain placebo effects, in which the positive effects on health are mediated by psychosocial mechanisms, which transduce meaning from the individual's cultural context and in turn activate intervening psychophysiological processes.

Fourth, they clarified that what is construed as placebo effects in clinical trials is actually a composite of veritable mind–body effects and outcome artifacts; confounding the apparent placebo effect are phenomena such as the natural history of disease, patient or investigator bias, and regression to the mean. If there is to be a "science" of the placebo, it is critical to distinguish these artifacts from true mind–body placebo effects. Clarity about these separable phenomena is sure to improve the design of clinical trials.

As hoped, the process of articulating the nature and uses of the placebo led to a set of recommendations for further research. Over the ensuing months, NIH staff toiled to coalesce these recommendations into a workable research strategy. In May 2001, however, as we were nearing the culmination of this effort, Hróbjartsson and Gøtzsche, in a widely publicized report, called the very existence of the placebo effect into question. Based on a systematic review of clinical trials in which patients were randomly assigned to either placebo or no treatment, they concluded in a special article in the *New England Journal of Medicine* that there is little evidence in general that placebos had powerful clinical effects.[1] This provocative assertion in a prestigious journal necessitated a cogent response. How can we reconcile the conclusion of conference participants that the placebo effect is real and potentially powerful with Hróbjartsson's and Gøtzsche's conclusion that the placebo effect is a myth?

As several authors eloquently stated in their letters to the Editor of the *N Engl J Med*, there are reasons to reject the sweeping conclusions of these two researchers. They cite, for example, the inappropriate performance of a meta-analysis that pools data from trials addressing different questions; procedural problems; and the failure to control for the potential therapeutic effects of clinical attention received by patients in the placebo and no-treatment groups.[2] The *N Engl J Med* report, furthermore, ignored not only the many studies employing strictly controlled experimental conditions that show that powerful mind–body placebo responses do exist, but also the fact that we are beginning to understand some of the underlying explanatory mechanisms.

Nevertheless, we welcome the uncertainty that Hróbjartsson and Gøtzsche raised. Healthy skepticism is critical to ensure that scientists remain ever vigilant in seeking the truth. Thus, rather than providing the closing argument in the case of the placebo, we believe they have made obvious the need for further research. As though in anticipation of this challenge, the interdisciplinary research agenda (fully described in Chapter 15 of this book) addressed each of the core issues raised by Hróbjartsson and Gøtzsche, and then some. In this regard, the conference was noteworthy in bringing together social and biological scientists, many of whom had not thought about the methodological problems that need to be solved to ensure rigorous and ethical clinical trial design, and clinical trialists, many of whom had not thought about placebo effects in their own right. The pooling of expertise created a forum where each group of scientists could offer fresh insights on elucidating placebo effects, improving clinical trial methodology, and exploring the opportunities to apply the placebo effect in clinical practice.

To implement the research recommendations, and in keeping with an undeferred commitment, NIH staff developed three trans-institute initiatives to:

1 study the use of placebos in clinical trials
2 elucidate the underlying mechanisms of the placebo effect
3 investigate applications of placebo effects in clinical practice.

As this is being written, the financial resources to support the research agenda are being husbanded and the initiatives are being released to the public. The impact of such research can be substantial.

The advent of the placebo controlled clinical trial ushered in the golden age of evidence-based medicine. But with so many effective therapies now available, the recently revised Helsinki Declaration raises ethical and methodological challenges for the conduct of clinical trials, on which we remain critically reliant to provide evidence of safety and efficacy of new therapies. Design of clinical trials will benefit from a fuller understanding of the underlying mechanisms of placebo effects and their interactions with test therapies. The fruits of this basic research are needed also to help engender new strategies to exploit placebo mechanisms as therapeutic allies

# Appendix

## Members of Breakout Groups

**Ader, Robert**
George L Engel Professor of Psychosocial Medicine
Director, Center for Psychoneuroimmunology Research
Director, Behavioral and Psychosocial Medicine
University of Rochester School of Medicine and Dentistry
Rochester, NY, USA

**Benedetti, Fabrizio**
Professor of Physiology and Neuroscience
Department of Neuroscience
Rita Levi-Montalcini Center for Brain Repair
University of Turin Medical School
Turin, Italy

**Bernal, Guillermo**
Professor
Department of Psychology
Director, University Center for Psychological Services and Research-CUSEP
University of Puerto Rico, Rio Piedras Campus
San Juan, Puerto Rico

**Bootzin, Richard R**
Professor
Department of Psychology
University of Arizona
Tucson, AZ, USA

**Borkovec, Thomas D**
Distinguished Professor of Psychology
Department of Psychology
Pennsylvania State University
University Park, PA, USA

**Brody, Howard**
Professor
Departments of Family Practice and Philosophy
Center for Ethics and Humanities in the Life Sciences
Michigan State University
East Lansing, MI, USA

**Brown, Walter A**
Clinical Professor
Department of Psychiatry
Brown Medical School
Tufts University School of Medicine
Providence, RI, USA

**Califf, Robert M**
Professor of Medicine
Associate Vice Chancellor for Clinical Research
Director, Duke Clinical Research Institute
Durham, NC, USA

**Castonguay, Louis G**
Associate Professor
Department of Psychology
Pennsylvania State University
University Park, PA, USA

**Chesney, Margaret A**
Professor in Residence
Department of Medicine
University of California, San Francisco
San Francisco, CA, USA

**Contoreggi, Carlo**
Chief, Clinical Imaging Service
Brain Imaging Branch
National Institute on Drug Abuse
National Institutes of Health
Baltimore, MD, USA

**Czajkowski, Susan M**
Social Scientist Analyst
Division of Epidemiology and Clinical Applications
Behavioral Medicine Scientific Research Group
National Heart Lung and Blood Institute
National Institutes of Health
Bethesda, MD, USA

**Davis, Clarence E**
Professor and Chair
Department of Biostatistics
School of Public Health
University of North Carolina at Chapel Hill
Chapel Hill, NC, USA

**Feigal, David W Jr**
Director
Center for Devices and Radiological Health
US Food and Drug Administration
Rockville, MD, USA

**Fischbach, Gerald D***
Director
National Institute of Neurological Disorders and Stroke
National Institutes of Health
Bethesda, MD, USA

**Fischbach, Ruth L**♦
Senior Advisor for Biomedical Ethics
National Institutes of Health
Bethesda, MD, USA

**Fox, Kenneth L**
Assistant Professor of Pediatrics
Boston University School of Medicine
Lecturer on Social Medicine
Harvard Medical School
Boston, MA, USA

**Gracely, Richard H**
Chief, Clinical Measurement and Mechanisms Unit
Pain and Neurosensory Mechanisms Branch
National Institute of Dental and Craniofacial Research
National Institutes of Health
Bethesda, MD, USA

*Currently Vice President for Health and Biomedical Sciences, Dean of the Faculty of Health Sciences, Dean of the Faculty of Medicine, Columbia University, New York, NY, USA
♦Currently Professor of Bioethics, Columbia University, College of Physicians and Surgeons, New York, NY, USA

**Hahn, Robert A**
Senior Scientist
Guide to Community Preventive Services Activity
Division of Prevention Research and Analytic Methods
Centers for Disease Control and Prevention
Atlanta, GA, USA

**Harrington, Anne**
Professor of the History of Science
Harvard University
Cambridge, MA, USA

**Holman, Halsted**
Berthold & Belle N. Guggenhime Professor of Medicine
Stanford University School of Medicine
Stanford, CA, USA

**Jonas, Wayne B**
Associate Professor
Department of Family Medicine
Uniformed University of the Health Sciences
Bethesda, MD, USA

**Kaptchuk, Ted J**
Assistant Professor of Medicine
Harvard Medical School
Cambridge, MA, USA

**Kirsch, Irving**
Professor
Department of Psychology
University of Connecticut
Storrs, CT, USA

**Kitt, Cheryl A**
Program Director for Pain Research
National Institute of Neurological Disorders and Stroke
National Institutes of Health
Bethesda, MD, USA

**Levine, Robert J**
Professor, Department of Medicine
Lecturer, Department of Pharmacology
Co-Chairperson, Yale University Interdisciplinary Program for Bioethics
Yale University
New Haven, CT, USA

**Miller, Frank G**
Special Expert
National Institute of Mental Health
Department of Clinical Bioethics
Warren Grant Magnuson Clinical Center
National Institutes of Health
Bethesda, MD, USA

**Moerman, Daniel E**
William E. Stirton Professor of Anthropology
Department of Behavioral Sciences
University of Michigan-Dearborn
Dearborn, MI, USA

**Moore, Rhonda J**
Fellow
Department of Epidemiology
University of Texas M. D. Anderson Cancer Center
Houston, TX, USA

**Moseley, J Bruce**
Clinical Associate Professor
Baylor Sports Medicine Institute
Baylor College of Medicine
Houston, TX, USA

**Onken, Lisa S**
Associate Director for Behavioral Treatment Research
Chief, Behavioral Treatment Development Branch
Division of Treatment Research and Development
National Institute on Drug Abuse
National Institutes of Health
Bethesda, MD, USA

**Petry, Nancy**
Associate Professor of Psychiatry
Department of Psychiatry
University of Connecticut Health Center
Farmington, CT, USA

**Pocock, Stuart J**
Professor of Medical Statistics
London School of Hygiene and Tropical Medicine
London, England

**Price, Donald D**
Professor
Department of Oral and Maxillofacial Surgery, College of Dentistry
Department of Neuroscience, College of Medicine
University of Florida
Gainesville, FL, USA

**Propert, Kathleen J**
Associate Professor of Biostatistics
Department of Bioethics and Epidemiology
University of Pennsylvania School of Medicine
Philadelphia, PA, USA

**Rose, Robert M**
Director of the Mind, Brain, Body & Health Initiative
John D. and Catherine T. MacArthur Foundation
Chicago, IL, USA

**Rothman, Kenneth J**
Professor
Department of Epidemiology and Biostatistics, Boston University School of Public Health
Section of Preventive Medicine, Department of Medicine, Boston University School of Medicine
Boston, MA, USA

**Sankar, Pamela**
Assistant Professor of Bioethics
Center for Bioethics
University of Pennsylvania
Philadelphia, PA, USA

**Siegel, Shepard**
University Professor
Department of Psychology
McMaster University
Hamilton, Ontario, Canada

**Spiegel, David**
Professor and Associate Chair of Psychiatry and Behavioral Sciences
Stanford University School of Medicine
Stanford, CA, USA

**Spielberg, Stephen P**
Vice President for Pediatric Drug Development
Janssen Research Foundation
Titusville, NJ, USA

**Spiro, Howard Marget**
Professor Emeritus
Department of Internal Medicine
Yale University
New Haven, CT, USA

**Stefanek, Michael**
Chief, Basic Biobehavioral Research Branch
Behavioral Research Program
Division of Cancer Control and Population Sciences
National Cancer Institute
National Institutes of Health
Bethesda, MD, USA

**Sternberg, Esther M**
Chief, Section on Neuroendocrine Immunology and Behavior
Director, Integrative Neural Immune Program
National Institute of Mental Health
National Institutes of Health
Bethesda, MD, USA

**Temple, Robert J**
Associate Director for Medical Policy
Center for Drug Evaluation and Research
US Food and Drug Administration
Rockville, MD, USA

**Thayer, Julian F**
Special Expert
Laboratory of Personality and Cognition
Gerontology Research Center
National Institute on Aging
National Institutes of Health
Baltimore, MD, USA

**Weijer, Charles**
Associate Professor of Medicine
Dalhousie University
Halifax, Nova Scotia, Canada

**Weinstein, John N**
Senior Research Investigator
Laboratory of Molecular Pharmacology
National Cancer Institute
National Institutes of Health
Bethesda, MD, USA

**Wendler, Dave S**
Head, Unit on Vulnerable Populations
Section on Human Subjects Research
Department of Clinical Bioethics
Warren Grant Magnuson Clinical Center
National Institutes of Health
Bethesda, MD, USA

**Wittes, Janet**
President
Statistics Collaborative
Washington, DC, USA

**Woolley, Sabra F**
Program Director, Health Promotion Research
Behavioral Research Program
Division of Cancer Control and Population Sciences
National Cancer Institute
National Institutes of Health
Bethesda, MD, USA

**Wristers, Kimberly**
Assistant Professor of Medicine
Houston Center for Quality of Care and Utilization Studies
Baylor College of Medicine
Houston, TX, USA

# Index

Page numbers in **bold** type refer to figures; those in *italics* refer to tables or boxed material.


abciximab 259
active controlled trials 209–25, 230
  appropriate use 237–9
  "double dummy" procedure 250
  ethical issues 210–16
  incentives for study quality 222
  inferential issues 216–23
active treatment
  effects, correlation with placebo effects 5–6
  placebo effects 5
  prescribed as placebo 18, 58, 297–8
acupuncture 83, 118, 179, 193
acute coronary syndromes 252, 257–8
addiction 58
add-on therapy 224, 232, 239, 253
adherence, treatment
  in non-inferiority trials 246, 247
  placebo effect and 6, 91, *92*, 127
adrenergic receptors 177
adrenocorticotropin hormone (ACTH) **172**, 176
adverse effects
  non-inferiority trials 239, 240
  placebos *see* "nocebo" effects; risks of placebos
  reporting 246
advertising, power of 4, 78–9, 100
aerobic exercise 4–5, 79
Africa, sub-Saharan 24–5, 69, 71, 267–8
AIDS 48, 69
  *see also* HIV infection
alcoholic beverages 142, 152
alcoholism 8, 116, 117, 142
allergy, to flowers 143
alteplase 27
alternative medicine *see* complementary and alternative medicine
Alzheimer's disease 305
American Academy of Pediatrics 66–7
American Medical Association
  Code of Ethics (1847) 56
  Principles of Medical Ethics (1980) 55, 56
amiodarone 91, *92*
amphetamine 11, 147, 148
amygdala 291
  in analgesia 13, 178, **186**, 188
  in conditioning of immune response 175, 176
analgesia
  brain stimulation produced (SPA) 185–7, 192–3
  counterirritation 193–4
  desire for 197
  endogenous systems 190–4
  learning 184–5
  neural pathways 175, 185–8
  placebo *see* placebo analgesia
  stress 13–14, 185, 198
analgesics 21, 266
  branded *v* unbranded 4, 78–9, 100
  physician effects 5, 81–3
  placebo 298
  sequence effects 145–6, 194–5
  *see also* cream, placebo; ketorolac; morphine
angina 145, 258–9
  abandoned treatments 94–5
  bilateral internal mammary artery ligation 84
  bypass surgery *v* angioplasty 23, 240
  laser treatment 84–6, 253
  randomized withdrawal design 224
angiotensin-converting enzyme inhibitors (ACEIs) 220, *221*
animal studies
  conditioning 10–11, 137–8, 173–4, 287
  endogenous analgesia systems 190–1
  learning analgesia 184–5
  neuroendocrine pathways 179
  *see also* dogs; rats
antacids 89
antibiotics 40–1, *92*
  equivalence trials 230–1
  as placebos 18, 58, 127, 297–8
anticoagulation 23, 240, 255
antidepressant drugs 103
  assay sensitivity problem 21, 219–20, 221
  effects, correlation with placebo effects 100

research recommendations 298
response expectancies 9, 122
risks of placebo controls 21–2
anti-epileptic drugs 224
antihistamines 21, 266
antihypertensives
assay sensitivity problem 21
placebo controlled trials 22, 266, 279
*see also* hypertension
antipsychotic drugs 21–2
anxiety 114–15, 287–8
placebo analgesia and 198
*see also* generalized anxiety disorder
arginine vasopressin (AVP) **172**
arthritis 170–1, 289
arthroscopy, knee 86–7
aspirin 79, 145–6, 240, 257–8
assay sensitivity 22, 217–21
establishing 219–21
non-inferiority (equivalence) trials 21, 210, 216, 217–18
study defects undermining *222*
ASSENT-2 trial 257
asthma 174, 289
atrial fibrillation 224
atropine 148
attention deficit hyperactivity disorder (ADHD) 118
attention placebo controls 110
attribution theory 122–3
autoimmune diseases 170–1, 173–4
autonomic nervous system 12, 173
in CAM therapy effects 178–9
in immunological conditioning 175, 176–7
autonomy, patient 212, 215, 233
aversion learning 136, 140, 174, 190
AZT (zidovudine) 24–5, 71, 267–9

β endorphin 193
β-adrenergic activity 177
Babinski, Joseph 38–9
back pain, low 95–7
Bandura, Albert 119, 120
Beecher, Henry K 41–2, 63, 87, 159
behavioral environments 288
behavioral therapy 8, 117
placebo controlled trials 306–10
bereavement 100
Bernheim, Hippolyte 38, 39
best interests, study participants 214, 215, 232
best proven therapeutic method
identifying 232
Levine's interpretation 274–6
standard 212, 229–30, 266–70
bias
observer (investigator) 16, 27, 112–13, 252–3
patient 15–16, 113
response 118
therapist 112–13
bilateral internal mammary artery ligation (BIMAL) 84
biofeedback 174
biological therapies 258–9
birthdays 47
blinding 228, 304
*see also* double blind studies
blindness, psychogenic 3, 47–8
brain
endogenous pain-inhibitory systems 184, 185–8
imaging *see* neuroimaging
immune system interaction 170, 171–3
mediators and pathways 289
stimulation produced analgesia (SPA) 185–7, 192–3
branding 4, 78–9, 100
Brazil 90
bright light therapy 113–14
bulbocapnine 138

Cabot, Richard 40
caffeine 9, 121, 141, 146–7
CAM *see* complementary and alternative medicine
Cambodian refugees 3, 47–8
cancer
chemotherapy 135–6, 137, 214
equivalence trials 230–1
Cannon, Walter Bradford 48
capsaicin 199
capsules *see* tablets/capsules
cardiac placebo effects 144–5
care, duty to 270–4
carotid endarterectomy 240
carotid stenting 240
Cartesian dualism 6, 313
catalepsy, conditional 138, 147
catecholamines 177
Catholic Charismatic rituals 6
causal attributions 122–3
central nervous system (CNS)
centers involved in conditioning 175
imaging *see* neuroimaging
immune system interaction 170, 171–3
mediators and pathways 289
cerebral cortex **186**
Charcot, Jean Martin 37–8, 39
chemical sensitivity, multiple (MCS) 10, 134, 140–1
chemotherapy, cancer 135–6, 137, 214
children, as research subjects 66–7, 304–5
Chinese traditional beliefs 5, 80
Chinese traditional medicine 83
chiropractic 95–7
chloral hydrate 122–3
chlorpromazine 11, *92*, 148
cholecystokinin (CCK) 178, 190–1
antagonists 99, 190–1
cholesterol, high blood 16, 159, 160–2
cholesterol-lowering drugs 91, *92*, 165
cholestyramine 165
cigarettes, placebo 142
cimetidine **83**, 87, 89, 100, **101**
classical conditioning *see* Pavlovian conditioning
clinical events
committees 252
non-fatal 252

clinical practice
placebo responses 94–7, 110
placebo use in 17–18, 35–6, 54–63
barriers to 297
bypassing informed consent 56–7
by deception 17–18, 55–6, 59–60
definitions 54–5
historical aspects 40
non-deceptive approaches 60–1
recommendations 59–60
research needs 29, 61–3, 293–9
risks from 18, 57–60
clinical research
*Declaration of Helsinki see Declaration of Helsinki*
placebo effects 110
therapeutic and non-therapeutic 276–7
clinical trials 2–3, 17, 28
analysis 20–1
classification 250
design *see* study design
in developing countries 24–5, 69–71, 266–70, 279, 305
large-scale pragmatic 25–7, 249–61
participants *see* study participants
placebo controlled *see* placebo controlled trials
clinicians *see* physicians
clofibrate 91, *92*
clonidine 121–2
cocaine 142–3
coffee 9, 10, 121, 141
cognition 6–10, 117–23, 287–8
Cohen, Sanford 48
color of tablets/capsules 4, 78, 88–9
communication, verbal and non-verbal 295
compensatory conditional responses (CRs) 11–12, 147–52
drug tolerance and 149–51
in Pavlovian conditioning 149
placebo effects and 151
unresolved issues 151–2
withdrawal symptoms and 150–1
complementary and alternative medicine (CAM)
CNS pathways 178–9
meaning responses 95–7
research recommendations 294, 298–9
role of placebo effect 17–18, 36, 125
compliance, treatment *see* adherence, treatment
conditional response (reflex) (CR) 10, 135
compensatory *see* compensatory conditional responses
conditional stimulus (CS) 10, 135
conditioning
arguments against 100–1
biological mechanisms 171–9
classical (Pavlovian) *see* Pavlovian conditioning
operant 174
*v* expectancy 14–15, 195–6
confidence intervals 241, 242–3
conflicts of interest 67
confounded treatment procedures 113–14
confounding 227–8
consent, informed *see* informed consent
constipation 165
constructive designs 307–8
coronary angiograms 277
coronary angioplasty 240
coronary artery bypass surgery 240
coronary artery catheters 277
coronary stenting 259
corticotropin releasing hormone (CRH) **172**, 176, 177
costs
best proven therapeutic method 267, 268
non-inferiority trials 23, 240
placebo controlled trials 27, 254–5
Council of International Organizations of Medical Sciences (CIOMS) 25, 268, 275
counterirritation analgesia 193–4
cream, placebo 14–15, 195–6, 199–200
cross-cultural studies 296
"crossover designs" 146
cultural influences 70, 171, 288
placebo responses 90–1
research recommendations 290, 296
*see also* meaning response
culture bound syndromes 91
cyclophosphamide
animal studies 10–11, 144, 152, 173–4, 175
in multiple sclerosis 10, 143–4, 174
cytokines 170, **172**, 176

δ 22–3, 241–5
data, missing 247, 252
death
cause of 252
postponement 47
as study endpoint 252
voodoo 48
*see also* mortality
deception
in clinical practice 17–18, 40, 55–6, 59–60
in clinical research 64, 121
*Declaration of Helsinki* 19–20, 28, 265–70
1975 revision 210–12
on conflicts of interest 67
developing countries and 25, 28, 70, 266–70
fifth revision (1996) 19, 266–70
history 274–6
on informed consent 233
Levine on 274–8
on patients *v* volunteers 233–4
Rothman on 23–4, 229, 232
routine violations 277–8
sixth revision (2000) 19, 67–8, 212–13, 270
Temple on 20–1, 22, 210–16
delinquency 117
delirium 179

demoralization 118–19
dental pain 5, 81–2
depression
  drug treatment *see* antidepressant drugs
  placebo response rates 114–15, 258
  safety of placebos 21–2
  therapeutic relationship 116
design, clinical trial *see* study design
desire for relief 197, 202, 287–8
developing countries 24–5, 28, 69–71, 266–70, 279, 305
diabetes 254
diclofenac 239
disclosure
  conflicts of interest 67
  emotional experiences 93, 99–100, 123, 174
discomfort, study participants 213–15, 224, 234–5
disease
  complex 170–1
  natural history 15, 112
  placebo effect and 6
diskectomy, lumbar 86
dismantling designs 307–8
documentation
  informed consent procedures 72
  placebo use in clinical practice 18, 59–60
dogs
  cardiac placebo effects 144
  morphine studies 10, 11, 137, 138, 147
  Pavlov's studies 134–5, 137–8
Dominican Republic 71
dorsal horn 178, 186, 187–8, 190–1
double blind, double dummy design 26–7
double blind studies 112–13
  informed consent 64–5
  investigator bias 16
  *v* deceptive administration 121
  double dummy procedures 250, 255
drugs
  administration cues 135–6, 148–9
  illicit use 142–3
  new 82, **83**
dualism, Cartesian 6, 313
Duke Clinical Research Institute (DCRI) 258
duodenal ulcer *see* peptic ulcer disease
duty to care 270–4
dwarfism, psychosocial 47
dying patients 47

"early escape" 213, 224
effect size 223
efficacy (self-efficacy) expectations 8, 119–20
electric shock 14, 195
electrocardiogram 144
emotional experiences, writing about 93, 99–100, 123, 174
endorphins 13, 185, 193
endoscopies, repeated 277
endpoints (outcome measures)
  in clinical effectiveness trials 27, 251–3
  measurability 251–2
  minimizing discomfort/harm 224
  non-inferiority trials 246
  objectivity 26, 228, 252–3, 260
enkephalin 187
environmental cues 10, 184–5
environmental factors 170–1, 288
epidemiology 276
epinephrine 148, 177
eptifibatide 259
equipoise, clinical 24, 68, 229, 254, 271–2, 301
equivalence trials *see* non-inferiority (equivalence) trials
errors
  in equivalence trials 231
  measurement 162
  medical 57
  type 1 238, 245
  type 2 238
ethical issues 16–27, 28–9, 53–73
  placebo controlled trials 210–16, 254
  principles 283–5
ethical review committees *see* Institutional Review Boards
ethnic studies 296
evaluative trials 250
exercise, aerobic 4–5, 79
expectancy 173–5
  and motivation 197
  placebo analgesia and 196–7, 202
  response *see* response expectancy
  theory 153
  *v* conditioning 14–15, 195–6
expectations
  efficacy (self-efficacy) 8, 119–20
  outcome 8, 119–20
  research agenda 287–8, 304
explanatory mechanisms 6–12, 77–103, 284, 314
  historical aspects 49–50
  meaning responses 98–103
  research needs 128–9, 286–91
  social learning perspective 108–29
explanatory trials 250
extinction 11, 137, 145–6

"fallacy of the package deal" 277
family, role of 296
FDA *see* Food and Drug Administration
fear 175, 184, 185
fentanyl 82
fibrinolytic therapy 254, 256–7
fiduciary obligation 270–4
flowers, allergy to 143
Food, Drug and Cosmetic Act, 1962 amendments 2, 275
Food and Drug Administration (FDA) 219, 221, 258, 259–60
footshock, inescapable 13–14, 185, 190

$GABA_A$ agonist 148
Galton, Sir Francis 160
gender differences 88, *92*

generalization, stimulus 11, 136–7
generalized anxiety disorder 100, 103
genetic studies 170–1
genomics 291
Germany 90
glucocorticoids **172**, 173, 176
glucose administration 148, 149
glycoprotein IIb/IIIa inhibitors 258, 259–60
good of personal care, duty to provide 270–1
GUSTO-I trial 256–7
GUSTO-IIa trial 257–8
GUSTO-III trial 27, 257

$H_2$ receptor antagonists 266
*see also* cimetidine; ranitidine
harmful effects of placebos *see* risks of placebos
Hawthorne effect 159, 285
headache
branded *v* unbranded analgesics 4, 78–9, 100
migraine 164
placebo controlled trials 234
healing, placebo effect and 124–5
healthy volunteers 68, 215–16, 233–4
heart failure 220, *221*
*Helicobacter pylori* 90, 242
"hello-goodbye" effect 113
Helsinki Declaration *see Declaration of Helsinki*
heparin 257–8
hepatitis B vaccination 99–100
herpes simplex virus (HSV) infection 95
*Herzinsuffienz* 90
"highest attainable and sustainable therapeutic method" 269–70, 279
Hill, Sir Austin Bradford 43
hippocampus 175
historical background 2–3, 35–51
HIV infection
perinatal transmission 24–5, 71, 267–9
*see also* AIDS
holidays, cultural or religious 47
homeopathy 36
homeostasis 125
hope 8, 118–19
hospital window, view through 3, 47
hot flushes, postmenopausal 121–2
hyperalgesia 99, 149, 151
hyperglycaemia 148, 149
hypertension
correlation of drug and placebo effects 100
physician's *v* patient's views 83–4
related placebo effects 289
safety of placebos 22, 254
*see also* antihypertensives
hypnosis 38, 287–8
hypochondriasis 39
hypoglycaemia 148, 152
hypothalamic-pituitary-adrenal (HPA) axis 12, **172**, 173, 176
hypothalamus 13, 175, **186**
hysteria 37–8, 39

imaging 242
*see also* neuroimaging
imipramine 219–20
immune response
conditioned 10–11, 138, 143–4, 152, 173–5
cultural influences 99–100
immunology, psychoneuroendocrine 12–13, 169–80, 289–90
inclusion criteria 159–60, 227
incurable patients 40
infectious diseases 69
inflammation 177
inflammatory disease 170–1
information
on risks of placebos 65–6, 72
withholding 55–6, 302
informed consent
in clinical practice 56–7
in clinical trials 64–7, 212, 273
in developing countries 69
research agenda 72, 302, 304–5
sufficiency 232–3
infusions, placebo 255
injection, compulsive 142
insomnia 113–14, 122–3, 288
Institutional Review Boards (IRBs) 63–4, 272
informed consent issues 65, 67, 72
protection of individual rights 68
in research agenda 303, 304
sufficiency of approval 233
insular cortex 175
insulin
induced hypoglycaemia 148, 152
shock therapy 138, 146
intention to treat analysis 246–7
interactive designs 307–8
interactive, multi-dimensional model (Bootzin) 9–10, 126–8
internal mammary artery ligation, bilateral (BIMAL) 84
International Code of Medical Ethics 275
International Conference on Harmonization (ICH) 26, 213–16, 256
*International Ethical Guidelines for Biomedical Research Involving Human Subjects* 25, 65, 268, 275
investigational tools 290–1
investigators
conflicts of interest 67
motivation 253
(observer) bias 16, 27, 112–13, 252–3
research agenda 303
"rogue" 214–15
separation of physician role 273–4, 279
IRBs *see* Institutional Review Boards
ischemia, recurrent 252
ISIS-2 study 27, 256

Jehovah's Witnesses 278

ketoprofen 239
ketorolac 14, 178, 199, 239
knee arthroscopy 86–7

large-scale multi-site trials 24–5
laser treatment, angina 84–6, 253
lead-in periods 222
learning
  analgesia 184–5
  aversion 136, 140, 174, 190
  research recommendations 286–7
  social 6–10, 108–29
  *see also* conditioning
leukopenia 143, 174
life-threatening conditions 19, 20
light therapy 113–14
limbic system 291
Lipid Research Clinics Coronary Primary Prevention Trial 165
literature, popular and professional 62–3
liver biopsies 277
locus coeruleus 176
luteinizing hormone 142
lymphatic cancer 5, 80
lymph nodes 176–7
lymphocytes 173, 177

magnetic resonance imaging (MRI), functional 290
"malingering" 97
masking *see* blinding
meaning response 3–6, 81–103, 114
  in clinical *v* experimental settings 94–7
  definition 3, 78
  dimensions 81–3
  mechanisms 98–103
  in other medical systems 97–8
  patients *v* physicians 83–4
  surgery 84–7
  variability 87–94
  adherence and 91, *92*
  cultural factors 90–1
  disclosure 93
  formal factors 88–9
  self-assessed health 93–4
  *see also* cultural influences
measurement
  artifacts 15–16
  error 162
  placebo analgesia 202–3
  reactivity 113
medical care
  standards in developing countries 70–1
  *see also* treatment
medical education 61–2, 294–5
medical practice
  definition 275
  *see also* clinical practice
meditation 178–9, 287–8
medulla, ventromedial (RVM) 178, **186,** 187, 188–90
memory distortion 15, 200–1, 203, 287–8
Meniere's disease 86
*The Merck Manual* 97
methodological aspects 16–27, 111–14
  conditioning studies 138
  research needs 308
  *see also* study design
methylphenidate 118
"me too" drug development 23, 239
mice 138, 144
microarray chip technology 291
migraine headache 164
mind–body–brain interactions 313–14
mind–body dualism 6, 313
missing data 247, 252
morphine 101–2, 191
  compensatory conditioned responses 11, 149, 151
  conditioning 10, 14, 137, 138, 178, 199
  immune effects 173, 177
mechanism of action 186–7
  reverse tolerance 11, 147
mortality
  self-assessed health and 93–4
  trials, large simple 256–7
  *see also* death
motivation 197, 253
multiple chemical sensitivity (MCS) 10, 134, 140–1
multiple sclerosis (MS) 10, 143–4, 174
myocardial infarction (MI)
  adherence and placebo effects 91, *92*
  study endpoints 252
  thrombolysis after *see* thrombolysis
myths, popular 5–6

naloxone 13, 101–2, 187, 190, 192
  in acupuncture analgesia 179, 193
  physician effects 81–2
  in placebo analgesia 99, 178, 199
  reversibility test 192, 201–2
naltrexone 178
narcotic analgesics *see* opioids
National Institute of Allergy and Infectious Diseases 36
National Institutes of Health (NIH) 1, 36–7, 313–16
natural history, disease 15, 112
nausea
  postoperative 221
  pretreatment 135–6
Navajo medicine 6, 98
"needle freaks" 142
neural pathways, mediating 171–3
neuroendocrine mediators 169–80
neuroendocrine stress response **172,** 173, 176
neuroimaging 13, 128, 179
  functional 202
  research recommendations 290–1
neuropeptides 12, 173, 177, 289
neuroticism 39
neurotransmitters 176, 289
*New England Journal of Medicine* 1, 267, 314–15
nicotine 142
nineteenth century 2, 37–8
nitroglycerin 144–5
"nocebo" effects 3, 58, 78, 284
  conditioning and 151
  research needs 293
  *see also* risks of placebos
noise, placebo effect as 43

nomifensine 219–20
non-inferiority (equivalence) trials 20, 210, 236–48
 appropriate goals 22–3, 241–5
 assay sensitivity 21, 210, 216, 217–18
 comparing therapies 222–3
 credible uses *223*
 defects undermining sensitivity *222*, 231, 245
 disadvantages 222–3, 230–2, 245–7, 254
 sample sizes 219, 221, 230, 231–2, 241–5
 significance testing and 231
 terminology 236
 types 239–41
 *v* superiority trials 216, 218
non-inferiority margin (M) 217, 219, 223, 241
non-steroidal anti-inflammatory drugs (NSAID) 239
norepinephrine 177
no-treatment controls 15, 43, 112
 regression to mean 165
nucleus raphe magnus (NRM) 187
nucleus reticularis gigantocellularis (NRG) 187
nucleus reticularis paragigantocellularis (NRP) 187
number of tablets/capsules 4, 89
Nuremberg Code 19, 232, 274

observer (investigator) bias 16, 27, 112–13, 252–3
obsessive-compulsive disorder 115
odors 140, 142–3
*off cells* 188–90
older people 287
omeprazole 242
*on cells* 188–90
ondansetron 221
open-label designs 26–7
operant conditioning 174
opioid antagonists 178, 192
 *see also* naloxone
opioids 101–2
 descending pain modulatory system 188–90
 endogenous 13, 185–8, 192
  in acupuncture analgesia 179, 193
  in placebo analgesia 198–200, 201–2
  in stimulation produced analgesia 193
 immune effects 177–8
 mechanisms of action 185–8, 191
 receptors 187
 *see also* morphine
oral hypoglycemic drugs 266
osteoarthritis, knee 86–7
outcome
 expectations 8, 119–20
 measures *see* endpoints
overdose, drug 150

pain 13–15
 dental 5, 81–2
 descending modulatory pathways 13, 188–90
 endogenous inhibitory systems 184–94
 mechanisms involving meaning responses 99
 relief *see* analgesia
 *see also* analgesics
panic disorder 115
parametric designs 307–8
parents 66–7, 304
Parkinson's disease 115
patent medicine 40
paternalism 69
pathogenesis 276
pathophysiology 276
patients
 autonomy 212, 215, 233
 bias 15–16, 113
 care *see* clinical practice
 meanings, *v* those of physicians 83–4
 not seeking treatment 24
 participation in clinical trials 18, 215–16, 233–4
placebo 16
 relationship with physician 8, 115–17, 295
 selection 245–6
 *see also* study participants
Pavlovian conditioning 10–12, 114, 133–53, 173
 compensatory conditional responses 147–52
 examples of placebo effects 139–45
 history 134–5
 with long delay 136
 as mechanism of placebo effect 139
 modulation of drug effects and 146–7
paradigm 135–7
pharmacological responses 137–8
placebo analgesia 148–9, 185, 194–6
 rapid 136
 research recommendations 286–7
 sequence effects and extinction 145–6
Pavlov, Ivan Petrovich 134–5, 137–8, 153
peptic ulcer disease 87, 89, 90, 266
 abandoned treatment 95
 correlation of drug/placebo effects 100, **101**
 new drugs 82, **83**
 placebo controlled trials 254
percutaneous myocardial laser revascularization (PMLR) 86, 253
periaqueductal-periventricular grey (PAG-PVG) 13, 186–7, 188
 in conditioning 175, 190
 in placebo analgesia 178
 stimulation studies 187, 192–3
peripheral nerves 12, 173, 177
personality 6–10, 114–15
pertussis vaccines, acellular 240
pharmacologic conditioned responses 11–12, 152
pharmacology of placebos 42
pharmacotherapeutic conditioned responses 11–12, 152

photodynamic therapy 95
physicians (clinicians)
  duty to care 270–4
  effects of giving placebos on 58–9
  influence on placebo response 5, 60, 81–3
  meanings, *v* those of patients 83–4
  obtaining informed consent 233, 273
positive attitudes 8, 81, 95, 116, 120
  professional guidelines 274–5
  referral to CAM practitioners 298–9
  relationship with patients 8, 115–17, 295
  research agenda 303
  separation of investigator role 273–4, 279
  training 61–2, 294–5
  *v* chiropractors 97
  *see also* investigators; therapeutic relationship
physiologic responses 12
"pithiatism" 39
placebo
  "attention" 110
  in clinical practice *see* clinical practice, placebo use in
  concept 283–4
  definitions 54–5, 109, 314
  historical background 2–3, 35–51
  manufacturing and packaging 255
  matching 250
  nature 2–16
placebo analgesia 14–15, 99, 183–203
  biological mechanisms 171, 178, 184–94
  conditioned 148–9, 184–5, 194–6
  factors influencing magnitude 194–201
  future directions 201–3, 289, 291
  measurement 202–3
  *see also* analgesics
placebo controlled trials (PCTs) 19–20, 28–9, 63–73
  alternative designs 129, 224
  appropriate use 223–5, 237–9
    decision criteria 251–60
  arguments against 23–4, 229–33
  arguments for 21–3, 227–9
  assay sensitivity and *see* assay sensitivity
  behavioral interventions 306–10
  in developing countries 69–71
  historical background 41–4
  large-scale pragmatic 249–61
  Levine on 264–79
  research recommendations 30, 71–3, 260–1, 300–5
  Rothman on 68, 227–35
  Temple on 20–1, 68, 209–25
  *v* open-label designs 25–7
  when effective therapy exists 21–4, 68–9, 212–13, 237–8, 254, 264–79
placebo effect 2–16, 284–5, 314
  biological mediators/pathways 169–80, 183–203, 289–90
  controlling for 228–9
  correlation with drug effect 100–2
  definitions 1, 44, 77–8, 109, 133–4
  evidence for 1
  explanatory mechanisms *see* explanatory mechanisms
  historical background 35–51
  measurement artifacts and 15–16
  methodological issues *see* methodological aspects
  negative *see* "nocebo" effect
  popular myths 5–6
  regression to mean and 164–5
  research needs 29, 286–99
  self-elicited 296–7
  variability 5, 6, 230
  *see also* meaning response
POINT study 239
positron emission tomography (PET) 290
postoperative nausea and vomiting 221
postoperative recovery 47
pragmatic trials 250
premenstrual syndrome 114–15
proglumide 99, 101–2
propoxyphene 194–5
propranolol *92*
proteomics 291
proxies, consent by 66–7, 304–5
psoriasis 174
psychiatric disorders
  consent issues 66–7, 305
  drugs for 9
psychological wellbeing 79
psychoneuroendocrine immunology 12–13, 169–80, 289–90
psychophysiology 12–15
psychosocial dwarfism 47
psychotherapy 8, 118, 287–8
  placebo controlled trials 110, 306–10
  specific and non-specific (common) factors 111, 124
  therapeutic relationship 116–17
  verbal dynamic 8, 117
PURSUIT trial 257–8
p values 231

quality of life 252–3
quarantine 234

random assignment 227–8
randomized controlled trials (RCTs) 77–8
  *see also* clinical trials
randomized open-label designs 26–7
randomized withdrawal design 224
ranitidine **83**, 87, 89, 100, **101**
rats
  analgesia 185, 191
  conditioning 10–11, 138, 139, 147, 152
record-keeping *see* documentation
reference point, placebo 229–30
refugees, Cambodian 3, 47–8
regression to mean 16, 112, 158–65
  definition 159–60
  illustrations 162–4

mathematics 160–2
and placebo effects 164–5
regulatory authorities
approved drugs 238
attitudes to placebo controlled trials 255–60
non-inferiority trials 230–1, 243–4
*see also* Food and Drug Administration
religious holidays 47
research
clinical *see* clinical research
principles 283–5
recommendations 29–30, 286–310
subjects *see* study participants
researchers *see* investigators
response bias 118
response expectancy 9, 14, 120–3
placebo analgesia 196–7, 199–200
*v* conditioning 14–15, 195–6
restriction 227
reteplase 27, 257
rheumatoid arthritis 174
risks of placebos
in clinical practice 18, 57–60
in clinical trials 21–3, 213–15, 234–5, 254, 266
informing study subjects about 65–6, 72
*see also* "nocebo" effects
rituals 6

safety
new drugs 23
non-inferiority studies 239
placebos *see* risks of placebos
salivation, conditioned 135, 137, 147
sample size, non-inferiority trials 219, 221, 230, 231–2, 241–5
schizophrenia 21–2
science, interests of 214, 215, 232, 271
scientific trials 250
scopolamine 139
sedatives 88
seizure, time to first 224
selective serotonin reuptake inhibitors (SSRIs) 298
self-assessed health 93–4
self-efficacy expectations 8, 119–20
self-esteem 79
self-placebo response 296–7
sensitization 11, 147
sequence effects 11, 145–6, 194–5
sham procedures 250, 301
"sightings" 3, 46–9
signal detection theory 117–18, 129
significance, statistical 231, 241
sleeping pills 88, 151
slippery slope 215
social influences 3–6, 288
mapping 290
*see also* meaning response
social learning 6–10, 108–29
society, interests of 214, 215, 232, 234
sociosomatics 80
somatotopic representation 199, 200
somatotropin deficiency, reversible 47
spinal cord dorsal horn 178, 186, 187–8, 190–1
spinal manipulation therapy 95–7
spinal nociceptive reflexes 202
spleen 176–7
spouse, role of 296
statistical analysis, non-inferiority trials 246–7
statistical significance 231, 241
stimulants 88
stimulation produced analgesia (SPA) 185–7, 192–3
stimulus generalization 11, 136–7
stimulus substitution model 196
streptokinase 27, 256
stress
analgesia 13–14, 185, 198
neuroendocrine response **172**, 173, 176
stroke 23, 252
study design 20–1, 129, 224
behavioral interventions 307–8
non-inferiority trials 222, 231
research agenda 303–4, 308
sequence effects and 146
study participants
best interests 214, 215, 232, 234
biases 15–16
in developing countries 70
early escape 213, 224
ethics of recruitment 18
informed consent 64–7, 212
motivation 253
non-inferiority trials 245–6
numbers *see* sample size
patients *v* volunteers 68, 215–16, 233–4
research agenda 301–2
risks of placebo controls 21–3, 213–15, 224, 234–5, 254
selection for extreme values 160, 164–5
vulnerable/impaired capacity 66–7, 70, 304–5
*see also* patients
substance P 177
suggestion 38–40, 134
suggestive therapeutics 39
suicide 22
superiority trials 20, 21, 210
behavioral interventions 306
*v* non-inferiority trials 216, 218
*see also* placebo controlled trials
surgery, meaning response 84–7
symptomatic treatment 211, 212, 213, 215–16, 278
symptoms, measurement 252–3
systemic lupus erythematosus 144

tablets/capsules
color 4, 78, 88–9
number 4, 89
type 89
taste aversion 174, 175
Taylor, Bishop Jeremy 55
tea 146–7
technologies, investigational 290–1
tenecteplase 257

testosterone, plasma 142
textbooks, medical 61
theory testing research 128–9
therapeutic misconception 211, 274
therapeutic relationship 8, 115–17, 295
therapeutic research 276–7
therapist
  bias 112–13
  equivalence of competence 309
  process research 309–10
therapy *see* treatment
thermal sensitivity 118, 199–200
thrombolysis
  anticoagulation after 23, 240
  large trials 27, 256–7
  non-inferiority trials 219, 223
thymus 176–7
tissue plasminogen activator (t-PA) 257
tolerability 23
tolerance 150
  reverse 11, 147
tourniquet pain 14, 199
traditional beliefs, Chinese 5, 80
traditional Chinese medicine 83
training, medical 61–2, 294–5
tranquilizers 88, 103
transcutaneous electrical nerve stimulation (TENS) 179, 193
transmyocardial laser revascularization (TMR) 84–6, 253
treatment
  abandoned 94–5
  active *see* active treatment
  add-on 224, 232, 239, 253
  combinations 253
  confounded procedures 113–14
  delay 21–2, 254
  duration, in non-inferiority trials 246
  "highest attainable and sustainable method" 269–70, 279
  interactions between 303–4
  life-saving 213
  meaning 78–9, 81–3
  non-specific elements 110–11
  pre-existing proven effective 68–9, 212–13, 237–8, 254
  *see also* best proven therapeutic method
  preventing serious harm 19, 213–15
  specific 110–11
  symptomatic 211, 212, 213, 215–16, 278
  *see also* no-treatment controls
trust, failure of 57
truth-telling 17, 18, 55
tuberculin reaction 174
twentieth century
  early decades 38–40
  second half 40–4, *45*, *49*
type 1 error 238
type 2 error 238

ulcerative colitis 116
unconditional response (reflex) (UCR) 10, 135, 149
unconditional stimulus (UCS) 10, 135
utilitarianism 232

vaccination 99–100, 234
variability
  meaning response 87–94
  placebo effects 5, 6, 230
vasoactive intestinal polypeptide 177
ventromedial medulla (RVM) 178, **186**, 187, 188–90
Viagra 88
vitamin tablets 88–9
volunteers, healthy 68, 215–16, 233–4
vomiting, postoperative 221
voodoo death 48
vulnerable research populations 66–7, 70, 304–5

"wash out" periods 146
withdrawal
  randomized 224
  symptoms 150–1
Wolf, Stewart 42
World Health Organization (WHO) 25, 268
World Medical Association 1, 274–5, 276
  *see also Declaration of Helsinki*

zidovudine (AZT) 24–5, 71, 267–9